13th Workshop Conference Hoechst

BIOCHEMICAL BASIS OF CHEMICAL CARCINOGENESIS

13th Workshop Conference Hoechst
Grainau
October 6–9, 1982

Biochemical Basis of Chemical Carcinogenesis

Editors

Prof. Dr. med. Helmut Greim
Gesellschaft für Strahlen- und Umweltforschung Neuherberg, F.R.G.

Dr. Reinhard Jung
Pharma Forschung Toxikologie Hoechst AG Frankfurt, F.R.G.

Prof. Dr. Martin Kramer
Pharma Forschung Toxikologie Hoechst AG Frankfurt, F.R.G.

Prof. Dr. med. Hans Marquardt
Pharmakologisches Institut Universitäts-Krankenhaus Eppendorf Hamburg, F.R.G.

Prof. Dr. Franz Oesch
Pharmakologisches Institut der Universität Mainz Mainz, F.R.G.

Raven Press ■ New York

Raven Press, 1140 Avenue of the Americas, New York, New York 10036

Made in the United States of America

Library of Congress Cataloging in Publication Data

Workshop Conference Hoechst (13th : 1982 : Grainau, Germany)
  Biochemical basis of chemical carcinogenesis.

  Includes index.
  1. Carcinogenesis—Congresses. 2. Carcinogens—Metabolism—Congresses. 3. Carcinogens—Metabolic detoxication—Congresses. I. Greim, Helmut. II. Title.
[DNLM: 1. Carcinogens—Metabolism—Congresses. 2. Cell transformation, Neoplastic—Drug effects—Congresses.
3. DNA repair—Congresses. 4. Neoplasms, Experimental—Chemically induced—Congresses. 5. Precancerous conditions—Enzymology—Congresses. W3 W051M 13th 1982b
QZ 202 W9235 1982b]
RC268.5.W63   1982   616.99'4071   83-48664
ISBN 0-89004-961-0

Opening Address

On behalf of the Pharmaceutical Research Department of the Hoechst Company I welcome you to Grainau to our Workshop Conference on chemical carcinogenesis. First of all I wish to thank my colleagues of the program committee for having made such an excellent program. I also wish to thank all the speakers for coming. Hoechst has sponsored such a workshop conference with the intention of stimulating research to elucidate the various steps by which chemicals may induce cancer. If one accepts the multistage model of chemical carcinogenesis one has to accept also that many enzymatic reactions are involved in this process which are dose dependent or even saturable. In this conference the various stages of chemical carcinogenesis will be discussed. We will begin with the activation of chemicals to an electrophyllic metabolite. This first step depends on the chemical structure of the compound. The extent and the quality of activation, inactivation and sequestration depend on the enzyme pattern and may therefore vary according to systems, species, and even individuals. There is some evidence that initiation alone is not carcinogenic. Further progression of the process needs promotion. Promoting agents have a threshold concentration or dose. DNA bound to a carcinogen or an alkyl moiety may undergo repair. There is evidence that repair processes might be saturable; in other words, repair capacity can be limited.

All these examples indicate that there is a good probability that threshold limits do exist for chemical carcinogenesis. It is my firm belief that in risk assessment the feeding of rodents with high concentrations of chemical compounds will become obsolete. This procedure is, scientifically speaking, rather poor. We need to better understand the biochemical process that leads to carcinogenesis. Quantitative aspects are of paramount importance in this connection. I hope the Workshop Conference will reach this goal or can at least come close to it.

M. Kramer

Preface

This volume was developed to provide a basis for elucidating the various steps by which chemicals may induce cancer, using as its basis the multi-stage model of chemical carcinogenesis that assumes that many enzymatic reactions are involved in this process which are dose-dependent or saturable.

Beginning with a discussion of the activation of chemicals to an electrophyllic metabolite, chapters discuss enzyme patterns as they vary with systems, species and individuals, the relationship between initiation and promotion, promoting agents and their mechanisms of action, and the repair of DNA following activation- and promotion-induced changes in gene structure.

This volume will be of interest to all scientists involved in basic research on cancer, cellular and molecular biologists, and molecular geneticists.

In memoriam
Charles Heidelberger

Contents

Contributors

Herman Autrup
Laboratory of Human Carcinogenesis
National Cancer Institute
Bethesda, Maryland 20205

Joseph Backer
Division of Environmental Sciences and
  Cancer Center
Institute of Cancer Research
Columbia University
New York, New York 10032

M. A. Bedell
Chemical Industry Institute of Toxicology
Department of Pathology
Research Triangle Park,
  North Carolina 27709

K. C. Billings
Chemical Industry Institute of Toxicology
Department of Pathology
Research Triangle Park,
  North Carolina 27709

K. W. Bock
Department of Pharmacology and
  Toxicology
University of Göttingen
Kreuzbergring 57
D-3400 Göttingen
Federal Republic of Germany

B. S. Bock-Hennig
Department of Pharmacology and
  Toxicology
University of Göttingen
Kreuzbergring 57
D-3400 Göttingen
Federal Republic of Germany

Carmia Borek
Radiological Research Laboratory
Departments of Radiology and Pathology
Columbia University
College of Physicians and Surgeons
New York, New York 10032

Sarah A. Bruce
Division of Biophysics
School of Hygiene and Public Health
The Johns Hopkins University
615 N. Wolfe Street
Baltimore, Maryland 21205

Peter A. Cerutti
Department of Carcinogenesis
Swiss Institute for Experimental Cancer
  Research
CH-1066 Epalinges s/Lausanne
Switzerland

M. C. Dyroff
Chemical Industry Institute of Toxicology
Department of Pathology
Research Triangle Park,
  North Carolina 27709

G. Fischer
Department of Pathology
University of Göttingen
Kreuzbergring 57
D-3400 Göttingen
Federal Republic of Germany

Sebastiano Gattoni-Celli
Division of Environmental Sciences and
  Cancer Center
Institute of Cancer Research
Columbia University
New York, New York 10032

H. R. Glatt
Institute of Pharmacology
University of Mainz
Obere Zahlbacher Strasse 67
D-6500 Mainz
Federal Republic of Germany

Roland C. Grafstrom
Laboratory of Human Carcinogenesis
National Cancer Institute
Bethesda, Maryland 20205

Helmut Greim
Department of Toxicology
Institute for Biochemistry and Toxicology
Gesellschaft für Strahlen-und
Umweltforschung
D-8042 Neuherberg, Post
Oberschleissheim
Federal Republic of Germany

Khin Khin Gyi
College of Medicine
University of Vermont
Burlington, Vermont 05401

Curtis C. Harris
Laboratory of Human Carcinogenesis
National Cancer Institute
Bethesda, Maryland 20205

E. Herchenhan
Department of Neuropathology
Institute of Pathology
Universität Freiburg
Federal Republic of Germany

Sigrun Hesse
Department of Toxicology
Institute of Toxicology and Biochemistry
Gesellschaft für Strahlen-und
Umweltforschung
D-8042 Neuherberg
Federal Republic of Germany

Wendy Hsiao
Division of Environmental Sciences and
Cancer Center
Institute of Cancer Research
Columbia University
New York, New York 10032

Alan Jeffrey
Division of Environmental Sciences and
Cancer Center
Institute of Cancer Research
Columbia University
New York, New York 10032

Bengt Jernström
Department of Forensic Medicine
Karolinska Institutet
S-1040 Stockholm, Sweden

Paul Kirschmeier
Division of Environmental Sciences and
Cancer Center
Institute of Cancer Research
Columbia University
New York
New York 10032

P. Kleihues
Department of Neuropathology
Institute of Pathology
Universität Freiburg
Federal Republic of Germany

Michael Lambert
Division of Environmental Sciences and
Cancer Center
Institute of Cancer Research
Columbia University
New York
New York 10032

Maurice Lambiotte
Départment Unité de Génétique Cellulaire
Institut de Recherches en Biologie
Moleculaire du C.N.R.S.
Université Paris VII
Paris, France

J. G. Lewis
Chemical Industry Institute of Toxicology
Department of Pathology
Research Triangle Park
North Carolina 27709

W. Lilienblum
Department of Pharmacology and
Toxicology
University of Göttingen
Kreuzbergring 57
D-3400 Göttingen
Federal Republic of Germany

C. Lindamood III
Chemical Industry Institute of Toxicology
Department of Pathology
Research Triangle Park
North Carolina 27709

Veronica M. Maher
Carcinogenesis Laboratory
Fee Hall
Department of Microbiology and
    Department of Biochemistry
Michigan State University
East Lansing, Michigan 48824–1316

Hans Marquardt
Department of Toxicology
University of Hamburg Medical School and
    Fraunhofer Institute of Toxicology and
    Aerosol Research
Grindelallee 117
D-2000 Hamburg 13
Federal Republic of Germany

J. Justin McCormick
Carcinogenesis Laboratory
Fee Hall
Department of Microbiology and
    Department of Biochemistry
Michigan State University
East Lansing, Michigan 48824–1316

Elena C. McCoy
Center for Environmental Health Sciences,
    and
Department of Epidemiology and
    Community Health
Case Western Reserve University
School of Medicine
Cleveland, Ohio 44106

I. Mertes
Institute of Pharmacology
University of Mainz
Obere Zahlbacher Strasse 67
D-6500 Mainz
Federal Republic of Germany

Manfred Metzler
Institute of Pharmacology and Toxicology
University of Würzburg
Versbacher Strasse 9
D-8700 Würzburg
Federal Republic of Germany

Michitoshi Nakamura
Developmental Pharmacology Branch
National Institute of Child Health and
    Human Development
National Institutes of Health
Bethesda, Maryland 20205

Shuji Nakano
School of Medicine
Kyushu University
Fukuoka 812, Japan

Daniel W. Nebert
Developmental Pharmacology Branch
National Institute of Child Health and
    Human Development
National Institutes of Health
Bethesda, Maryland 20205

Masahiko Negishi
Developmental Pharmacology Branch
National Institute of Child Health and
    Human Development
National Institutes of Health
Bethesda, Maryland 20205

Hans-Günter Neumann
Institute of Pharmacology and Toxicology
University of Würzburg
Versbacherstr. 9
8700 Würzburg
Federal Republic of Germany

Hugo J. Niggli
Department of Carcinogenesis
Swiss Institute for Experimental Cancer
    Research
CH-1066 Epalinges s/Lausanne
Switzerland

F. Oesch
Institute of Pharmacology
University of Mainz
Obere Zahlbacher Strasse 67
D-6500 Mainz
Federal Republic of Germany

Anthony E. Pegg
Department of Physiology and Specialized
    Cancer Research Center
The Pennsylvania State University
College of Medicine
Hershey, Pennsylvania 17033

P. Petrovic
Institute of Pharmacology
University of Mainz
Obere Zahlbacher Strasse 67
D-6500 Mainz
Federal Republic of Germany

K. L. Platt
Institute of Pharmacology
University of Mainz
Obere Zahlbacher Strasse 67
D-6500 Mainz
Federal Republic of Germany

Anita B. Roberts
Laboratory of Chemoprevention
Division of Cancer Cause and Prevention
National Cancer Institute
National Institutes of Health
Bethesda, Maryland 20205

A. Seidel
Institute of Pharmacology
University of Mainz
Obere Zahlbacher Strasse 67
D-6500
Federal Republic of Germany

Abulkalam M. Shamsuddin
Laboratory of Human Carcinogenesis
National Cancer Institute
Bethesda, Maryland 20205;
Department of Pathology
University of Maryland School of Medicine
Baltimore, Maryland 21201

Jaswant Singh
Regional Research Laboratory
CSIR
Jammu Tawi
India

Nuntia T. Sinopoli
Laboratory of Human Carcinogenesis
National Cancer Institute
Bethesda, Maryland 20205

Jack Spira
Department of Tumor Biology
Box 60400
104 01 Stockholm
Sweden

Michael B. Sporn
Laboratory of Chemoprevention
Division of Cancer Cause and Prevention
National Cancer Institute
Bethesda, Maryland 20205

Karl-Heinz Summer
Institute of Biochemistry and Toxicology
Department of Toxicology
Gesellschaft für Strahlen- und
Umwelforschung
D-8042 Neuherberg-München
Federal Republic of Germany

J. A. Swenberg
Chemical Industry Institute of Toxicology
Department of Pathology
Research Triangle Park,
North Carolina 27709

Heinz Walter Thielmann
German Cancer Research Centre
Institute of Biochemistry
D-6900 Heidelberg
Federal Republic of Germany

S. S. Thorgeirsson
Laboratory of Carcinogen Metabolism
National Cancer Institute
National Institutes of Health
Bethesda, Maryland 20205

Benjamin F. Trump
Department of Pathology
University of Maryland School of Medicine
Baltimore, Maryland 21201

Paul O. P. Ts'o
Division of Biophysics
School of Hygiene and Public Health
The Johns Hopkins University
615 N. Wolfe Street
Baltimore, Maryland 21205

Robert H. Tukey
Developmental Pharmacology Branch
National Institute of Child Health and
Human Development
National Institutes of Health
Bethesda, Maryland 20205

Hiroaki Ueo
School of Medicine
Kyushu University
Fukuoka 812
Japan

D. Ullrich
Department of Pharmacology and
  Toxicology
University of Göttingen
Kreuzbergring 57
D-3400 Göttingen
Federal Republic of Germany

A. Uozumi
Department of Neuropathology
Institute of Pathology
Freiburg University
Federal Republic of Germany

C. Veit
Department of Neuropathology
Institute of Pathology
Universität Freiburg
Federal Republic of Germany

K. Vogel
Institute of Pharmacology
University of Mainz
Obere Zahlbacher Strasse 67
D-6500 Mainz
Federal Republic of Germany

Robert A. Weinberg
Whitehead Institute for Biomedical
  Research
Center for Cancer Research and
  Department of Biology
Massachusetts Institute of Technology
Cambridge, Massachusetts 02139

I. Bernard Weinstein
Division of Environmental Sciences and
  Cancer Center
Institute of Cancer Research
Columbia University
New York, New York 10032

Friedrich J. Wiebel
Institute of Biochemistry and Toxicology
Department of Toxicology
Gesellschaft für Strahlen- und
  Umweltforschung
D-8042 Neuherberg-München
Federal Republic of Germany

O. Wiestler
Department of Neuropathology
Institute of Pathology
Universität Freiburg
Federal Republic of Germany

T. Wölfel
Institute of Pharmacology
University of Mainz
Obere Zahlbacher Strasse 67
D-6500 Mainz
Federal Republic of Germany

Thomas Wolff
Institute of Biochemistry and Toxicology
Department of Toxicology
Gesellschaft für Strahlen- und
  Umweltforschung
D-8042 Neuherberg-München
Federal Republic of Germany

Maria Zajac-Kaye
Center for Experimental Cell Biology
Mt. Sinai School of Medicine
New York, New York 10029

Biochemical Basis of Chemical Carcinogenesis,
edited by H. Greim, R. Jung, M. Kramer,
H. Marquardt, and F. Oesch.
Raven Press, New York © 1984.

Scope of the Application of the Biochemical Basis of Chemical Carcinogenesis Towards a More Rational Risk Estimation

F. Oesch

*Institute of Pharmacology, University of Mainz,
D-6500 Mainz, Federal Republic of Germany*

During the last two decades we have become increasingly aware that in the majority of cases for carcinogenic and mutagenic effects of chemical compounds, it is not the parent compound that is directly responsible, but our exposure to reactive metabolites which are generated from chemically inert precursors (5–8). Therefore we now realize that for a rational estimation of the risk of such compounds to man it is necessary to know the control of these reactive metabolites (8). On the one hand, these are under the control of the activating enzymes which produce them, as is by now realized by most toxicologists. On the other hand, there are also inactivating enzymes. Many toxicologists are still of the opinion that these are less important because once generated by the activating enzymes, the reactive species represents the factor which is responsible for the toxic effect. But in fact, such inactivating enzymes can be crucial when it is a question of whether or not a toxic effect will occur (2,9,10). Finally, in the last few years we have begun to realize that a further set of enzymes is very important: the sequestering enzymes. These are enzymes which shunt the metabolism to non-toxic pathways in competition with activating enzymes. We are now beginning to realize that these are of great importance. There are very widely used toxicological tests, such as bacterial mutagenicity tests, that rely on activation by mammalian enzymes that are added to organisms that do not have these enzymes (1). At least in part, inactivation enzymes are also added. However, the sequestration enzymes, most of which need co-factors, which in these tissue preparations are highly diluted (usually far below their K_m value), are typically operating to such a small extent that, in practice, they exhibit no action in these tests. This leads to a highly distorted picture of toxicity results (3). This third set of enzymes is therefore also of great importance for a rational risk extrapolation.

Many researchers studying DNA binding and repair as well as consequent effects, start their experiments with the ultimate reactive species in order not to introduce confusion into their systems resulting from the complexity of metabolism. Although this method may provide a clearer picture and this approach is valuable, if the

1

interest is confined to those steps of the carcinogenic process which occur after the generation of the reactive metabolite, for risk extrapolation and toxicological studies it is necessary to know about the differences in toxic effects which are introduced by differences in metabolism (2,8–10). During the last decade it has been established that the enzymes which control the reactive species differ greatly among toxicological test systems, and between animal species and man (4,9,11,12).

In this regard, it is important to understand that enzymes behave as enzymes. This is biochemically trivial, but it is not appreciated by all toxicologists. Enzymes are saturable and their substrates have K_m values. Examples are known in which a given compound may be metabolized by a high-velocity but low-capacity enzyme, and also by a high-capacity but low-velocity enzyme. At low concentrations, therefore, the pathway of the first type of enzyme will predominate and, if the dose is very much below the K_m value of the second type of enzyme, the second pathway may not be taken to any measurable extent. If the doses are higher by orders of magnitude they may then be so much above the saturation of the first enzyme that the first pathway may now contribute much less than 1% to the total metabolism. If one of the pathways leads to a highly toxic metabolite and the other represents an inactivation pathway the toxicological consequences can be dramatic. Furthermore, there are examples in which the same enzyme which catalyzes the first step of metabolism of a given compound is also responsible for a much later step of further metabolism of a metabolite. Depending on the K_m values of the mother compound and that of the metabolite for the enzyme, situations exist in which at low concentrations of the mother compound the metabolite is efficiently converted by the enzyme, whereas higher concentrations of the mother compound can inhibit this conversion of the metabolite. If this further conversion of the metabolite leads to a highly toxic secondary or tertiary metabolite, the toxicity will paradoxically be reduced (or totally absent) at higher doses of the mother compound—an example of which I shall discuss later in this volume (see chapter by Oesch et al. on dihydrodiol dehydrogenase).

Typically the reactive species reacts with many different targets within the cell. One important target is DNA. There are positions on the bases which are important for the base pairing; if this is disturbed, the typical result is miscoding. Other positions which are not in that area are quite often the major binding positions. Various chemical carcinogens can be converted by enzymes to several reactive metabolites which lead to different binding products and are toxicologically very different. Again, the pattern of activating and inactivating enzymes will decide which of the binding products will predominate. Thus, it may be misleading if a certain level of total DNA binding is introduced as critical, as is done with the covalent-binding index. Such a quantitative level, above which danger is predicted and below which safety is inferred, is hazardous when information on the position, chemical nature and biological persistence of the adducts is absent. Some of these lesions can be enzymically repaired and others cannot (or at least firm evidence for their enzymic repair is lacking); some organs are very efficient in repair and others are not; some repair processes are beneficial, whereas others are error-prone and increase mutagenicity. Again, quantitative knowledge of all these processes is important for a rational risk estimation.

Finally, what happens after binding to DNA and other possible critical targets in the cell has occurred? What is the relationship of activation of oncogenes to what is called "initiation" by chemical carcinogens? What are the products of the oncogenes and how are they involved in the process of carcinogenesis? After "initiation" has taken place, what is then the role in molecular terms of "promotion"? All of these questions, which we are only beginning to answer, will be addressed in this volume.

It is hoped that despite the very many details that remain unknown or in doubt we can begin to build on facts, which are by now known with certainty, in order to allow for a stepwise approach to a more rational risk estimation for man.

REFERENCES

1. Ames, B. N., Durston, W. E., Yamasaki, E., and Lee, F. D. (1973): *Proc. Natl. Acad. Sci. USA,* 70:2281–2285.
2. Bücker, M., Glatt, H. R., Platt, K. L., Avnir, D., Ittah, Y., Blum, J., and Oesch, F. (1979): *Mutat. Res.,* 66:337–348.
3. Glatt, H. R., Billings, R., Platt, K. L., and Oesch, F. (1981): *Cancer Res.,* 41:270–277.
4. Glatt, H. R., Lorenz, J., Fleischmann, R., Remmer, H., Ohnhaus, E. E., Klatenbach, E., Tegtmeyer, F., Rüdiger, H., and Oesch, F. (1980): In: *Microsomes, Drug Oxidations, and Chemical Carcinogenesis, Vol. 2,* edited by M. J. Coon, A. H. Conney, R. W., Estabrook, H. V. Gelboin, J. R. Gillette, and P. J. O'Brian, pp. 651–654. Academic Press, New York.
5. Jerina, D. M., Lehr, R., Schaefer-Ridder, M., Yagi, H., Karle, J. M., Thakker, D. R., Wood, A. W., Lu, A. Y. H., Ryan, D., West, S., Levin, W., and Conney, A. H. (1977): In: *Origins of Human Cancer, Vol. 4,* edited by H. H. Hiatt, J. D. Watson, and J. A. Winsten, pp. 639–658. Cold Spring Harbor Laboratory, Cold Spring Harbor, New York.
6. Miller, J. A., and Miller, E. C. (1977): In: *Origins of Human Cancer, Vol. 4,* edited by H. H. Hiatt, J. D. Watson, and J. A. Winsten, pp. 605–628. Cold Spring Harbor Laboratory, Cold Spring Harbor, New York.
7. Oesch, F. (1973): *Xenobiotica,* 3:305–340.
8. Oesch, F. (1979): *Arch. Toxicol.,* Suppl. 2:215–227.
9. Oesch, F. (1980): *Arch. Toxicol.,* Suppl. 3:179–194.
10. Oesch, F., and Glatt, H. R. (1976): In: *Screening Tests in Chemical Carcinogenesis,* edited by R. Montesano, H. Bartsch, and L. Tomatis, pp. 255–274. IARC, Lyon.
11. Oesch, F., Schmassmann, H. U., Ohnhaus, E., Althaus, U., and Lorenz, J. (1980): *Carcinogenesis,* 1:827–835.
12. Walker, C. H., Bentley, P., and Oesch, F. (1978): *Biochim. Biophys. Acta,* 539:427–434.

Biochemical Basis of Chemical Carcinogenesis,
edited by H. Greim, R. Jung, M. Kramer,
H. Marquardt, and F. Oesch.
Raven Press, New York © 1984.

Role of Glutathione S-Transferases: Detoxification of Reactive Metabolites of Benzo(a)pyrene-7,8-dihydrodiol by Conjugation with Glutathione

*Sigrun Hesse and **Bengt Jernström

*Department of Toxicology, Institute of Toxicology and Biochemistry, GSF, D-8042
Neuherberg, Federal Republic of Germany; and **Department of Forensic Medicine,
Karolinska Institutet, S-1040 Stockholm, Sweden

Currently DNA is believed to be the target site of attack by chemical carcinogens. Covalent binding to DNA of a carcinogen is thought to initiate critical permanent alterations in the genetic materal which may result in the formation of tumors. Most chemical carcinogens require metabolic activation yielding electrophiles, i.e., intermediates which are the actual binding species. However, the cell possesses various protective mechanisms to inactivate the reactive metabolites before binding to the macromolecular target sites can occur. One of the most important defense mechanisms is based on the detoxification by the glutathione (GSH) S-transferase system.

POSSIBLE ROLES OF GSH S-TRANSFERASES IN THE INACTIVATION OF CHEMICAL CARCINOGENS

Different modes of interaction between GSH S-transferases and chemical carcinogens are possible:

1. GSH S-transferases may noncovalently bind the carcinogenic metabolites, e.g., of azo dyes, polycyclic aromatic hydrocarbons, aromatic amines (16,24). Such non-covalent binding traps electrophiles and decreases their steady state levels. Furthermore, it facilitates the transport of the lipophilic molecules within the cell (26) and their elimination. However, a faster transport also more readily delivers the electrophiles to the nuclear target sites (23) increasing the risk of binding.

2. GSH S-transferases covalently bind reactive metabolites, as shown for dimethylamino-azobenzene and 3-methylcholanthrene (24). This reaction may efficiently trap the toxic metabolites; however, it leads also to the irreversible inactivation of the enzyme.

3. GSH S-transferases catalyze the conjugation between electrophilic metabolites and GSH. The intracellular concentrations of GSH are high. This has been partic-

ularly shown for the rat liver, which exhibits high levels of GSH S-transferases. However, the extent of a substrate's conjugation depends also on the nature of the electrophilic metabolite and may vary greatly. Some ultimate carcinogens, e.g., those formed during the activation of *N*-hydroxyacetyl-2-aminofluorene or dimethylamino-azobenzene are strong electrophiles but, nevertheless, only weakly react with GSH and are poorly detoxified (10,15). In contrast, other reactive products, such as the ultimate carcinogenic epoxides of benzo*(a)*pyrene (BP) and aflatoxin B$_1$ are readily conjugated with GSH and largely inactivated (4,10).

The efficiency of the inactivation by GSH depends on three major parameters: (a) the rate of the nonenzymatic reaction between reactive metabolites and GSH, (b) the property of the reactive metabolite, to be a good or poor substrate for GSH S-transferases, and (c) the accessibility of the reactive metabolites for GSH and GSH S-transferases. Most of the transferase activity (ca. 80 to 90%) is localized in the cytosol, whereas electrophiles are preferentially formed in the endoplasmic reticulum or the nuclear membrane. Thus, it is open to question whether the reactive metabolites are accessible to GSH and the transferases. If the electrophiles are highly lipophilic they are especially unlikely to come into contact with GSH and the enzymes. Recent observations have shown that GSH S-transferases may also be localized in membranes, i.e., the endoplasmic reticulum comprising about 10% of the total transferase activity (6,21). The importance of these membrane-bound transferases for the detoxification of carcinogens remains to be established.

ROLE OF GSH S-TRANSFERASES IN THE INACTIVATION OF BP-METABOLITES

In the following, BP will serve to demonstrate the multiplicity of possible interactions of the GSH S-transferases with the metabolism of a carcinogen (Fig. 1).

BP, 3-hydroxy-BP and the dihydrodiols (in the positions 4,5-, 7,8-, 9,10-) bind non-covalently to the transferases (17). Among the epoxides tested, BP-4,5-epoxide is a good substrate for GSH S-transferase (22), whereas BP-7,8-epoxide reacts only poorly (13). The anti-isomer of BP-7,8-dihydrodiol-9,10-epoxide (BP-diol-epox-

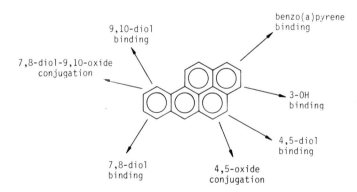

FIG. 1.   Sites of interactions of GSH S-transferases with the metabolism of benzo*(a)*pyrene.

ide), the presumed ultimate carcinogenic form of BP, has also been shown to be a substrate for the GSH S-transferases (3). The efficient trapping of this metabolite in the cell is of particular interest since this reaction may directly control the degree of DNA-modification.

Inactivation of Reactive Metabolites of BP-7,8-Dihydrodiol by Conjugation with GSH

The studies presented below concern the question whether and to what extent the conjugation of BP-diol-epoxides with GSH may prevent their DNA binding.

Our results showed that the binding of BP metabolites to DNA was dependent on the content of GSH in incubation mixtures containing isolated rat liver nuclei, BP, reduced nicotinamide-adenine dinucleotide phosphate (NADPH), and a cytosolic fraction (Table 1). Two metabolite-DNA adducts were detectable: one arising from metabolites of BP-7,8-dihydrodiol, most probably isomers of BP-diol-epoxide (9), and another from metabolites of 9-hydroxy-BP (9-OH-BP). When we decreased the levels of GSH in the incubation mixture by 70 to 80% the amount of DNA adducts of BP-7,8-dihydrodiol metabolites increased almost fourfold whereas the binding of the 9-OH-BP-metabolites increased only about twofold. The results indicated that GSH conjugation specifically inhibits the binding of BP-7,8-dihydrodiol metabolites. This was confirmed by replacing the cytosolic fraction by purified GSH S-transferases as shown in the following.

The GSH S-transferases in the rat liver constitute a family of at least six enzymes with overlapping substrate specificities. The various transferases may have different activities towards a given substrate. In the present studies we investigated four different purified GSH S-transferases (B, C, D, A) for their capability to reduce the formation of BP-7,8-dihydrodiol-derived DNA adducts.

TABLE 1. *Effect of glutathione on binding of BP-7,8-dihydrodiol metabolites formed by nuclei from benzo(a)pyrene in the presence of cytosol* [a]

Additions	BP-7,8-diol metabolites bound (pmoles/mg DNA/30 min)
Cytosol from control rats (0.2 mM GSH)	0.4
Cytosol from DEM-treated rats (0.05 mM GSH)	1.5
+ 0.1 mM GSH	1.0
+ 0.2 mM GSH	0.5

Data from ref. 9.

[a]Incubations contained 250×10^6 nuclei, TKM-buffer (50 mM Tris, 25 mM KCl, 5 mM $MgCl_2$, pH 7.5),1 mM NADPH, 20 μM ^{3}H-BP (1.7 Ci/mmoles) and cytosolic fraction corresponding to 8 mg protein in a final volume of 10 ml and were carried out for 30 min at 37°C. Nuclei and cytosolic fraction were obtained from livers of 3-methylcholanthrene-treated rats. To reduce the content of cytosolic GSH, rats were pretreated with diethylmaleate (DEM) 1 hr before death. BP-modified DNA was isolated, hydrolyzed and desoxyribonucleosides were separated by Sephadex LH20 chromatography as described by Guenthner et al. (8).

Using BP as a substrate, GSH and GSH S-transferases may react with either BP-diol-epoxide or with its precursor BP-7,8-oxide. Both reactions would lead to a decrease in BP-7,8-dihydrodiol-derived DNA adducts. To find out whether one of the epoxides is preferentially conjugated, we carried out two sets of incubations, using either BP or BP-7,8-dihydrodiol as substrate. As shown in Fig. 2, purified GSH S-transferase B decreased the amount of BP-7,8-dihydrodiol-derived DNA adducts in the presence of relatively low GSH concentrations (0.2 mM) by 60 to 70% when incubated with nuclei, NADPH and BP-7,8-dihydrodiol. Increasing the concentration of GHS up to 1 mM decreased the binding further but failed to inhibit it completely. However, the concentration of GSH S-transferase B in the incubation mixture was only ~10 μM, i.c., 1/10 of that in rat liver cells (27). Thus, one might expect that GSH conjugation is efficient in intact cells *in vivo* and no significant DNA binding occurs.

The decrease in DNA adducts was inversely correlated with the formation of GHS conjugates supporting the concept that reactive BP-7,8-diol metabolites are trapped by conjugation with GSH (Fig. 2). Inhibition of DNA binding with GSH alone in the absence of GSH S-transferases was negligible (Fig. 2, Table 2). This

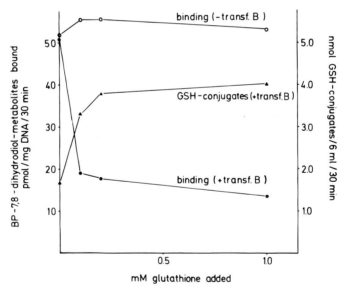

FIG. 2. Effect of GSH and GSH S-transferase B on the binding of BP-7,8-dihydrodiol metabolites and formation of GSH conjugates during metabolism of ³H-BP-7,8-dihydrodiol with rat liver nuclei. Incubations with 125 × 10⁶ nuclei and 3 μM ³H-BP-7,8-dihydrodiol (0.23 Ci/mmole) in a total volume of 6 ml were carried out as given in Table 1 of this chapter. GSH S-transferase B was provided by Dr. Brian Ketterer, London. GSH conjugates were determined as described by Jernström et al. (14). Binding in the absence of GSH and GSH S-transferase B corresponds to 51.8 pmoles/mg DNA/30 min. Twenty-five milligrams of protein were added to incubations containing GSH S-transferase B. *Empty circles,* binding in the absence of GSH S-transferase B; *solid circles,* binding in the presence of GSH S-transferase B; *triangles,* GSH conjugates. (Data from ref. 10.)

TABLE 2. *Effects of GSH and GSH S-transferases on DNA binding of BP-7,8-dihydrodiol metabolites during metabolism of benzo(a)pyrene or BP-7,8-dihydrodiol[a]*

| | DNA-binding | |
Conditions	Benzo(a)pyrene (%)	BP-7,8-dihydrodiol (%)
Nuclei	100	100
+ GSH	79 ± 2 (4)	93 ± 12 (3)
+ transferase B + GSH	32 ± 5 (3)	25 ± 9 (4)
+ transferase A + GSH	63 (2)	65 (2)
+ transferase C + GSH	54 (1)	41 (2)
+ transferase E + GSH	26 (1)	15 ± 4 (3)

Data from ref. 10.
[a]Incubations were carried out as given in Table 1 and Fig. 2 of this chapter. The purified GSH S-transferases were provided by Dr. Brian Ketterer, London. DNA binding in control incubations with nuclei alone: 5 pmoles/mg DNA/30 min (with 20 μM BP) and 120 pmoles/ mg DNA/30 min (with 8 μM BP-7,8-dihydrodiol). Two milligrams of protein of each GSH S-transferase were added. Number of experiments is given in parentheses.

TABLE 3. *Effect of glutathione and GSH S-transferase E and A on DNA binding and GSH conjugate formation of BP-7,8-dihydrodiol metabolites formed by nuclei*

Conditions	Binding (pmoles/mg DNA/30 min)	Conjugation (nmoles/mg DNA/30 min)
Nuclei	119	0.7
+ transferase E	17	8.1
+ transferase A	103	1.0

Data from ref. 10.

indicates that the nonenzymatic reaction between BP-7,8-dihydrodiol metabolites and GSH is poor, in agreement with earlier observations by Cooper et al. (3).

GSH S-transferase E appeared to be more active than transferase B in inhibiting the binding of BP-7,8-dihydrodiol metabolites, whereas transferase C and even more transferase A were less active (Table 2). Transferase E also formed relatively large amounts of the conjugates, whereas transferase A which had the lowest inhibitory activity produced only traces of conjugates (Table 3).

As demonstrated in Table 2 the differences in the inhibitory capacity of the various purified transferases were similar for the two substrates, BP-7,8-dihydrodiol and BP. The results suggest that the major substrate for GSH-conjugation most likely is the BP-diol-epoxide rather than its precursor BP-7,8-epoxide.

Observations with freshly isolated hepatocytes (7,13) showed that conjugation with GSH effectively traps reactive species formed from BP-7,8-dihydrodiol also in the intact cell. Jernström et al. (14) and Glatt et al. (7) have recently shown that in cells obtained from 3-methylcholanthrene induced rats the binding of BP-7,8-dihydrodiol metabolites to DNA (14) as well as the mutagenicity (7) depend on the levels of GSH. Furthermore, Jernström et al. (14) showed that the formation of conjugates was decreased in parallel to the increased DNA binding which they attributed to the GSH-depletion in the hepatocytes.

In vivo BP-diol-epoxide-DNA-adducts were either not detectable in the liver (2) or were present in only very low amounts (18) compared to other organs. This is in agreement with the fact that BP is not carcinogenic for the liver (11). Our results obtained *in vitro* indicate that detoxification by GSH may play an important role in the protection of the rat liver against the genotoxicity of BP.

This might be different for extrahepatic tissues which contain considerably lower activities of the GSH S-transferases. *In vivo* investigations in the lung and fore-stomach of mice have shown that the induction of GSH S-transferases by antioxidants and other compounds is associated with a lower formation of BP-diol-epoxide-DNA-adducts (1) and also with the inhibition of BP-induced neoplasia (12,25). But a causal relationship has so far not been established.

Although the liver seems to be well protected against carcinogenic BP-diol-epoxides it is susceptible to another carcinogenic epoxide, aflatoxin B_1-2,3-epoxide. This presumed ultimate carcinogenic form of aflatoxin B_1 is substrate for cytosolic GSH S-transferases *in vitro* (4) like BP-diol-epoxide. The DNA binding of this metabolite is reduced in the presence of GSH and cytosolic transferases in microsomal incubations (19). Furthermore, observations of Degen and Neumann (5) suggest that the low susceptibility of mice for aflatoxin B_1-induced tumor formation may be attributable to the high potential for GSH conjugation with aflatoxin. However, the fact that aflatoxin B_1 is a very potent liver carcinogen shows that the efficiency of the GSH-dependent inactivation *in vivo* is limited.

At present no *in vivo* data are available to indicate that the different sensitivity of the rat liver against BP and aflatoxin B_1 may be due to differences in the GSH-conjugation of the ultimate carcinogenic metabolites. The *in vitro* data strongly suggest that GSH conjugation plays an important role in the inactivation of both metabolites. However, repair and other factors will determine whether initial lesions lead to the expression of cancer.

CONCLUSIONS

The efficiency of GSH conjugation in the detoxification of reactive metabolites depends on the substrate specificities of the GSH S-transferases and cannot be predicted from the electrophilic character of the substrate. Our studies using nuclei and purified transferases of rat liver indicate that conjugation with GSH efficiently traps the ultimate reactive species of BP. This might contribute to the understanding of the lack of hepato-genotoxicity of BP in the rat. However, *in vivo* data are lacking which show a causal relationship between the formation of BP-induced tumors in susceptible organs and an inadequate GSH conjugation. Furthermore, aflatoxin B_1 is also subject to an effective GSH conjugation *in vitro* (4,5), but, nevertheless, it is a potent hepato-carcinogen. Thus, the *in vitro* experiments suggest that GSH and GSH S-transferases play an important role in the inactivation of ultimate carcinogenic metabolites, such as those formed from BP or aflatoxin B_1. However, it remains to be elucidated whether and under what conditions the *in vivo* detoxification by GSH conjugation is a decisive factor in the prevention of tumor initiation.

ACKNOWLEDGMENTS

The authors are grateful to Dr. Brian Ketterer, London, G.B., who generously provided the purified GSH S-transferases. We are also indebted to Prof. Sten Orrenius for his encouragement and continuous interest in this work and to Dr. Peter Moldéus for fruitful collaboration and discussions. The excellent technical assistance of Ms. Margareta Martinez and the expert secretarial help of Ms. Ursula Welscher are gratefully acknowledged.

REFERENCES

1. Anderson, M. W., Boroujerdie, M., and Wilson, A. G. E. (1981): Inhibition *in vivo* of the formation of adducts between metabolites of benzo*(a)*pyrene and DNA by butylated hydroxyanisole. *Cancer Res.*, 41:4309–4315.
2. Boroujerdie, M., Kung, Hsiao-c., Wilson, A. G. E., and Anderson, M. W. (1981): Metabolism and DNA binding of benzo*(a)*pyrene *in vivo* in the rat. *Cancer Res.*, 41:951–957.
3. Cooper, C. S., Hewer, A., Ribeiro, O., Grover, P. L., and Sims, P. (1980): The enzyme-catalysed conversion of *anti*-benzo*(a)*pyrene-7,8-diol 9,10-oxide into a glutathione conjugate. *Carcinogenesis*, 1:1075–1080.
4. Degen, G. H., and Neumann, H.-G. (1978): The major metabolite of aflatoxin B$_1$ in the rat is a glutathione conjugate. *Chem.-Biol. Interact.*, 22:239–255.
5. Degen, G. H., and Neumann, H.-G. (1981): Differences in aflatoxin B$_1$-susceptibility of rat and mouse are correlated with the capability *in vitro* in inactivate aflatoxin B$_1$-epoxide. *Carcinogenesis*, 2:299–306.
6. Friedberg, T., Bentley, P., Stasiecki, P., Glatt, H. R., Raphael, D., and Oesch, F. (1979): The identification, solubilization, and characterization of microsome-associated glutathione S-transferases. *J. Biol. Chem.*, 254:12028–12033.
7. Glatt, H. R., Billings, R., Platt, K. L., and Oesch, F. (1981): Improvement of the correlation of bacterial mutagenicity with carcinogenicity of benzo(a)pyrene and four of its major metabolites by activation with intact liver cells instead of cell homogenate. *Cancer Res.*, 41:270–277.
8. Guenthner, T. M., Jernström, B., and Orrenius, S. (1980): On the effect of cellular nucleophiles on the binding of metabolites of 7,8-dihydroxy-7,8-dihydrobenzo*(a)*pyrene and 9-hydroxy-benzo(a)pyrene to nuclear DNA. *Carcinogenesis*, 1:407–418.
9. Hesse, S., Jernström, B., Martinez, M., Guenthner, T. M., and Orrenius, S. (1980): Inhibition of binding of benzo(a)pyrene metabolites to nuclear DNA by glutathione and glutathione S-transferase B. *Biochem. Biophys. Res. Commun.*, 94:612–617.
10. Hesse, S., Jernström, B., Martinez, M., Moldéus, P., Christodoulides, L., and Ketterer, B. (1982): Inactivation of DNA-binding metabolites of benzo(a)pyrene and benzo(a)pyrene-7,8-dihydrodiol by glutathione and glutathione S-transferases. *Carcinogenesis*, 3:757–760.
11. *IARC Monographs on the Evaluation of Carcinogenic Risk of the Chemicals to Man Vol 3*, 1973. International Agency for Research on Cancer, Lyon.
12. Ioannou, Y. M., Wilson, A. G. E., and Anderson, M. W. (1982): Effect of butylated hydroxyanisole on the metabolism of benzo(a)pyrene and the binding of metabolites to DNA, *in vitro* and *in vivo*, in the forestomach, lung and liver of mice. *Carcinogenesis*, 3:739–745.
13. Jerina, D. M. (1976): 18. Products, specificity, and assay of glutathione S-transferase with epoxide substrates. In: *Glutathione: Metabolism and Function*, edited by I. M. Arias and W. B. Jakoby, pp. 267–279. Raven Press, New York.
14. Jernström, B., Babson, J. R., Moldéus, P., Homgren, A., and Reed, D. J. (1982): Glutathione conjugation and DNA-binding of (±)-*trans*-7,8-dihydroxy-7,8-dihydrobenzo(a)pyrene and (±)-7β,8α-dihydroxy-9α,10α-epoxy-7,8,9,10-tetrahydrobenzo(a)pyrene in isolated rat hepatocytes. *Carcinogenesis*, 3:861–866.
15. Kadlubar, F. F., Ketterer, B., Flammang, T. J., and Christodoulides, L. (1980): Formation of 3-

(glutathione-S-YL)-N-methyl-4-aminoazobenzene and inhibition of aminoazo dye-nucleic acid binding in vitro by reaction of glutathione with metabolically-generated N-methyl-4-aminobenzene-N-sulfate. *Chem. Biol. Interact.*, 31:265–278.

16. Ketterer, B. (1982): The role of nonenzymatic reactions of glutathione in xenobiotic metabolism. *Drug Metabolism Reviews*, 13:161–187.

17. Ketterer, B., and Tipping, E. (1978): An appraisal of the likely roles of ligandin (glutathione S-transferase B) in hepatocarcinogenesis. In: *Conjugation Reactions in Drug Biotransformation*, edited by A. Aito, pp. 91–100. Elsevier/North-Holland, New York, Amsterdam, Oxford.

18. Kleihues, P., Doerjer, G., Ehret, M., and Guzman, J. (1980): Reaction of benzo(a)pyrene and 7,12-dimethylbenz(a)anthracene with DNA of various rat tissues *in vivo*. *Arch. Toxicol.* Suppl. 3:237–246.

19. Lotlikar, P. D., Insetta, S. M., Lyons, P. R., and Eun-Chung Jhee (1980): Inhibition of microsome-mediated binding of aflatoxin B_1 to DNA by glutathione S-transferase. *Cancer Lett.*, 9:143–149.

20. Meerman, J. H. N., Beland, F. A., Ketterer, B., Srai, S. K. S., Bruins, A. P., and Mulder, G. J. (1982): Identification of glutathione conjugates formed from N-hydroxy-2-acetylaminofluorene in the rat. *Chem.-Biol. Interact.*, 39:149–168.

21. Morgenstern, R., DePierre, J. W., and Ernster, L. (1979): Activation of microsomal glutathione S-transferase activity by sulfhydryl reagents. *Biochem. Biophys. Res. Commun.*, 81:657–663.

22. Nemoto, N., Gelboin, H. V., Habig, W. H., Ketley, J. N., and Jakoby, W. B. (1975): K-region benzo(a)pyrene-4,5-oxide is conjugated by homogeneous glutathione S-transferases. *Nature*, 255:512.

23. Smith, G. J., and Litwack, G. (1980): Roles of ligandin and the glutathione S-transferases in binding steroid metabolites, carcinogens and other compounds. In: *Reviews in Biochemical Toxicology 2*, edited by E. Hodgson, J. R. Bend, and R. M. Philpot, pp. 1–47. Elsevier/North-Holland, New York, Amsterdam, Oxford.

24. Smith, G. J., Ohl, V. S., and Litwack, G. (1977): Ligandin, the glutathione S-transferases, and chemically induced hepatocarcinogenesis: A review. *Cancer Res.*, 37:8–14.

25. Sparnins, V. L., and Wattenberg, L. W. (1981): Enhancement of glutathione S-transferase activity of the mouse forestomach by inhibitors of benzo(a)pyrene-induced neoplasia of the forestomach. *J. Natl. Cancer Inst.*, 66:769–771.

26. Tipping, E., and Ketterer, B. (1981): The influence of soluble binding proteins on lipophile transport and metabolism in hepatocytes. *Biochem. J.*, 195:441–452.

27. Tipping, E., Moore, B. P., Jones, C. A., Cohen, G. M., Ketterer, B., and Bridges, J. W. (1980): The non-covalent binding of benzo(a)pyrene and its hydroxylated metabolites to intracellular proteins and lipid bilayers. *Chem.-Biol. Interact.*, 32:291–304.

Biochemical Basis of Chemical Carcinogenesis,
edited by H. Greim, R. Jung, M. Kramer,
H. Marquardt, and F. Oesch.
Raven Press, New York © 1984.

Role of Glucuronidation and Sulfation in the Control of Reactive Metabolites

*K. W. Bock, *B. S. Bock-Hennig, **G. Fischer,
*W. Lilienblum, and *D. Ullrich

*Department of Pharmacology and Toxicology, and **Department of Pathology,
University of Göttingen, D-3400 Göttingen, Federal Republic of Germany

Most chemical carcinogens must be converted to electrophilic ultimate carcinogens which initiate primary lesions in target cells, most probably alterations of cellular DNA (29). Based on this concept many toxicologists have been preoccupied with enzymes controlling electrophilic metabolites. Although the role of these enzymes is not disputed it is increasingly recognized that UDP-glucuronosyltransferases (GTs) and sulfotransferases, enzymes controlling nucleophilic proximal carcinogens and cytotoxins, often play a major role in chemical carcinogenesis. It is also important to note that drug metabolizing enzymes not only control the initiation of primary lesions but also the resistance of preneoplastic cells to carcinogens and the generation of promoters at stages subsequent to initiation (42).

Conjugation with glucuronic acid or sulfate leads to polar metabolites which are efficiently eliminated either via the bile or the urine. Sulfotransferases and GTs can replace each other in the conjugation of phenols, sulfotransferases usually exhibiting higher affinity but lower capacity. The two enzymes also show different cellular localization and inducibility. Sulfotransferases are localized in the cytosol whereas GTs are bound to the endoplasmic reticulum and nuclear membranes; GTs, in contrast to sulfotransferases, are markedly inducible by xenobiotic inducers (14,30).

MECHANISMS BY WHICH GLUCURONIDATION AND SULFATION CONTROL THE GENERATION OF REACTIVE METABOLITES

Formation of Reactive (Unstable) Sulfates and Glucuronides

In general, glucuronides and sulfates are biologically and chemically less reactive than their parent compounds, with the exception of certain conjugates of N-hydroxyarylamines. The sulfate ester of N-hydroxy-2-acetylaminofluorene and deacetylated metabolites are probably proximal carcinogens and cytotoxins in 2-acetylaminofluorene carcinogenesis (28–30). The N-O-glucuronide of N-hydroxyphenacetin is probably a proximal carcinogen responsible for cancer of the urinary tract in people who abused phenacetin-containing analgesic mixtures (11). The role of glucuronidation has been clearly established in urinary bladder carcinogenesis caused by 2-naphthylamine (29). The *N*-glucuronide of *N*-hydroxy-2-naphthylamine, which is readily formed in liver, is transported to the kidney where it enters the urine. Under the acidic conditions of urine (pH 5-6) the *N*-glucuronide decomposes to the ultimate carcinogen, an aryl nitrenium ion. This aryl nitrenium ion is probably not the ultimate mutagen responsible for 2-naphthylamine mutagenicity in the Ames test (9). Moreover it remains to be elucidated which ultimate reactant is responsible for preneoplastic liver lesions produced by the administration of 2-naphthylamine following partial hepatectomy (39).

Enzymic Release of Proximal Carcinogens from Glucuronides at Sites Distant from Their Formation

Glucuronides with high molecular weights (>300 in rats or >400 in man) are preferentially secreted from liver into the intestine. Hydrolysis of the glucuronides, e.g., of 3-hydroxybenzo*(a)*pyrene glucuronide (21), by bacterial β-glucuronidase may lead to the release of proximal carcinogens in the intestine. Biliary excretion may be the major factor for the high incidence of intestinal neoplasms produced by subcutaneous injection of 3-methyl-2-naphthylamine and 3,2-dimethyl-4-aminobiphenyl to male rats (41).

Inhibition of Recycling to Ultimate Carcinogens and of Toxic Oxidation-Reduction Cycles

Intensive studies of benzo*(a)*pyrene metabolism revealed various phenols, quinones, and diols as major primary metabolites (Fig. 1). Further oxidation of benzo*(a)*pyrene-7,8-diol leads to generation of bay region diol epoxides which probably represent ultimate carcinogens (37). Conjugation of benzo*(a)*pyrene-7,8-diol decreases the formation of these diol epoxides. Since benzo*(a)*pyrene-7,8-diol is a poor substrate of GT and sulfotransferase these enzymes cannot completely prevent the formation of diol epoxides (33). Phenols are rapidly conjugated. The glucuronidation rate of 3-hydroxybenzo*(a)*pyrene [about 1 nmole/min/mg protein (2)] corresponds with its rate of formation in rat liver microsomes in the aryl hydrocarbon hydroxylase assay [0.7 nmole/min/mg protein (22)]. The toxicity of phenols is probably caused by oxidation products. Although quinones are not substrates of GT, they can be rapidly reduced by various oxido-reductases [cytochrome P-450 reductase (3) and DT diaphorase (23)]. Quinones have been shown to be cytotoxic by undergoing oxidation-reduction cycles whereby superoxide radicals and semiquinone radicals are generated (24). In these cycles quinols are formed which are rapidly trapped by glucuronidation (3). In this way glucuronidation may efficiently prevent toxic oxidation-reduction cycles. On the other hand, benzo*(a)*pyrene quinones have been shown to inhibit cytochrome P-450 dependent oxidation of benzo*(a)*pyrene (36). By conversion of quinones to quinol glucuronides this product inhibition is removed leading to enhanced benzo*(a)*pyrene oxidation (1,36). This

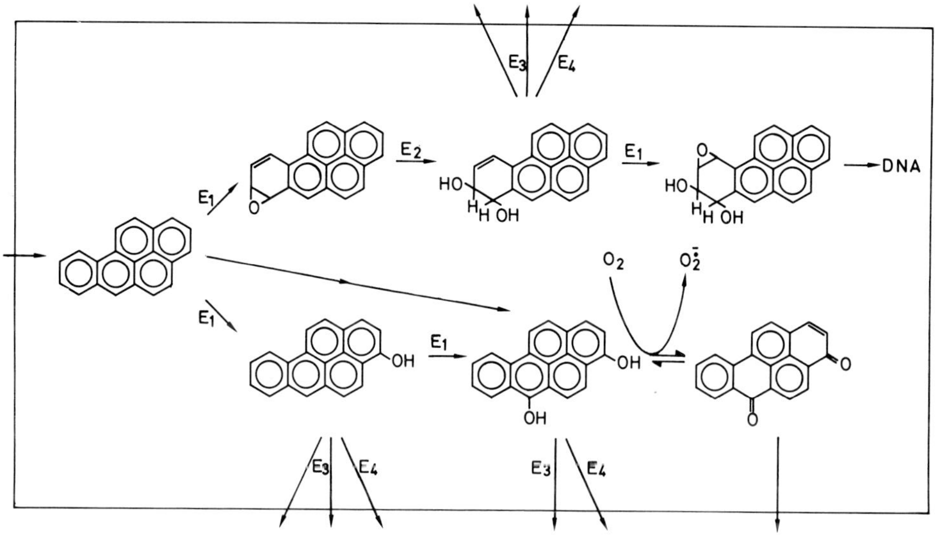

FIG. 1. Selected pathways of benzo(a)pyrene metabolism leading to mutagenic and cytotoxic metabolites. E_1, cytochrome P-450; E_2, epoxide hydrolase; E_3, UDP-glucuronosyltransferase; E_4, sulfotransferase.

may be the reason why at high concentrations, DNA-binding (36) and benzo(a)pyrene mutagenicity (27) are increased in the presence of glucuronidation.

Generation of reactive metabolites is critically dependent upon a complex balance between activating and inactivating enzymes. To understand the balance it is important to know the independently regulated enzyme entities (forms) and their inducibility. In the following two enzyme forms which are pivotal in the control of benzo(a)pyrene metabolism, cytochrome P_1-450 and GT_1, will be discussed. Since drug metabolism in the intact cell is controlled by numerous other enzymes, studies *in vitro* will be compared with results obtained in intact cell systems where all enzymes are operating in a concerted manner.

INDUCTION OF CYTOCHROME P_1-450 AND OF GT_1 AND ITS IMPLICATIONS FOR BENZO(A)PYRENE MUTAGENICITY

Multiplicity of cytochromes P-450 is firmly established (25), and there is also accumulating evidence for a multiplicity of GTs (8). Thorgeirsson and Nebert (38) defined cytochrome P_1-450 as that form of aromatic hydrocarbon (Ah)-inducible cytochrome P-450 which is most closely associated with arylhydrocarbon hydroxylase activity. Similarly, we define GT_1 as that Ah-inducible form of GT most closely associated with the conjugation of planar phenols such as p-nitrophenol or 3-hydroxybenzo(a)pyrene (8) and benzo(a)pyrene-3,6-quinol (3). The term recommended for GT_1 is p-nitrophenol-GT, in which a commonly used model substrate is used as the basis for terminology (8). Cytochrome P_1-450 and GT_1 appear to exist in a variety of species, including man (5,7,32).

There has been some uncertainty about how to interpret GT activities since glucuronide formation is regulated by a variety of factors, e.g., phospholipid-dependence and latency of GT activity (14). However, recent advances in electroimmunochemical quantitation of GT suggest that enzyme activity is a reasonable index of the enzyme level (6). Moreover, in studies with isolated hepatocytes from untreated controls and from 3-methylcholanthrene- and phenobarbital-treated rats we could demonstrate that the conjugation of GT_1-substrates, such as 3-hydroxy-benzo(a)pyrene, is selectively enhanced in hepatocytes from 3-methylcholanthrene-treated rats (Fig. 2), suggesting that the enzyme level is a major determinant of glucuronide formation in the intact cell.

Evidence obtained with inbred strains of mice suggests that the inducibility of both cytochrome P_1-450 and GT_1 by 3-methylcholanthrene-type inducers is regulated by the same genetic locus, which has been termed Ah locus (34). This suggests that the induction of both enzymes is mediated by the same receptor protein, which resembles steroid receptors in many ways. Nebert was able to demonstrate that high inducibility, regulated by the Ah locus, was associated either with increased susceptibility to toxic reactions [such as benzo(a)pyrene initiated subcutaneous fibrosarcomas] or with increased resistance to toxicity at a more physiological type of exposure, such as oral administration of benzo(a)pyrene (31).

We studied the role of GT_1 inducibility in the control of reactive mutagenic metabolites using the Ames test (4). Addition of co-factors of glucuronidation to the Ames test reduced benzo(a)pyrene mutagenicity (Table 1,A). Interestingly both the generation of mutagenic metabolites and their reduction by glucuronidation were most pronounced using liver homogenates from 3-methylcholanthrene-treated rats, nicely illustrating the potential of a coordinate induction of cytochrome P_1-450 and GT_1. However, at high benzo(a)pyrene concentrations its mutagenicity was enhanced by glucuronidation (Table 1,B and ref. 27). This is probably due to removal of inhibitory quinones, as discussed above.

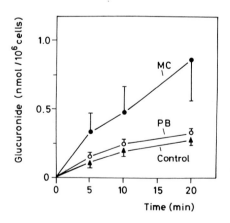

FIG. 2. Glucuronidation of 3-hydroxy-benzo(a)pyrene in isolated hepatocytes from untreated controls and from phenobarbital- or 3-methylcholanthrene-treated cells. Rat hepatocytes (2×10^6 cells/ml) were incubated in the presence of 20 nmoles 3-hydroxybenzo(a)pyrene. After termination of the reaction by addition of acetone, metabolites were separated by TLC in ethyl acetate/methanol/H_2O/formic acid (100/25/10/1, v/v/v/v) and 3-hydroxybenzo(a)pyrene glucuronide was eluted and quantified fluorimetrically as described (2).

TABLE 1. *Effects of glucuronidation on benzo*(a)*pyrene mutagenicity in the Ames test*[a]

Treatment *in vivo*	Revertant colonies		
	− UDPGA[b] (control)	+ UDPGA[c] (+ UDPNAG)[d]	(% of control)
(A) Untreated (2.5)[c]	34 ± 16	12 ± 7	35
Phenobarbital (2.5)	61 ± 10	40 ± 8	66
3-Methylcholanthrene (2.5)	495 ± 20	72 ± 25	15
(B) Arochlor 1254 (2.5)	283 ± 79	54 ± 19	19
Arochlor 1254 (10)	142 ± 70	201 ± 53	142
Arochlor 1254 (25)	123 ± 21	223 ± 24	181

[a]S-9 preparations from untreated, phenobarbital- and 3-methylcholanthrene-treated rats were compared. Each plate contained 10^8 bacteria and S-9 mix (1mg protein). In experiments with glucuronidation, UDP-gluouronic acid (3 mM) and UDP-N-acetylglucosamine (3 mM) were included. Backround revertants (20/plate) were subtracted. Each value is the mean ± S.D. of 6 determinations.
[b]UDPGA, UDP-glucuronic acid.
[c]UDPNAG, UDP-N-acetylglucosamine.
[d]Benzo(a)pyrene concentration (μg/plate).

TABLE 2. *Differential induction of benzo(a)pyrene monooxygenase and UDP-glucuronosyltranferase activities by various inducing agents in rat liver microsomes*

Inducer	Monooxygenase (Benzo(a)pyrene)	UDP-glucuronosyltransferase	
		(1-Naphthol)	(Morphine)
	Untreated controls (nmoles/min/mg protein)		
	2.8 ± 0.5	66 ± 10	10.7 ± 2.7
	(-fold increase over control)		
1) 3-Methylcholanthrene	4.4	3.2	1.3
β-Naphthoflavone	3.1	2.9	1.0
2) Phenobarbital	1.5	1.3	4.1
DDT	1.2	1.2	2.3
1+2) Aroclor 1254	3.6	6.4	2.7
3) Ethoxyquin	1.0	3.0	4.2
Trans-stilbene oxide	0.8	1.8	3.0

Data from ref. 22.

In addition to coordinated induction by 3-methylcholanthrene-type inducers, there is also evidence for independent control of cytochrome P_1-450 and GT_1. Selective induction of GT_1 is observed after the administration of trans-stilbene oxide or anticarcinogenic antioxidants such as ethoxyquin (Table 2). Other enzymes, such as epoxide hydrolase and GSH S-transferase are also known to be induced by these agents (12). The altered pattern of drug metabolizing enzymes after treatment with trans-stilbene oxide or ethoxyquin is consistent with increased resistance to chemical carcinogens. It is similar to the altered enzyme pattern seen in putative preneoplastic hepatocytes (see below).

An inactivating role of glucuronidation and sulfation was also demonstrated in studies with enzyme inhibitors such as salicylamide. In the presence of salicylamide covalent binding of benzo(a)pyrene metabolites to DNA (10) and the release of mutagenic metabolites from the perfused rat liver were enhanced (4).

"PERMANENT INDUCTION" OF GT$_1$ IN PRENEOPLASTIC HEPATOCYTES

The balance between activating and inactivating drug metabolizing enzymes not only controls initiation but also resistance of preneoplastic cells to chemical carcinogens and the generation of promoters at stages following initiation. GT$_1$ activities are selectively enhanced (fivefold) in preneoplastic liver nodules (Fig. 3 and ref. 6). In the same nodules epoxide hydrolase and GSH S-transferase were also increased [sevenfold and fivefold, respectively (17)]. However cytochrome P-450 dependent activities were decreased. This altered pattern of drug metabolizing enzymes is consistent with increased resistance to chemical carcinogens. Resistance

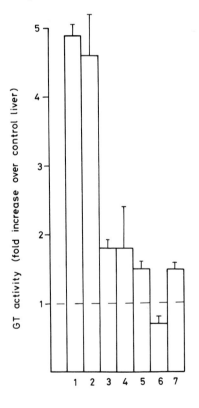

FIG. 3. Differentially increased UDP-glucuronosyltransferase activities in preneoplastic liver nodules. Liver nodules were produced by feeding alternatively a basal diet containing 2-acetylaminofluorene (0.05%, w/v) and basal diet alone for 22 weeks. UDP-glucuronosyltransferase activities were determined in nodular microsomes as described (6). Substrates tested were (1) 1-naphthol, (2) 3-hydroxybenzo(a)pyrene, (3) 4-hydroxybiphenyl, (4) morphine, (5) chloramphenicol, (6) bilirubin, (7) estrone.

of malignant cells is indicated by studies on the cytotoxicity of 7,12-dimethyl-benzanthracene in cell cultures (20). Resistance was associated with increased generation of glucuronides.

Using antibodies to GT_1 we developed a method for histochemical detection of GT_1 (Fig. 4). Positive staining of GT_1 was found in the same foci which were ATPase negative and γ-glutamyltranspeptidase positive. Increased GT_1 in preneoplastic foci was substantiated by biochemical analysis of samples obtained after microdissection showing that GT_1 activities were fivefold higher in the focal area compared with the surrounding tissue (18,19). Hence GT_1 may be considered as a preneoplastic marker enzyme. Increased GT_1 activity should lead to a shift of conjugation from sulfation to glucuronidation. This shift has been observed in human organ cultures from bronchial carcinomas and colonic tumor tissues (13). This marker, therefore, may be of general importance and may be useful to analyze persistence or remodeling of the altered phenotype observed after cessation of carcinogenic stimuli (15,16).

The reason why GT_1 activity is permanently increased remains unclear. Since increased GT_1 activity persists in hyperplastic nodules and hepatomas after many years of transplantation it has been operationally termed "permanent induction" (26). In addition it remains unclear why cytochrome P-450 dependent reactions are decreased under conditions leading to a marked increase of a battery of other drug metabolizing enzymes.

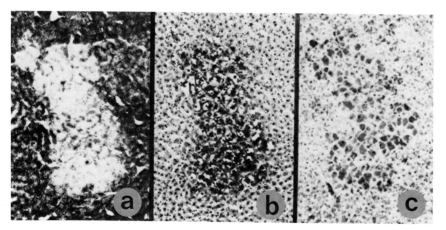

FIG. 4. Immunohistochemical detection of ATPase **(a)**, γ-glutamyltranspeptidase **(b)**, and UDP-glucuronosyltransferase **(c)** in putative preneoplastic liver lesions. Focal lesions were produced by continuous feeding of a diet containing 2-acetylaminofluorene (0.03%, w/v) for 25 weeks, followed by feeding the diet without the carcinogen for 10 weeks. Serial sections from the two major liver lobes were prepared at −20°C on a cryostat microtome. Standard methods were used to visualize ATPase negative foci (40) and γ-glutamyltranspeptidase positive foci (35). UDP-glucuronosyltransferase positive foci were detected by an indirect method in which rabbit anti-GT_1 immunoglobulins (6) were incubated with peroxidase-labeled swine anti-rabbit IgG (19). The tissue was counterstained with hematoxylin and eosin.

CONCLUSIONS

1. Glucuronidation and sulfation control the generation of ultimate carcinogens and cytotoxins in many ways:

   a. formation of reactive conjugates,
   b. enzymic release of proximal carcinogens from conjugates,
   c. inhibition of recycling to ultimate carcinogens,
   d. inhibition of toxic oxidation-reduction cycles.

2. Studies with enzyme inducers and inhibitors demonstrate an inactivating role of glucuronidation in benzo(a)pyrene mutagenicity. However, at high concentrations glucuronidation leads to increased benzo(a)pyrene mutagenicity.
3. In the model of liver carcinogenesis UDP-glucuronosyltransferase is "permanently induced" in putative preneoplastic foci, hyperplastic nodules, and certain hepatomas, whereas cytochrome P-450 dependent monooxygenase activities are decreased. This altered pattern of drug metabolizing enzymes is consistent with increased resistance to chemical carcinogens.

ACKNOWLEDGMENTS

We are grateful to the Deutsche Forschungsgemeinschaft and the Stiftung Volkswagenwerk for financial support.

REFERENCES

1. Bock, K. W. (1978): Increase of liver microsomal benzo(a)pyrene monooxygenase activity by subsequent glucuronidation. *Naunyn-Schmiedeberg's Arch. Pharmacol.*, 304:77–79.
2. Bock, K. W., and Lilienblum, W. (1979): Activation and induction of rat liver microsomal UDP-glucuronyltransferase with 3-hydroxybenzo(a)pyrene and N-hydroxy-2-naphthylamine as substrates. *Biochem. Pharmacol.*, 28:695–700.
3. Bock, K. W., Lilienblum, W., and Pfeil, H. (1980): Conversion of benzo(a)pyrene-3,6-quinone to quinol glucuronides with rat liver microsomes or purified NADPH-cytochrome c reductase and UDP-glucuronosyltransferase. *FEBS Lett.*, 121:269–272.
4. Bock, K. W., Bock-Hennig, B. S., Lilienblum, W., and Volp, R. F. (1981): Release of mutagenic metabolites of benzo(a)pyrene from the perfused rat liver after inhibition of glucuronidation and sulfation by salicylamide. *Chem.-Biol. Interact.*, 36:167–177.
5. Bock, K. W., Lilienblum, W., and Pfeil, H. (1982): Functional heterogeneity of UDP-glucuronosyltransferase activities in C57BL/6 and DBA/2 mice. *Biochem. Pharmacol.*, 31:1273–1277.
6. Bock, K. W., Lilienblum, W., Pfeil, H., and Eriksson, L. C. (1982): Increased uridine diphosphate-glucuronyltransferase activity in preneoplastic liver nodules and Morris hepatomas. *Cancer Res.*, 42:3747–3752.
7. Bock, K. W., Lilienblum, W., and von Bahr, Ch. (1984): Studies of UDP-glucuronyltransferase activities in human liver microsomes. *Drug Metal. Disp. (in press)*.
8. Bock, K. W., Burchell, B., Dutton, G. J., Hänninen, O., Mulder, G. J., Owens, I. S. Siest, G., and Tephly, T. R.: UDP-glucuronosyltransferase: Guidelines for consistent interim terminology and assay conditions. *Biochem. Pharmacol.*, 32:953–955.
9. Bock-Hennig, B. S., Ullrich, D., and Bock, K. W. (1982): Activating and inactivating reactions controlling 2-naphthylamine mutagenicity. *Arch. Toxicol.*, 50:259–266.
10. Burke, M. D., Vadi, H., Jernström, B., and Orrenius, S. (1977): Metabolism of benzo(a)pyrene with isolated hepatocytes and the formation and degradation of DNA-binding derivatives. *J. Biol. Chem.*, 252:6424–6431.

11. Camus, A.-M., Friesen, M., Croisy, A., and Bartsch, H. (1982): Species-specific activation of phenacetin into bacterial mutagens by hamster liver enzymes and identification of N-hydroxyphenacetin O-glucuronide as a promutagen in the urine. *Cancer Res.*, 42:3201–3208.
12. Cha, Y.-N., and Heine, H. S. (1982): Comparative effects of dietary administration of 2(3)-tert-butyl-4-hydroxyanisole and 3,5-di-tert-butyl-4-hydroxytoluene on several hepatic enzyme activities in mice and rats. *Cancer Res.*, 42:2609–2615.
13. Cohen, G. M., Gibby, E. M., and Mehta, R. (1981): Routes of conjugation in normal and cancerous tissue from human lung. *Nature*, 291:662–664.
14. Dutton, G. J. (1980): *Glucuronidation of Drugs and Other Compounds.* CRC Press, Inc., Boca Raton, Florida.
15. Enomoto, K., Ying, T. S., Griffin, M. J., and Farber, E. (1981): Immunohistochemical study of epoxide hydrolase during experimental liver carcinogenesis. *Cancer Res.*, 41:3281–3287.
16. Enomoto, K., and Farber, E. (1982): Kinetics of phenotypic maturation of remodeling of hyperplastic nodules during liver carcinogenesis. *Cancer Res.*, 42:2330–2335.
17. Eriksson, L. C., Aström, A., de Pierre, J. W., and Bock, K. W. (1981): Induction of drug metabolizing enzymes in preneoplastic liver nodules. *Biochem. Soc. Trans.*, 9:271.
18. Fischer, G., Schauer, A., and Katz, N. R. (1982): Facilitation of microdissection by use of a new microscopic and micromanipulatory unit. *Naturwissenschaften*, 69:146.
19. Fischer, G., Ullrich, D., Katz, N. R., Bock, K. W., and Schauer, A. (1983): Immunohistochemical and biochemical detection of UDP-glucuronyl transferase in putative preneoplastic liver foci. *Virchows Arch.*, 42:193–200.
20. Iype, T. P., Tomaszewski, J. E., and Dipple, A. (1979): Biochemical basis for cytotoxicity of 7,12-dimethyl-benz(a)anthracene in rat liver epithelial cells. *Cancer Res.*, 39:4925–4929.
21. Kinoshita, N., and Gelboin, H. V. (1978): β-Glucuronidase catalysed hydrolysis of benzo(a)pyrene-3-glucuronide and binding to DNA. *Science*, 199:307–309.
22. Lilienblum, W., Walli, A. K., and Bock, K. W. (1982): Differential induction of rat liver microsomal UDP-glucuronosyltransferase activities by various inducing agents. *Biochem. Pharmacol.*, 31:907–913.
23. Lind, Ch., Vadi, H., and Ernster, L. (1978): Metabolism of benzo(a)pyrene-3,6-quinone and 3-hydroxybenzo(a)pyrene in liver microsomes from 3-methylcholanthrene-treated rats. *Arch. Biochem. Biophys.*, 190:97–108.
24. Lorentzen, R. J., Lesko, S. A., McDonald, K., and Ts'o, P. O. P. (1979): Toxicity of metabolic benzo(a)pyrenediones to cultured cells and the dependence upon molecular oxygen. *Cancer Res.*, 39:3194–3198.
25. Lu, A. Y. H., and West, S. B. (1980): Multiplicity of mammalian microsomal cytochromes P-450. *Pharmacol. Rev.*, 31:277–295.
26. Lueders, K. K., Dyer, H. M., Thompson, E. B., and Kuff, E. L. (1970): Glucuronyltransferase activity in transplantable rat hepatomas. *Cancer Res.*, 30:274–279.
27. Malaveille, C., Brun, G., Hautefeuille, A., and Bartsch, H. (1980): Effect of glutathione and uridine 5-disphosphoglucuronic acid on benzo(a)pyrene mutagenesis in the salmonella/microsome assay. In: *Mechanism of Toxicity and Hazard Evaluation*, edited by B. Holmstedt, R. Lauwerys, M. Mercier, and M. Roberfroid, pp. 175–180. Elsevier/North-Holland Biomedical Press, Amsterdam.
28. Meerman, J. H. N., Beland, F. A., and Mulder, G. J. (1981): Role of sulfation in the formation of DNA adducts from N-hydroxy-2-acetylaminofluorene in rat liver in vivo. Inhibition of N-acetylated aminofluorene adduct formation by pentachlorophenol. *Carcinogenesis*, 2:413–416.
29. Miller, E. C. (1978): Some current perspectives on chemical carcinogenesis in humans and experimental animals. *Cancer Res.*, 38:1479–1496.
30. Mulder, G. J. (1981): *Sulfation of Drugs and Related Compounds.* CRC Press, Inc., Boca Raton, Florida.
31. Nebert, D. W. (1980): The Ah locus. A gene with possible importance in cancer predictability. *Arch. Toxicol. [Suppl. 2]*:195–207.
32. Nebert, D. W., and Negishi, M. (1982): Multiple forms of cytochrome P-450 and the importance of molecular biology and evolution. *Biochem. Pharmacol.*, 31:2311–2317.
33. Nemoto, N. (1981): Glutathione, glucuronide, and sulfate transferase in polycyclic aromatic hydrocarbon metabolism. In: *Polycyclic Hydrocarbons and Cancer, Vol. 3*, edited by H. V. Gelboin, and P. O. P. Ts'o, pp. 213–258. Academic Press, New York.

34. Owens, I. S. (1977): Genetic regulation of UDP-glucuronosyltransferase induction by polycyclic aromatic compounds in mice. *J. Biol. Chem.*, 252:2827–2833.
35. Rutenberg, A. M., Kim, H., Fischbein, J. W., Hanker, J. S., Wasserkrug, H. L., and Seligman, A. M. (1969): Histochemical and ultrastructural demonstration of γ-glutamyl transpeptidase activity. *J. Histochem. Cytochem.*, 17:517–526.
36. Shen, A. L., Fahl, W. E., Wrighton, S. A., and Jefcoate, C. R. (1979): Inhibition of benzo(a)pyrene and benzo(a)pyrene-7,8-dihydrodiol metabolism by benzo(a)pyrene quinones. *Cancer Res.*, 39:4123–4129.
37. Sims, P., Grover, P. L., Swaisland, A., Pal, K., and Hewer, A. (1974): Metabolic activation of benzo(a)pyrene proceeds by a diol-epoxide. *Nature*, 252:326–327.
38. Thorgeirsson, S. S., and Nebert, D. W. (1977): The Ah locus and the metabolism of chemical carcinogens and other foreign compounds. *Adv. Cancer Res.*, 25:149–193.
39. Tsuda, H., Lee, G., and Farber, E. (1980): Induction of resistant hepatocytes as a new principle for a possible short-term in vivo test for carcinogens. *Cancer Res.*, 40:1157–1164.
40. Wachstein, M., Meisel, E., and Niedzwiedz, A. (1960): Histochemical demonstration of mitochondrial adenosine triphosphatase with the lead adenosine triphosphate technique. *J. Histochem. Cytochem.*, 8:387–388.
41. Williams, G. M., Chandrasekaran, V., Katayama, S., and Weisburger, J. H. (1981): Carcinogenicity of 3-methyl-2-naphthylamine and 3,2-dimethyl-4-amino-biphenyl to the bladder and gastrointestinal tract of the Syrian golden hamster with atypical proliferative enteritis. *J. Natl. Cancer Inst.*, 67:481–486.
42. Ying, T. S., Sarma, D. S. R., and Farber, E. (1981): Role of acute hepatic necrosis in the induction of early steps in liver carcinogenesis by diethylnitrosamine. *Cancer Res.*, 41:2096–2102.

Biochemical Basis of Chemical Carcinogenesis,
edited by H. Greim, R. Jung, M. Kramer,
H. Marquardt, and F. Oesch.
Raven Press, New York © 1984.

Dihydrodiol Dehydrogenase: A New Level of Control by Both Sequestration of Proximate and Inactivation of Ultimate Carcinogens

F. Oesch, H. R. Glatt, K. Vogel, A. Seidel, P. Petrovic,
and K. L. Platt

*Institute of Pharmacology, University of Mainz,
D-6500 Mainz, Federal Republic of Germany*

PURIFICATION OF DIHYDRODIOL DEHYDROGENASE TO APPARENT HOMOGENEITY

The cytosolic $NADP^+$-dependent dihydrodiol dehydrogenase converts benzene dihydrodiol (1,2-dihydroxy-cyclohexa-3,5-diene) to catechol (2). Considering that some dihydrodiols derived from polycyclic aromatic hydrocarbons are biotransformed in the presence of cytosolic fraction of liver homogenates, the suggested biotransformation products being catechols (8,23), it appeared possible that this enzyme may also be capable of oxidizing dihydrodiol metabolites of polycyclic hydrocarbons. We have, therefore, purified a dihydrodiol dehydrogenase to apparent homogeneity from the cytosolic fraction of rat liver homogenate to investigate if this enzyme plays a role in the control of mutagenic metabolites derived from polycyclic aromatic hydrocarbons.

The purification steps shown in Table 1 led to an apparently homogeneous enzyme: $(NH_4)_2SO_4$ fractionation, DEAE-cellulose chromatography, interfacial salting-in and gel filtration through Sephadex G-100 superfine. The end product, which was purified over 500-fold with a yield of about 14% when compared to rat liver $100,000 \times g$ supernatant, was judged to be homogeneous by several independent criteria: A single symmetrical peak was obtained when the final enzyme preparation was reapplied to a Sephadex G-100 superfine column. The specific enzyme activity was the same in all fractions containing protein. Also a single symmetrical peak appeared when the preparation was analyzed in the analytical ultracentrifuge. A single protein-staining band was obtained by SDS-polyacrylamide gel electrophoresis, even when large amounts of protein were applied to the gels. When antiserum raised against the preparation in New Zealand White rabbits was tested in a double diffusion assay a single precipitation band was obtained (38).

TABLE 1. *Purification to apparent homogeneity of rat liver cytosolic dihydrodiol dehydrogenase*

Purification step	Total units[a]	Specific activity[b]	Purification factor	Purification factor/step	Total yield	Yield/ step
100,000 × g supernatant	1,140	0.010	1	1	100	100
Ammonium sulfate precipitation	950	0.065	6.5	6.5	83	83
DEAE-cellulose chromatography	380	0.516	52	8	33	40
Interfacial salting-in	280	2.500	250	4.8	25	73
Gel filtration on Sephadex G-100 superfine	160	5.525	553	2.2	14	57

Data from ref. 38, with permission.

[a]One unit of activity is defined as the amount of enzyme which formed 1 μmole of NADPH/min.

[b]Specific activity is expressed as units/min/mg of protein.

A molecular weight of 35,000 was calculated both by gel filtration and SDS-polyacrylamide gel electrophoresis in the presence of standard proteins of known molecular weight. These findings suggest that in the active state the dihydrodiol dehydrogenase consists of a single subunit. It was shown by fluorimetric titrations of the enzyme with NADPH that it bound 1 mole of coenzyme per 35,000 daltons. Thus, each enzyme molecule contains one coenzyme binding site and presumably one active center. pH Gradients between pH 5 to 8 and pH 6.0 to 6.5 were used to estimate the isoelectric point of the dihydrodiol dehydrogenase. An isolectric point of 6.2 was found in all experiments. Over a wide range of substrate and coenzyme concentrations, plots of reciprocal velocity versus reciprocal benzene dihydrodiol and NADP$^+$ concentrations were linear. K_m values for benzene dihydrodiol and NADP$^+$ were estimated to be 2.2 mM and 7.7 μM, respectively. The apparent V_{max} of this reaction was found to be 6.67 μmoles/mg of enzyme per minute. In agreement with the relatively low isoelectric point, the amino acid composition of dihydrodiol dehydrogenase showed relatively high concentrations of acidic and neutral amino acids.

SUBSTRATE SPECIFICITY OF THE APPARENTLY HOMOGENEOUS DIHYDRODIOL DEHYDROGENASE

In Tables 2 and 3 the compounds are listed which were tested as substrates for the apparently homogeneous dihydrodiol dehydrogenase. Except for quinones derived from polycyclic hydrocarbons, all the test substances were dissolved in water or ethanol. Quinones derived from polycyclic hydrocarbons were dissolved in acetone. Substrate concentrations were in the range of 1 to 10 mM. Since most of the compounds precipitated in the assay mixture (due to their limited solubility in water) the exact concentrations could not be determined. To obtain a better suspension of

TABLE 2. *Substrate specificity of purified rat liver cytosolic dihydrodiol dehydrogenase for xenobiotics*

Substances	% Activity[a]
Miscellaneous	
Benzene dihydrodiol	100
Indanol	27
1,2-Diphenyl-1,2-dihydroxyethane	1.4
p-Nitrobenzaldehyde	38
m-Nitrobenzaldehyde	10
Cyclohexanone	5.6
DL-Glyceraldehyde	2.7
Indanone	0.3
4-Carboxybenzaldehyde	0.3
Daunorubicin	0.12
o-Quinones	
Phenanthrene-9,10-quinone	110
Benzo(a)pyrene-4,5-quinone	69
Benzo(a)pyrene-7,8-quinone	1.6
Chrysene-5,6-quinone	0.8
Dibenz (a,h)anthracene-5,6-quinone	0.1
p-Quinones	
p-Benzoquinone	40
1,4-Naphthoquinone	3.4
Phenanthrene-1,4-quinone	2.8
Menadione (vitamin K_3)	0.6
Anthraquinone	n.d.[b]
Benz(a)anthracene-7,12-quinone	n.d.
Dibenz(a,h)anthracene-7,12-quinone	n.d.
Polynuclear polycyclic quinones	
Benzo(a)pyrene-1,6-quinone	n.d.
Benzo(a)pyrene-3,6-quinone	n.d.
Benzo(a)pyrene-6,12-quinone	n.d.

Data from ref. 39, with permission.
[a]100% represents 3.5 μmoles NADP(H) converted/min × mg protein. Oxidation reactions were carried out with NADP, reduction reactions with NADPH as cofactor.
[b]n.d., not detectable.

the substrates, the assay mixture contained in those cases bovine serum albumin at a concentration of 1 mg/ml.

The fact that the enzyme consists of a single polypeptide with a molecular weight of about 35,000 and that dihydrodiol dehydrogenase is able to convert aromatic aldehydes, the antibiotic daunorubicin and indanol, shows striking similarities with other dehydrogenases and aldo-keto reductases reported in literature (7,12,13, 34,41,42).

Furthermore, the enzyme converted o-quinones derived from polycyclic aromatic hydrocarbons and p-quinones possessing an aromatic system only on one side of the quinone structure (39).

Of the steroids tested only those were oxidized which contained a 3α-hydroxy group. Only steroids which contained a 3-keto group and no double bond at the Δ^4

TABLE 3. *Substrate specificity of purified rat liver cytosolic dihydrodiol dehydrogenase for steroids*

Hydroxysteroids	% Activity[a]	
	NADP+	NAD+
Etiocholan-3α-ol-17-one	108	143
Etiocholan-3β-ol-17-one	n.d.[b]	n.d.
Estradiol	n.d.	n.d.
Pregnenolone	n.d	n.d.
Androsterone	73	197
5β-Pregnan-3α,17β-diol-20-one	100	270
Sodium desoxycholate	14	5
5β-Cholanic acid-3α,7α,12α-triol	9	8
Ketosteroids	NADPH	NADH
5β-Androstan-3,17-dione	70	100
5α-Androstan-3,17-dione	30	41
5α-Androstan-17β-ol-3-one	13	66
Etiocholan-17β-ol-3-one	87	72
5β-Cholanic acid-3,7,12-trione	52	50
Prednisone	n.d.	n.d.
20β-Hydroxy-Δ4-pregnen-3-one	n.d.	n.d.
Testosterone	n.d.	n.d.
Corticosterone	n.d.	n.d.

Data from ref. 38, with permission.
[a]The rate of reaction for each substrate is reported relative to that of benzene dihydrodiol with NADP+ as coenzyme taken as 100% (5.6 μmoles of NAD(P)H/min/mg of protein), and relative to that of 5β-androstan-3,17-dione with NADH as coenzyme taken as 100% in case of reduction of the 3-keto group (6.1 μmoles of NAD+/min/mg of protein).
[b]n.d., not detectable.

position could be reduced. The other steroids which were tested with hydroxy groups in position 3β, 11β, 17α, 17β, 20α, 20β, 21, and 22 were not substrates. In addition to the enzyme's endogenous steroid metabolizing role, the results of the substrate specificity study indicate that it plays also an important role in the metabolism of foreign compounds (38,39).

REDUCTION OF BACTERIAL MUTAGENICITY BY THE APPARENTLY HOMOGENEOUS DIHYDRODIOL DEHYDROGENASE

Two metabolic pathways mainly contribute to the mutagenicity of benzo(a)pyrene (5) as observed in the mammalian enzyme-mediated *Salmonella* mutagenicity test (1):

1. When liver microsomes from control mice are used activation to benzo(a)pyrene-4,5-oxide is predominant (5,33).

2. When low doses of benzo(a)pyrene are activated by microsomes from mice in which cytochrome P-448 is induced (by treatment with polycyclic hydrocarbons

or with Aroclor 1254 then vicinal dihydrodiol bay region epoxides are mainly responsible for the mutagenicity (5).

In the latter situation simple epoxides again become the major mutagenic metabolites if epoxide hydrolase is inhibited, or at benzo(*a*)pyrene concentrations which are high enough to inhibit oxidation of the dihydrodiols. The *Salmonella typhimurium* strain TA 1537 is much more susceptible to benzo(*a*)pyrene 4,5-oxide than to the vicinal dihydrodiol bay region epoxides (5) whereas the strains TA 98 or TA 100 are highly susceptible to both groups of mutagenic metabolites.

The effect of dihydrodiol dehydrogenase in these two metabolic situations is shown in Fig. 1. When benzo(*a*)pyrene was activated by liver microsomes from 3-methycholanthrene-treated mice, addition of pure dihydrodiol dehydrogenase clearly reduced the mutagenicity (17). Doses of dihydrodiol dehydrogenase up to 0.5 units per plate increased the effect, whereas further addition of dihydrodiol dehydrogenase had no significant effect. When using about 15 times more enzyme than that present in the amount of liver equivalent to the microsomes used for activation maximal reduction of mutagenicity was achieved. Between various animal species (31,40) or after exposure to foreign compounds with inducing properties (10,30), similar or even greater differences in activities of foreign compound-metabolizing enzymes occur.

No effect of dihydrodiol dehydrogenase on the mutagenicity of benzo(*a*)pyrene was found when microsomes from control mice were used, in contrast to the experiments where microsomes from 3-methylcholanthrene-treated mice were used. This is readily understandable, as control mouse liver microsomes activate

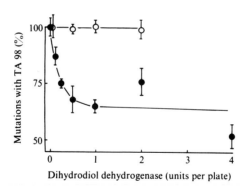

FIG. 1. Effect of dihydrodiol dehydrogenase on the mutagenicity of benzo(*a*)pyrene activated by liver microsomes from control *(empty circle)* or 3-methylcholanthrene-treated *(solid circle)* mice. Benzo(*a*)pyrene (5 μg, dissolved in 10 μl dimethylsulphoxide), 500 μl of a microsomal metabolizing system (1 mg liver microsomal protein from adult male C3H mice, 2 mM NADP+, 2 mM NADPH, 8 mM MgC1$_2$, 80 mM KCl, 50 mM Na phosphate, pH 7.4), 100 μl *his*− bacteria (1.7 × 10^8 *S. typhimurium* TA 98), various amounts of pure dihydrodiol dehydrogenase (in 100 μl 150 mM KC1) and 2,000 μl histidine-poor top agar (0.55% agar, 0.55% NaC1, 50 μM histidine, 50 μM biotin, 25 mM Na phosphate, pH 7.4, 45°C) were mixed in a test tube and poured onto a minimal agar plate. After incubation for 3 days in the dark, colonies (*his*+ revertants) were counted. Values are means ± S.E.M. of 3–10 parallel incubations. (Data from ref. 17, with permission.)

benzo*(a)*pyrene mainly to benzo*(a)*pyrene 4,5-oxide rather than to vicinal dihy-drodiol bay region epoxides (5,33). This is the metabolic situation where microsomal epoxide hydrolase markedly reduced the mutagenicity (5,32).

Little is known of the enzymic inactivation of vicinal diol epoxides, the metabolites of polycyclic hydrocarbons that seem to be responsible for most of the carcinogenic and mutagenic effects induced by polycyclic hydrocarbons (6,9,11, 14,21,22,26,27,29,35,37,43). Mutagenicity and DNA-binding experiments with *trans*-7,8-dihydro-7,8-dihydroxybenzo*(a)*pyrene indicate that some inactivation is caused by the presence of glutathione (16,18,20,25) but not by microsomal epoxide hydrolase (5,15,18,44). The inability of microsomal epoxide hydrolase to inactivate the *anti*-isomer of the corresponding bay region diol epoxide and the very weak effect on the activity of the *syn*-isomer (44) confirm the latter observation. These negative findings may result from the short half-life of the diol epoxide in an aqueous environment, although this may not necessarily be the same in a biological membrane. Not all vicinal diol epoxides are of low stability. The *anti*-isomer of a non-bay-region diol epoxide, *r*-8,t-9-dihydroxy-t-10,11,-oxy-8,9,10,11-tetra-hydrobenz*(a)*anthracene (BA-8,9-diol 10,11-oxide), has a half-life of many hours and is therefore useful for metabolic studies. It is mutagenic (28,45) and is often the major DNA-binding species formed from benz*(a)*anthracene *in vivo* and *in vitro* (11,27,37). It also serves as a model for less stable diol epoxides. The results reported below show that a diol epoxide can be metabolically inactivated. Inactivation was obtained with dihydrodiol dehydrogenase but not with microsomal or cytosolic epoxide hydrolase. If one assumes that the activities of the investigated enzymes *in vivo* are comparable to those that are present in our experiments *in vitro*, inactivation of the diol epoxide by dihydrodiol dehydrogenase would be slower than the rate of inactivation of the K-region oxide by microsomal epoxide hydrolase, but still sufficiently rapid to substantially affect diol epoxide concentrations in mammalian systems.

To study their role in metabolic inactivation, the three enzymes, microsomal and cytosolic epoxide hydrolase and cytosolic dihydrodiol dehydrogenase, were purified and bacterial mutagenicity was used as an indication of their effects on the muta-genicity of BA-8,9-diol 10,11-oxide and, for comparison, benz*(a)*anthracene 5,6-oxide (BA 5,6-oxide), the K-region epoxide. The test compounds were used at concentrations that are in the increasing portion of the concentration-mutagenicity curve (Fig. 2). As expected from its substrate specificity (3,24), microsomal epoxide hydrolase readily inactivated BA 5,6-oxide (Fig. 3). No significant effect on the mutagenicity of BA-8,9-diol 10,11-oxide was obtained even with a 100-fold excess over that required for complete inactivation of the K-region oxide. Relatively large amounts of cytosolic epoxide hydrolase were required to inactivate BA 5,6-oxide. Cytosolic epoxide hydrolase did not inactivate the diol epoxide as was the case with microsomal epoxide hydrolase. However, the diol epoxide was inactivated by dihydrodiol dehydrogenase and this inactivation required the presence of NADP (19). The inability of either NADP (Fig. 2) or of dihydrodiol dehydrogenase alone (Fig. 3) to inactive the vicinal diol epoxide, and the lack of inactivation of BA 5,6-

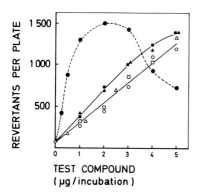

FIG. 2. Dose-dependent mutagenicity, in the absence of pure enzymes, of BA 5,6-oxide in phosphate-buffered KC1 *(solid circle)* and of BA-8,9-diol 10,11-oxide in phosphate-buffered KC1 *(empty circle, empty square, empty triangle)*; experiments performed on different days or in glycine buffer with *(solid square)* or without *(solid triangle)* NADP. Values are means of duplicate determinations, which differed by less than 10%. (Data from ref. 19, with permission.)

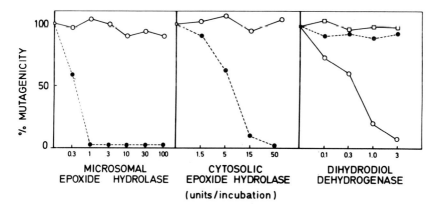

FIG. 3. Effect of purified enzymes on the mutagenicity of BA 5,6-oxide *(solid circle)* and BA-8,9-diol 10,11-oxide (*empty circle:* in the presence of NADP; *empty square:* in the absence of NADP) for *S. typhimurim* TA 100. The number of mutants above solvent control induced by 1 µg of BA 5,6-oxide or 3 µg of BA-8,9-diol 10,11-oxide in the presence of various amounts of purified enzymes is expressed as the percentage of the corresponding value without enzyme. The absolute values of colonies in the absence of enzyme were 92 to 150 for solvent controls, 920 to 1,060 for BA 5,6-oxide, and 560 to 860 (depending on the incubation conditions; see Fig. 1) for BA-8,9-diol 10,11-oxide. Triplicate incubations were performed. The coefficients of variation in the numbers of colonies were less than 10%. Enzyme units are described in the papers which describe their purification (4,38). One gram liver from an adult Sprague-Dawley rat contains approximately 300 units of microsomal epoxide hydrolase and 2.5 units of dihydrodiol dehydrogenase, whereas 1 g liver from an adult male rabbit contains about 250 units of cytosolic epoxide hydrolase. (Data from ref. 19, with permission.)

oxide by dihydrodiol dehydrogenase either with or without NADP, indicate that inactivation is not the result of nonspecific binding of the vicinal diol epoxide to protein or to NADP but rather a consequence of enzymic activity.

High concentrations of dihydrodiol dehydrogenase were necessary for inactivation of the diol epoxide, whereas a low concentration of microsomal epoxide hydrolase was sufficient for the inactivation of BA 5,6-oxide. A 50% inactivation of 1 µg of BA 5,6-oxide was achieved with either 0.4 unit of purified rat microsomal epoxide hydrolase, equivalent to 1.3 mg of liver, or with 7 units of purified rabbit cytosolic epoxide hydrolase, equivalent to 28 mg of liver, as can be seen in Fig. 3. These are relatively small quantities of enzyme. Microsomal epoxide hydrolase equivalent to 330 mg of rat liver and cytosolic epoxide hydrolase equivalent to 200 mg of rabbit liver did not inactivate this mutagen, whereas with dihydrodiol dehydrogenase an amount equivalent to 200 mg of liver was required for obtaining a 50% inactivation. The K-region epoxide is inactivated noticeably more efficiently than the vicinal diol epoxide, considering the concentrations of the enzymes present *in vivo*. This may be one of the reasons for the much stronger biological activities in mammalian systems of vicinal diol epoxides compared with K-region epoxide. An effective but moderate rate of inactivation of vicinal diol epoxides, furthermore, suggests that differences in enzyme activity among species, organs, and physiologic states are a likely cause for differences in susceptibility to the effects of polycyclic aromatic hydrocarbons. Very likely dihydrodiol dehydrogenase is more important for the inactivation of vicinal diol epoxides in general than either microsomal or cytosolic epoxide hydrolase.

ACKNOWLEDGMENT

The authors thank the Fonds der Chemischen Industrie for financial support.

REFERENCES

1. Ames, B. N., McCann, J., and Yamasaki, E. (1975): *Mutat. Res.*, 31:347–364.
2. Ayengar, P. K., Hayaishi, O., Nakajima, M., and Tomida, I. (1959): *Biochim. Biophys. Acta*, 33:111–119.
3. Bentley, P., Schmassmann, H. U., Sims, P., and Oesch, F. (1976): *Eur. J. Biochem.*, 69:97–103.
4. Bentley, P., and Oesch, F. (1975): *FEBS Lett.*, 59:291–295.
5. Bentley, P., Oesch, F., and Glatt, H. R. (1977): *Arch. Toxicol.*, 39:65–75.
6. Bigger, C. A. H., Tomaszweski, J. E., and Dipple, A. (1980): *Biochem. Biophys. Res. Commun.*, 80:229–237.
7. Billings, R. E., Sullivan, H. R., and McMahon, R. E. (1971): *J. Biol. Chem.*, 246:3512–3517.
8. Booth, J., and Sims, P. (1976): *Biochem. Pharmacol.*, 25:979–980.
9. Boyland, E., and Sims, P. (1967): *Int. J. Cancer*, 2:500.
10. Burk, M. D., and Mayer, R. T. (1974): *Drug Metab. Dispos.*, 2:583–588.
11. Cooper, C. S., MacNicoll, A. D., Ribeiro, O., Gervasi, G., Hewer, A., Walsh, C., Pal, K., Grover, P. L., and Sims, P. (1980): *Cancer Lett.*, 9:53–57.
12. Felsted, R. L., Gee, M., and Bachur, N. R. (1974): *J. Biol. Chem.*, 249:3672–3679.
13. Felsted, R. L., Richter, D. R., and Bachur, N. R. (1977): *Biochem. Pharmacol.*, 26:1117–1124.
14. Flesher, J. W., Harvey, R. G., and Sydnor, K. L. (1976): *Int. J. Cancer*, 18:351.
15. Glatt, H. R. (1976): *Thesis*, University of Basel.
16. Glatt, H. R., and Oesch, F. (1977): *Arch. Toxicol.*, 39:87–96.
17. Glatt, H. R., Vogel, K., Bentley, P., and Oesch, F. (1979): *Nature*, 277:319–320.
18. Glatt, H. R., Billings, R., Platt, K. L., and Oesch, F. (1981): *Cancer Res.*, 41:270–277.
19. Glatt, H. R., Cooper, C. S., Grover, P. L., Sims, P., Bentley, P., Merdes, M., Waechter, F., Vogel, K., Gùenthner, T. M., and Oesch, F. (1982): *Science*, 215:1507–1509.
20. Guenthner, T. M., Jernstöm, B., and Orrenius, S. (1980): *Carcinogenesis*, 1:407–416.
21. Hecht, S. S., LaVoie, E., Mazzorese, R., Amin, S., Bedenko, V., and Hoffmann, D. (1978): *Cancer Res.*, 38:2191–2199.
22. Huberman, E., Sachs, L., Yang, S. K., and Gelboin, H. V. (1976): *Proc. Natl. Acad. Sci. U.S.A.*, 73:607–612.

23. Jerina, D. M., Ziffer, H., and Daly, J. W. (1970): *J. Am. Chem. Soc.*, 92:1056–1061.
24. Jerina, D. M., Dansette, P. M., Lu, A. Y. H., and Levin, W. (1977): *Mol. Pharmacol.*, 13:342–351.
25. Ketterer, B. (1980): *Biochem. Biophys. Res. Commun.*, 94:612–617.
26. Levin, W., Thakker, D. R., Wood, A. W., Chang, R. L., Lehr, R. E., Jerina, D. M., and Conney, A. H. (1978): *Cancer Res.*, 38:1705–1714.
27. MacNicoll, A. D., Cooper, C. S., Ribeiro, O., Pal, K., Hewer, A., Grover, P. L., and Sims, P. (1981): *Cancer Lett.*, 11:243–248.
28. Malaveille, C., Kuroki, T., Sims, P., Grover, P. L., and Bartsch, H. (1977): *Mutat. Res.*, 44:313–321.
29. Newbold, R. F., Brookes, P. (1976): *Nature (Lond.)*, 261:52–53.
30. Oesch, F. (1976): *J. Biol. Chem.*, 251:79–87.
31. Oesch, F., Thoenen, H., and Fahrländer, H. (1974): *Biochem. Pharmacol.*, 23:1307–1317.
32. Oesch, F., Bentley, P., and Glatt, H. R. (1976): *Int. J. Cancer*, 18:448–452.
33. Oesch, F., and Glatt, H. R. (1976): In: *Screening Tests in Chemical Carcinogenesis*, edited by R. Montesano, H. Bartsch, and L. Tomatis, pp. 255–274. IARC, Lyon.
34. Sawada, H., Hara, A., Nakayama, T., and Kato, F. (1980): *J. Biochem.*, 87:1153–1165.
35. Sims, P., Grover, P. L., Swaisland, A. Pal, K., and Hewer, A. (1974): *Nature (Lond.)*, 252:326–327.
36. Slaga, T. J., Viaje, A., Berry, D. L., Bracken, W. M., Buty, S. G., and Scribner, J. D. (1976): *Cancer Lett.*, 2:115–119.
37. Vigny, P., Kindts, M., Duquesne, M., Cooper, C. S., Grover, P. L., and Sims, P. (1980): *Carcinogenesis*, 1:33–40.
38. Vogel, K., Bentley, P., Platt, K. L., and Oesch, F. (1980): *J. Biol. Chem.*, 255:9621–9625.
39. Vogel, K., Platt, K. L., Petrovic, P., Seidel, A., and Oesch, F. (1982): *Arch. Toxicol. [Suppl. 5]*:360–364.
40. Walker, C. H., Bentley, P., and Oesch, F. (1978): *Biochem. Biophys. Acta*, 539:427–434.
41. Wermuth, B., Münch, J. D. B., and Von Wartburg, J. P. (1977): *J. Biol. Chem.*, 252:3821–3828.
42. Wermuth, B., and Münch, J. D. B. (1978): *Biochem. Pharmacol.*, 28:1431–1433.
43. Wislocki, P. G., Wood, A. W., Chang, R. L., Levin, W., Yagi, H., Hernandez, O., Jerina, D. M., and Conney, A. H. (1976): *Biochem. Biophys. Res. Commun.*, 68:1006–1010.
44. Wood, A. W., Levin, W., Lu, A. Y. H., Yagi, H., Hernandez, O., Jerina, D. M., and Conney, A. H. (1976): *J. Biol. Chem.*, 251:4882–4892.
45. Wood, A. W., Chang, R. L., Levin, W., Lehr, R. E., Schaefer-Ridder, M., Karle, J. M., Jerina, D. M., and Conney, A. H. (1977): *Proc. Natl. Acad. Sci. U.S.A.*, 74:2746–2751.

Biochemical Basis of Chemical Carcinogenesis,
edited by H. Greim, R. Jung, M. Kramer,
H. Marquardt, and F. Oesch.
Raven Press, New York © 1984.

Quantitative Aspects in the Metabolic Activation of Aflatoxin B_1 and Carcinogenic Aromatic Amines

Hans-Günter Neumann

*Institute of Pharmacology and Toxicology, University of Würzburg,
8700 Würzburg, Federal Republic of Germany*

Chemical carcinogens damage cellular macromolecules and thereby directly determine cell transformation and indirectly determine the growth of tumors. This hypothesis has been the subject of many recent investigations. Particular efforts have been made in seeking quantitative correlations between the extent of DNA-modifications as the critical biochemical lesion and the biological response with tumor formation as the end point (12).

The extent of DNA modification depends on the availability of reactive metabolites at the reaction site. For many carcinogens, the balance of activating and inactivating metabolic pathways has turned out to be rather complex and, in addition to the activity of many enzymes involved, depends on numerous other pharmacokinetic parameters. It was therefore obvious to assume that the availability of reactive metabolites, which is controlled by these parameters, largely determines the extent of the primary DNA-lesions. These lesions were then found to be modulated by elimination which results from the spontaneous hydrolysis of base adducts or from their enzymatic repair. Persistent and pertinent DNA damage could therefore be expected to correlate best with the biological effect. However, it appears now that positive correlations of this kind are difficult to establish even in detailed *in vivo* studies of the quantitative relationships (26–28).

AFLATOXIN B_1

A good example supporting the apparent validity of this concept is aflatoxin B_1 (AFB_1). It produces liver tumors in many species, including man, but considerable species-related differences in susceptibility exist. In rats, liver tumors may be induced by low doses under the conditions of first-order kinetics of metabolic activation (1). Mice, in contrast, are virtually resistant. Initial binding of metabolites to liver DNA is 50 to 100 times greater in rats than in mice (19,39,40), and persistent adducts which accumulate upon repeated administration of AFB_1 are formed in the target tissue (6,13).

The species difference appears not to be due to the capability of rats to activate AFB_1 (15,32), but rather to the more efficient elimination of reactive intermediates by mice. From studies in our laboratory with liver preparations, we have concluded that both species may produce comparable amounts of AFB_1-8,9-epoxide (Fig. 1), the major DNA-binding metabolite (37,38). However, mice appear to more rapidly conjugate this reactive intermediate with GSH to form 8,9-dihydro-8-glutathionyl-9-hydroxy-AFB_1, the major water soluble metabolite (8), due to their higher GSH-S-transferase activity (Fig. 2) (7,9). This difference in the inactivation capacity may indeed contribute to the twice as rapid overall clearance of AFB_1 in mice (42); recent studies (17) support this proposal by demonstrating that an increase in GSH-S-transferase activity in rats by pretreatment with butylated hydroxyanisole decreases the binding of AFB_1-metabolites *in vitro* and *in vivo*.

The expected quantitative differences in DNA modification have also been found when target and nontarget tissues were compared. Thus, DNA-binding in rat liver is 10 times as high as in rat kidney, which is considered a nontarget tissue for tumor formation. In mice, however, the kidney is susceptible to toxic effects, and DNA-binding in the kidney is more than double that in the liver (6). It is remarkable, however, that the same pattern of base adducts has been found in all four tissues. The corresponding major adducts were also formed in cultured human bronchial and colonic tissues (3).

DNA is damaged to the greatest extent in susceptible tissues in the case of AFB_1, and the desired positive correlation with the biological effects appears to exist. However, it turns out that this is not a true tissue specific effect, because the same adducts are formed also in nonsusceptible tissues. It might be questioned whether

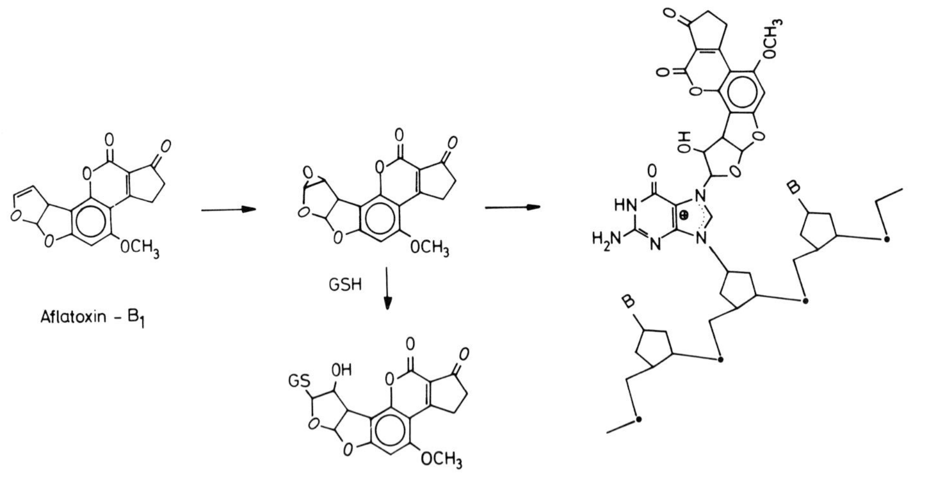

FIG. 1. Metabolic activation and inactivation of AFB₁. Present data (9) indicate that there is only one major reactive metabolite formed, AFB₁-8,9-epoxide, which binds to DNA, and only one major enzymic inactivation of the epoxide with glutathione. Minor pathways are omitted.

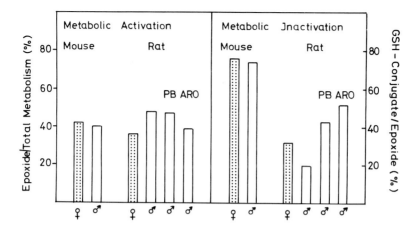

FIG. 2. *In vitro* activation and inactivation of AFB₁. Based on the working hypothesis, expressed in the legend of Fig. 1, the capacity of liver preparations to activate has been calculated as epoxide formed per total metabolism, and the capacity to inactivate as the fraction of epoxide conjugated. For details see ref. 9.

the quantitative differences are sufficient to explain the biological response. Cytotoxic effects might play a role in this response, as indicated by the observation that the minimum feeding time necessary to produce liver tumors in rats with 4 ppm AFB₁ coincides with the time necessary to evoke regenerative hyperplasia (11). An increase of the proliferation rate following partial hepatectomy enhances the effects of AFB₁ only if hepatocytes resistant to the cytotoxic effects have already developed, since AFB₁ inhibits DNA synthesis in normal cells (23).

AROMATIC AMINES

Aromatic amines exhibit a wide range of tissue, sex, and species specific carcinogenic effects which should be explained by the extent of biochemical lesion, if the hypothesis is correct. However, consistent correlations between DNA-damage and susceptibility have not emerged. Three examples will be discussed in more detail (Table 1).

Female Fischer or Sprague-Dawley rats are relatively resistant to liver tumor formation by 2-acetamidofluorene (AAF). However, the reaction of metabolites with DNA is comparable or even more extensive in females than in the susceptible male animals (35). Moreover, 7-F-AAF, which is a powerful hepatocarcinogen in both male and female Sprague-Dawley rats, and which is equally effective in females of this and the Fischer strain, binds less efficiently to DNA than AAF. Moreover, DNA-damage is 2.5 times lower in female Sprague-Dawley than in female Fischer rats (35).

Another example is 2-acetamidophenanthrene (AAP). It produces mammary and Zymbal's gland but no liver tumors in rats, yet initial binding to liver DNA is comparable or even greater than that of the liver carcinogen AAF. Among six base

TABLE 1. *Tissue-specific effects of aromatic amines*

Compound administered	Target tissue in rat	DNA binding index in rat liver	Cytotoxicity in liver
AAF	Liver	300	+
trans-AAS	Zymbal's gland	280	−
AAP	Mammary gland	110	−

adducts formed, four are rapidly eliminated ($t_{1/2} = 15$ h), but two are persistent: After 4 weeks one-third of the total initial adducts is still present (33).

Similarly, other aromatic amines possess binding indices (18) for rat liver DNA which do not correlate at all with their potencies to induce liver tumors (27). On the more refined level of base adduct analysis, aromatic amines are difficult to compare because their reactive metabolites attack a variety of different sites as well as different bases in DNA (16). Many of the adducts have been identified and most of them are likely to represent either promutagenic lesions influencing the tertiary structure of DNA or inhibiting DNA replication. It has not been possible to discriminate between the more or less critical adducts with respect to tumor formation (16,27). If persistency is chosen as a parameter, C8-(N-aminofluorenyl)-guanine should be more critical than the acetylated derivatives, C8-(N-acetamidofluorenyl)-guanine and N^2-(3-acetamidofluorenyl)-guanine in the case of AAF. The aminofluorenyl compound is the only base adduct which accumulates after repeated administration of AAF (5). However, after 4 biweekly doses, the levels of this adduct are considerably higher in the DNA of two nontarget tissues [liver (30.6 pmoles/mg DNA), kidney (17.2)] of females than in the target tissue [liver (9.4)] of male Sprague-Dawley rats (5).

TRANS-4-ACETAMIDOSTILBENE

We have extensively investigated possible correlations between tissue specific effects and the tissue susceptibility with trans-4-acetamidostilbene (trans-AAS). This carcinogen induces sebaceous gland tumors, particularly of the Zymbal's glands in rats. Other tissues can essentially be regarded as nontarget tissues. All tissues are exposed to the reactive metabolites. A rough estimate of the tissue dose is given by the protein-binding 3 days after dosing, when the level of unbound metabolites can be neglected (Table 2). After a single or after 12 twice-weekly doses of labelled trans-AAS tissue doses vary by a factor of no more than 10 with the target tissue value ranging at the lower end of the scale. In all tissues thus exposed, metabolites also react with DNA and DNA-damage accumulates during repeated administration (14). The nontarget tissues liver and kidney not only show the greatest initial DNA-binding but also accumulate these lesions to the greatest extent (Fig. 3) (14). The initial binding to DNA in the Zymbal's gland is lower than in these tissues (4).

TABLE 2. *Tissue dose and tissue susceptibility[a]*

				Tissue		
Doses	Liver	Kidney	Lung	Zymbal's gland	Glandular stomach	Mammary gland
1	2.4	1.8	0.7	0.4	0.3	0.2
12	7.2	7.0	3.0	1.4	1.3	0.8

[a]Total radioactivity (pmoles/mg wet wt) 3 days after single or 12 doses (twice weekly) of trans-AAS (5 μmoles/kg) to Wistar rats.

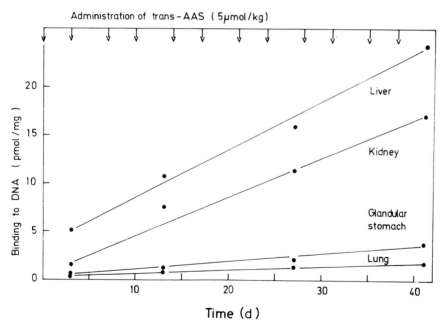

FIG. 3. Accumulation of DNA-damage in different rat tissues. (³H)-trans-AAS was orally administered to female Wistar rats and total DNA-binding of metabolites was measured 3 days after administration of 1, 4, 8, and 12 doses, respectively ($\overline{X}$, $n=3$, standard deviation<25%). Details are described in ref. 14.

We have previously shown that the metabolism follows first-order kinetics with the doses used in these experiments as well as in carcinogenicity studies (25,29). We can now demonstrate that some of the parameters which complicate the situation with other carcinogens do not influence the results with trans-AAS: during repeated administration [twice weekly over 6 weeks (14)] the initial binding of each dose remained constant, i.e., enzymes involved in metabolic activation or inactivation were neither induced nor inhibited by the treatment; the elimination rate of individual DNA adducts remained the same, i.e., repair activities were not changed; the pattern of adducts in liver-DNA was not altered(Fig. 4).

In addition, the pattern of nucleic acid adducts was very similar in all tissues which we analyzed so far, i.e., liver, kidney, lung, and glandular stomach (4). The possibility that tissue specific adducts will eventually turn out to be responsible for tissue specific effects is therefore considered to be very low. This is in agreement with an increasing number of observations on other carcinogens, such as AFB_1, as emphasized earlier in this paper.

According to all parameters measured, the liver and kidney should be most susceptible to tumor induction by trans-AAS if persistent DNA-damage measured by adduct formation were a sufficient determinant for tumor induction.

INITIATION-PROMOTION

At this point, it was considered most likely that DNA-lesions would correlate with tumor initiation rather than with complete carcinogenesis. Experiments were therefore carried out to demonstrate that trans-AAS treatment indeed produces critical lesions in rat liver and that these lesions require promotion to give rise to tumors. This was achieved either by partial hepatectomy or feeding of phenobarbital, DDT or diethylstilbestrol after trans-AAS pretreatment (Fig. 5) (14,28). The combination of partial hepatectomy and promoter feeding was particularly effective (Table 3). It is important to note that the trans-AAS treatment chosen for this experiment induced sebaceous gland tumors in modest yields, but produced neither enyzme deficient foci nor hyperplastic nodules in liver within the duration of the experiment. Preneoplastic lesions as well as hepatoma were observed within 24 weeks in some of the promoted groups, and by the end of 1 year the livers of all animals were affected if hyperplastic nodules were included. In addition, diethylstilbestrol promoted the development of mammary tumors. These tumors were not observed in any of the control animals and should therefore be related to trans-AAS treatment, which in the previous experiment led to the lowest exposure in this tissue.

The results obtained with a typical initiation-promotion protocol indicate that trans-AAS is an incomplete carcinogen for rat liver. This leads to the question why trans-AAS is not a complete liver carcinogen. Some clues may be obtained from a comparison of AAF with AAP and trans-AAS. These carcinogens are very similar in respect to metabolic activation in that they have similar DNA-binding indices in liver, but their carcinogenic and toxic effects are dissimilar. AAF is a complete

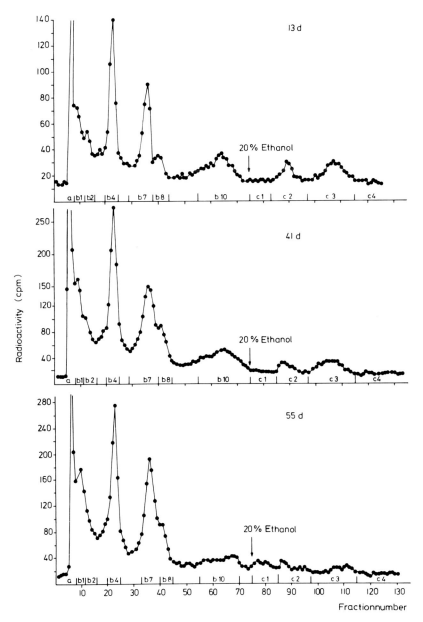

FIG. 4. Pattern of liver DNA-adducts at different time points during repeated administration. (³H)-trans-AAS (5 μmoles/kg) was administered twice weekly by gavage. Liver DNA was enzymically digested and the hydrolysate chromatographed on Sephadex LH-20. Shown is the elution profile of radioactivity. Peak designations correspond to those used in ref. 4.

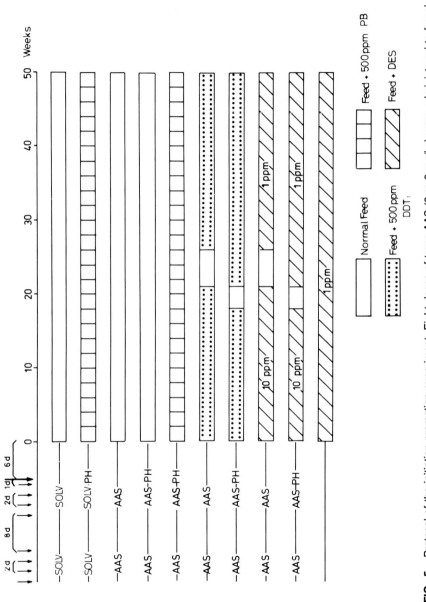

FIG. 5. Protocol of the initiation-promotion experiment. Eight doses of trans-AAS (8 × 6 mg/kg) were administered to female Wistar rats as indicated. In some groups partial hepatectomy (PH) was performed 1 day after the last dose. Tumor promoters were added to the feed 1 week after the last dose. PB, phenobarbital, DES, diethylstilbestrol.

TABLE 3. *Effects of partial hepatectomy and promoters on tumor incidence after trans-AAS[a]*

Treatment	No. incidence	Sebaceous glands		Liver			Mammary tissue
		Zymbal's gland	Lip	Hyperplastic nodule	Hepatoma	Cholangioma	
Solvent	0/10	—	—	—	—	—	—
So. + PH + PB	0/8	—	—	—	—	—	—
AAS	4/9	3	2	—	—	—	—
AAS + PH	8/9	1	—	6	2	—	2
AAS + PH + PB	11/11	3	2	4	7	1	—
AAS + DDT	6/6	1	—	2	4	2	1
AAS + PH + DDT	11/13	2	—	3	7	—	1
DES	0/10	—	—	—	—	—	—
AAS + DES	9/10	1	2	4	5	1	5
AAS + PH + DES	12/12	1	—	6	6	2	1

[a]The experiment was terminated after 54 weeks, except for the control groups. Tumors were histologically verified. Hyperplastic nodules are contained in the incidence rate. It was not attempted to specify the malignancy of liver tumors.

liver carcinogen. Trans-AAS has now been shown to initiate liver cells, and AAP appears to be less efficient even in this respect. Using the protocol proposed by Peraino (31) with DDT as a promoter AAP-pretreated animals developed no liver tumors (34). AAF appears to be unique among these compounds in being toxic to liver cells. With trans-AAS, on the other hand, necrosis of liver cells was not observed even with lethal doses (22), despite the great overall acute toxicity (LD_{50} = ca. 40 mg/kg). Adaptive hyperplasia may thus have a promotional effect in AAF carcinogenesis.

Obviously, it is now difficult to explain the differences in cytotoxicity of compounds which lead to a similar tissue exposure to reactive metabolites. It has been suggested that the cytotoxic effects of AAF are caused by the N-hydroxy-AAF-sulfate-ester. The role of sulfate esters of other hydroxamic acids, however, has not been studied to any extent. Some support may be derived from the finding that with AAP only deacetylated DNA-adducts were found, indicating that hydroxamic acid esters including the sulfate may not be direct precursors for macromolecular binding of this compound (33).

Cytotoxicity has been studied in cultures of diploid human fibroblasts (20). When these cells were exposed to the N-acetoxy derivatives of AAF, AAP, trans-AAS, and 4-acetylaminobiphenyl (AABP), graded survival rates were observed. In addition, the survival rate was considerably lower in repair deficient cells from xeroderma pigmentosum patients than in cells from healthy controls. This indicates that DNA-damage plays a role in cytotoxicity. The aminostilbene derivatives proved to be the most cytotoxic of the four compounds. A higher degree of initial DNA-modification was necessary for the other amines to obtain comparable survival rates (due to differences in repair). It can only be hypothesized that toxicity in this system is different from that *in vivo*. Possibly, the persistent DNA adducts have only little acute toxic impact on the non- or slowly dividing liver cells.

Another possibility is that protein, RNA and DNA damage *in vivo* is not truly reflected by the amount of adducts formed. Radicals and reactive oxygen may produce lesions which are not detected by measuring covalent binding of metabolites. Although the same metabolic intermediates may be precursors of the formation of reactive electrophiles, radicals and redox cycles, it has not been determined how the relative fractions of these different pathways depend on the molecular structure. A role for radicals is indicated (10,41), but studies comparing different aromatic amines in this respect are lacking.

Finally, differences in enzyme inducing activity should be considered. AAF clearly shares this typical property with many tumor promoters (2,21,36), whereas trans-AAS apparently does not induce drug metabolizing enzymes (24,28). It would be interesting to compare the affinities of these and other aromatic amines to receptor proteins, such as the cytosolic Ah receptor (30).

CONCLUSIONS

It is still true that tissue exposure to reactive chemicals or metabolites is a prerequisite for the biological effects of chemical carcinogens. Modification of nuclear DNA appears to be a critical biochemical lesion, but neither initial nor persistent modifications permit assessment of the risk of tumor development in a particular tissue. This is partially due to our present ignorance about the contribution of cytotoxic or true promotional effects by the exogenous carcinogen itself or its metabolites.

The data discussed for the aromatic amines indicate that measurement of the extent of metabolic activation does not provide easy access for evaluation of the cytotoxic or promotional potential of these compounds. It even appears possible that the structural requirements are more specific for promotional effects than for initiation by DNA damage.

ACKNOWLEDGMENTS

Work carried out in this laboratory was supported in part by the Deutsche Forschungsgemeinschaft. We are also indebted for support from the R. J. Reynolds Tobacco GmbH and the Dr. Robert Pfleger Stiftung, Bamberg.

REFERENCES

1. Appleton, B. S., Goetchius, M. P., and Campbell, T. C. (1982): Linear dose-response curve for the hepatic macromolecular binding of aflatoxin B₁ in rats at very low exposures. *Cancer Res.*, 42:3659–3662.
2. Aström, A., and DePierre, J. W. (1981): Characterization of the induction of drug-metabolizing enzymes by 2-diethylaminofluorene. *Biochem. Biophys. Acta*, 673:225–233.
3. Autrup, H., Essigmann, J. M., Croy, R. G., Trump, B. F., Wogan, G. N., and Harris, C. C. (1979): Metabolism of aflatoxin B₁ and identification of the major aflatoxin B₁-DNA adducts formed in cultured human bronchus and colon. *Cancer Res.*, 39:694–689.
4. Baur, H., and Neumann, H.-G. (1980): Correlation of nucleic acid binding by metabolites of trans-4-aminostilbene derivatives with tissue specific acute toxicity and carcinogenicity in rats. *Carcinogenesis*, 1:877–886.
5. Beland, F. A., Dooley, K. L., and Jackson, C. D. (1982): Persistence of DNA adducts in rat liver and kidney after multiple doses of the carcinogen N-hydroxy-2-acetylaminofluorene. *Cancer Res.*, 42:1348–1354.
6. Croy, R. G., and Wogan, G. N. (1981): Quantitative comparison of covalent aflatoxin-DNA adducts formed in rat and mouse livers and kidneys. *J. Natl. Cancer Inst.*, 66:761–768.
7. Degen, G. H. (1979): Metabolic inactivation of aflatoxin B₁-epoxide as a cause for the difference in aflatoxin-susceptibility of rat and mouse. An in vitro investigation. *Naunyn-Schmiedeberg's Arch. Pharmacol.*, 307:R 15.
8. Degen, G. H., and Neumann, H.-G. (1978): The major metabolie of aflatoxin B₁ in the rat is a glutathione conjugate. *Chem.-Biol. Interact.*, 22:239–255.
9. Degen, G. H., and Neumann, H.-G. (1981): Differences in aflatoxin B₁-susceptibility of rat and mouse are correlated with the capability in vitro to inactivate aflatoxin B₁-epoxide. *Carcinogenesis*, 2:299–306.
10. Floyd, R. A. (1981): Free radicals in arylamine carcinogenesis. *Natl. Cancer Inst. Monogr.*, 58:123–131.
11. Godoy, H. M., Judah, D. J., Arora, H. L., Neal, G. E., and Jones, G. (1976): The effects of prolonged feeding with aflatoxin B₁ on adult rat liver. *Cancer Res.*, 36:2399–2407.
12. Grover, P. L., editor (1979): *Chemical Carcinogens and DNA*. CRC Press, Inc. Boca Raton, Florida.
13. Hertzog, P. J., Smith, J. R. L., and Garner, R. G. (1980): A high pressure liquid chromatography study on the removal of DNA-bound aflatoxin-B₁ in rat liver and in vitro. *Carcinogenesis*, 1:789–793.
14. Hilpert, D. (1982): Die Rolle der Entstehung von DNA-Schäden sowie von Sekundäreffekten für

die carcinogene Wirkung von trans-4-acetylaminostilbene bei der Ratte. Dissertation of the Faculty of Natural Sciences, University of Würzburg.

15. Hsieh, D. P. H., Wong, Z. A., Wong, J. J., Michas, C., and Ruebner, B. H. (1977): Comparative metabolism of aflatoxin. In: *Mycotoxins in Human and Animal Health*, edited by J. V. Rodricks, C. W. Hesseltine, and M. A. Mehlman, pp. 37–50. Pathotox, Park Forest South, Illinois.

16. Kriek, E. (1980): Modification of DNA by carcinogenic aromatic amines in vivo and in vitro with possible promutagenic consequences. In: *Carcinogenesis: Fundamental Mechanism and Environmental Effects*, edited by B. Pullman, P. O. P. Ts'o, H. Gelboin, pp. 103–111. D. Reidel Publishing Company, Dordrecht, Holland, Boston, London.

17. Lotliker, P. D., Ihee, E. C., Clearfield, M. S., and Pandey, R. N. (1982): Effect of butylated hydroxyanisole (BHA) on the in vivo and in vitro hepatic aflatoxin B₁ (AFB₁)-DNA binding in rats. *Proceedings of the 13th International Cancer Congress*, 1982 Seattle. Abstract 3896.

18. Lutz, W. K. (1979): In vivo covalent binding of organic chemicals as a quantitative indicator in the process of chemical carcinogenesis. *Mutat. Res.*, 65:289–356.

19. Lutz, W. K., Jaggi, W., Lüthy, J., Sagelsdorff, P., and Schlatter, C. (1980): In vivo covalent binding of aflatoxin B₁ and aflatoxin M₁ to liver DNA of rat, mouse and pig. *Chem.-Biol. Interact.*, 32:249–256.

20. Maher, V. M., Heflich, R. H., and McCormick, J. J. (1981): Repair of DNA damage induced in human fibroblasts by N-substituted aryl compounds. *Natl. Cancer Inst. Monogr.*, 58:217–222.

21. Malejka-Giganti, D., McIver, R. C., Glasebrook, A. L., and Gutmann, H. R. (1978): Induction of microsomal N-hydroxylation of N-2-fluorenylacetamide in rat liver. *Biochem. Pharmacol.*, 27:61–69.

22. Marquardt, P., Neumann, H.-G., and Romen, W. (1982): Tissue specific, acute toxic effects of the carcinogen trans-4-dimethylaminostilbene. *J. Environ. Pathol. Toxicol.*, 5:411–424.

23. Neal, G. E., and Cabral, J. R. P. (1980): Effect of partial hepatectomy on the response of rat liver to aflatoxin B₁. *Cancer Res.*, 40:4739–4743.

24. Neumann, H.-G. (1973): The metabolism of repeatedly administered trans-4-dimethylaminostilbene and 4-dimethylaminobibenzyl. *Z. Krebsforsch.*, 79:60–70.

25. Neumann, H.-G. (1980): Biochemical effects and early lesions in regard to dose-response studies. *Oncology*, 37:255–258.

26. Neumann, H.-G. (1981): On the significance of metabolic activation and binding to nucleic acids of aminostilbene derivatives in vivo. *Natl. Cancer Inst. Monogr.*, 58:165–171.

27. Neumann, H.-G. (1983): The role of extent and persistence of DNA modifications in chemical carcinogenesis of aromatic amines. *Recent Results in Cancer Research*, 84:77–89.

28. Neumann, H.-G.: The role of tissue exposure and DNA-lesions for organ specific effects of carcinogenic trans-4-acetylaminostilbene in rats. *Environ. Health Perspect.*, 49:51–58.

29. Neumann, H.-G., Baur, H., and Wirsing, R. (1980): Dose-response relationships in the primary lesion of strong electrophilic carcinogens. *Arch. Toxicol. [Suppl.]*, 3:69–77.

30. Okey, A. B., Bondy, G. P., Mason, M. E., Kahl, G. F., Eisen, H. J., Guenthner, T. M., and Nebert, D. W. (1979): Regulatory gene product of the Ah locus. Characterization of the cytosolic inducer-receptor complex and evidence for its nuclear translocation. *J. Biol. Chem.*, 254:11636–11648.

31. Peraino, C., Fry, R. J. M., Staffeldt, E., and Christopher, J. P. (1975): Comparative enhancing effects of phenobarbital, amobarbital, diphenylhydantoin, and dichlorodiphenyltrichlorethane on 2-acetylaminofluorene-induced hepatic tumorgenesis in the rat. *Cancer Res.*, 35:2884–2890.

32. Roebuck, B. D., and Wogan, G. N. (1977): Species comparison of in vitro metabolism of aflatoxin B₁. *Cancer Res.*, 37:1649–1656.

33. Scribner, J. D., and Kopenen, G. (1979): Binding of the carcinogen 2-acetamidophenanthrene to rat liver nucleic acids: lack of correlation with carcinogenic activity, and failure of the hydroxamic acid ester model for in vivo activation. *Chem.-Biol. Interact.*, 15:201–209.

34. Scribner, J. D., and Mottet, N. K. (1981): DDT acceleration of mammary gland tumors induced in the male Sprague-Dawley rat by 2-acetamidophenanthrene. *Carcinogenesis*, 2:1235–1239.

35. Scribner, J. D., Scribner, N. K., and Koponen, G. (1982): Metabolism and nucleic acid binding of 7-fluoro-2-acetamidofluorene in rats: oxidative defluorination and apparent dissociation from hepatocarcinogenesis of 8-(N-arylamide)guanine adducts on DNA. *Chem.-Biol. Interact.*, 40:27–43.

36. Stout, D. L., and Becker, F. F. (1978): Alteration of the ability of liver microsomes to activate

N-2-fluorenylacetamid to a mutagen of Salmonella typhimurium during hepatocarcinogenesis. *Cancer Res.*, 38:2274–2278.

37. Swenson, D. H., Miller, E. C., and Miller, J. A. (1974): Aflatoxin B_1-2,3-oxide: evidence for its formation in rat liver in vivo and by human liver microsomes in vitro. *Biochem. Biophys. Res. Commun.*, 60:1036–1043.

38. Swenson, D. H., Lin, J. K., Miller, E. C., and Miller, J. A. (1977): Aflatoxin B_1-2,3-oxide as a probable intermediate in the covalent binding of alfatoxins B_1 and B_2 to rat liver DNA and ribosomal RNA in vivo. *Cancer Res.*, 37:172–181.

39. Ueno, I., Friedman, L., and Stone, C. L. (1980): Species difference in the binding of aflatoxin B_1 to hepatic macromolecules. *Toxicol. Appl. Pharmacol.*, 52:177–180.

40. Wogan, G. N., Croy, R. G., Essigmann, J. M., and Benne, R. A. (1980): Aflatoxin-DNA interactions: qualitative quantitative and kinetic features in relation to carcinogenesis. In: *Carcinogenesis: Fundamental Mechanisms and Environmental Effects*, edited by B. Pullman, P. O. P Ts'o, H. Gelboin, pp. 179–191. D. Reidel Publ. Co., Dordrecht, Holland, Boston, London.

41. Wong, P. K., Hampton, M. J., and Floyd, R. A. (1982): Evidence for lipoxigenase-peroxidase activation of N-hydroxy-2-acetylaminofluorene by rat mammary gland parenchymal cells. In: *Prostaglandins and Cancer*, edited by T. J. Powles, R. S. Bockman, K. V. Hohn, and P. Ramwell, pp. 167–179. First International Congress. Alan R. Liss, New York.

42. Wong, Z. A., and Hsieh, D. P. H. (1980): The comparative metabolism and toxicokinetics of alfatoxin B_1 in the monkey, rat and mouse. *Toxicol. Appl. Pharmacol.*, 55.115–125.

Biochemical Basis of Chemical Carcinogenesis,
edited by H. Greim, R. Jung, M. Kramer,
H. Marquardt, and F. Oesch.
Raven Press, New York © 1984.

Metabolic Determinants in the Carcinogenicity of Aromatic Amines

S. S. Thorgeirsson

Laboratory of Carcinogen Metabolism, National Cancer Institute, National Institutes of Health, Bethesda, Maryland 20205

Aromatic amines and amides have been extensively used as model compounds in the study of molecular events involved in chemical carcinogenesis (41). Of all the aromatic amines, 2-acetylaminofluorene (AAF) and its derivatives are the ones most often used in model experiments to determine the mechanism of action for this type of chemical carcinogen (22). In fact, studies by the Millers (22,23) on the metabolism and carcinogenic effects of AAF and other aromatic amines led to the hypothesis that most chemical carcinogens are metabolically converted into reactive electrophiles that interact covalently with critical cellular macromolecules and thereby initiate the carcinogenic process. This hypothesis has provided the framework for explaining the effects of this very diverse group of chemical carcinogens.

METABOLISM

Because it is extensively metabolized in the body before being excreted (Fig. 1), AAF provides a probe for examination of the roles of different metabolic pathways in the carcinogenic and mutagenic effects of AAF. Initial studies on the metabolism of AAF revealed that it was mainly metabolized by ring hydroxylation to less toxic, more water soluble phenolic compounds (23,25,41). However, Cramer et al. (6) discovered that rats fed AAF excreted a proportion of the dose as a conjugate of *N*-hydroxy-2-acetylaminofluorene (*N*-OH-AFF). This new *N*-hydroxylated metabolite was more carcinogenic than the parent amide, was often active locally, and was active in species such as the guinea pig which had been shown resistant to AAF induced carcinogenesis (22,24). These observations led to the hypothesis that *N*-hydroxylation was both the first and obligatory step in the metabolic activation of this compound. The importance of *N*-hydroxylation in the metabolic activation of aromatic amines and amides has now been thoroughly substantiated by numerous laboratories (15,22,36,41).

Early studies clearly showed that *N*-hydroxylation of AAF by mouse and hamster liver microsomes was a cytochrome P-450 dependent reaction (37). AAF *N*-hydroxylase activity was inhibited by carbon monoxide and an antibody against *N*ADPH

47

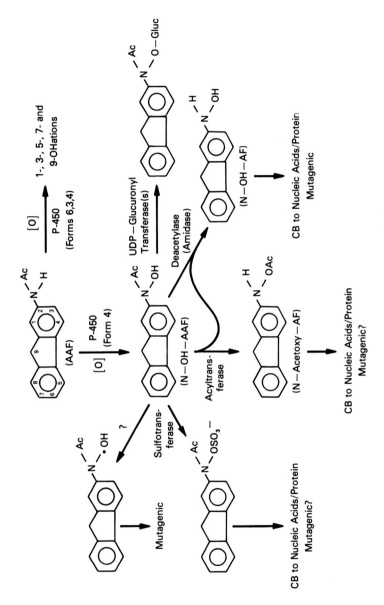

FIG. 1. Metabolic pathways for 2-acetylaminofluorene.

cytochrome *c* reductase, and prior treatment of animals with cobaltous chloride decreased cytochrome P-450 levels and the rate of N-hydroxylation. Similar studies using rat liver microsomes have also shown that AAF N-hydroxylation is cytochrome P-450 dependent (8,19).

AAF can be hydroxylated on the carbon atoms in the 1-, 3-, 5-, 7- and 9-positions on the fluorene ring (Fig. 2). *In vivo*, 7-OH-AAF is the major ring hydroxylated metabolite in all species so far examined (41). Further studies on the metabolism of AAF have revealed that 7-OH-AAF is also the major metabolite *in vitro*, but 9-OH-AAF is also produced in significant amounts (5,30,33,34). Evidence for the involvement of cytochrome P-450 in these reactions includes the following: (a) that *N*ADPH and O_2 are necessary for liver microsomal metabolism (6,32), (b) that induction with 3-methylcholanthrene (MC), phenobarbital and 2,3,7,8-tetracholanthrene (TCDD) causes increased metabolite production, both *in vivo* and *in vitro* (16,21,30,33), (c) that CO inhibits the formation of both the phenolic metabolites and 9-OH-AAF in liver microsomes (17,34), and (d) that purified reconstituted forms of cytochrome P-450 are capable of ring hydroxylation of AAF (14,17).

Several forms of cytochrome P-450 have been identified in the liver of laboratory animals such as the rat, mouse and rabbit. In addition to the constitutive forms of cytochrome P-450, there are other cytochrome P-450 isoenzymes that can be induced by various foreign chemicals. Although the exact number of cytochrome P-450 forms in any particular species has not been determined, the general consensus of most laboratories is that there are 20 or less forms (13,18). However, Nebert (27) has proposed that the organism is endowed with the genetic capacity for induction of hundreds or even thousands of cytochrome P-450 forms.

Evidence, derived primarily from the effects of inducing agents on the activity of AAF N-hydroxylation, has implicated specific forms (isoenzymes) of the cytochrome in AAF activation (1,2,35,36). Several isoenzymes of cytochrome P-450 have been purified and their significance in the metabolism of AAF investigated. Johnson et al. (14) demonstrated that four highly purified forms of rabbit hepatic cytochrome P-450 differ with respect to both rate and site specificity of AAF oxidation (Table 1). Form 4, the major isoenzyme of cytochrome P-450 induced by TCDD in adult rabbits, was the only form that catalyzed N-hydroxylation. This accounted for approximately 75% of the metabolites produced by the action of this cytochrome (Table 1). In contrast, Form 6, the major isoenzyme of cytochrome P-

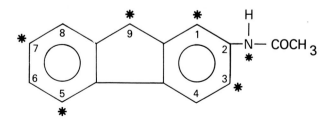

FIG. 2. Major sites of hydroxylations (*) on the 2-acetylaminofluorene molecule.

TABLE 1. *Metabolism of AAF by reconstituted forms of cytochrome P-450*

Metabolite formation	mole product formed/min/moles cytochrome P-450[b]		
	Form 3	Form 4	Form 6
7-OH-AAF	0.94 ± 0.07[a]	0.58 ± 0.13	1.13 ± 0.15
5-OH-AAF	0	0.13 ± 0.03	0
3-OH-AAF	0	0.04 ± 0.01	0
1-OH-AAF	0	0.14 ± 0.02	0
N-OH-AAF	0	2.09 ± 0.16	0

Data from ref. 14, with permission.
[a]Mean ± S.D. of triplicate experiments with two different preparations of each cytochrome.
[b]Form 2 exhibited no catalytic activity for AAF.

450 induced by TCDD in neonate rabbit liver, and Form 3, a constitutive form of the cytochrome, both catalyzed the hydroxylation of AAF exclusively in the 7-position. Form 2, the major phenobarbital-inducible cytochrome P-450 in rabbit liver, exhibited no catalytic activity with AAF as substrate. These *in vitro* data agree well with earlier work on the urinary excretion of AAF metabolites by the rabbit showing that 7-OH-AAF and N-OH-AAF were the major metabolites (9).

Since numerous factors determine the expression of cytochrome P-450, and since carcinogenesis is a multi-step process, it is difficult to predict the impact of metabolic differences arising from isoenzyme variability on N-arylamine-induced carcinogenesis. However, the proportion of the dose of carcinogen that is processed via the initial activation step, as in the case of AAF, is clearly dependent on the relative composition of the different forms of cytochrome P-450 in the organism.

As earlier stated, N-OH-AAF is more carcinogenic when compared to the parent amide. In addition, the higher yields of macromolecule-bound fluorene derivatives in the livers of rats given N-OH-AAF implicate it as an intermediate in the carcinogenicity and *in vivo* reactivity of AAF (11,20). However, N-OH-AAF, like AAF, has little ability to react under physiologic conditions with proteins or nucleic acids or their derivatives (3,12). Thus, further metabolic activation is necessary for conversion of N-OH-AAF to reactive electrophiles. The metabolic activation steps capable of generating both toxic and ultimate carcinogenic form(s) of this hydroxamic acid were initially thought to be catalyzed by the cytosolic enzymes sulfotransferase and N,O-acyltransferase (22) (Fig. 1). However, recent data, obtained in *in vitro* mutagenesis systems, indicate that the microsomal and nuclear associated deacylase (amidase) may play an important role in the metabolic activation of arylhydroxamic acids (38). Furthermore, UDP-glucocuronyltransferase and one electron oxidation, i.e., radical formation, may also participate in the metabolic activation of these compounds (4,7,10,15).

MUTAGENICITY AND CARCINOGENICITY

Since N-OH-AAF can be further activated via several metabolic pathways (Fig. 1) we have sought to determine the relative importance of each of the three major pathways, i.e., sulfotransferase, N,O-acyltransferase and deacetylase, in the mutagenic and possible carcinogenic effect of this compound. The model system used in these studies is the *Salmonella* mutagenesis system (38). The assumption is made in this model that bacterial mutation, i.e., *S. typhimurium* mutants that require histidine are assayed for reversion to prototrophy after exposure to N-OH-AAF and/ or its derivatives, corresponds to the initiating events in the carcinogenic process. Employing this model the following results were obtained:

1. No mutations were induced in the *Salmonella* mutagenesis system when the sulfate ester was formed *in situ* (26); in fact, the addition of 3'-phosphoadenosine-5'-phosphosulfate (PAPS) decreased the N-OH-AAF mutagenicity mediated by rat liver S-9 fractions (31). When partially purified rat liver sulfotransferase was used, the hydroxyapatite-purified fraction, which had the greatest sulfotransferase activity, was completely inactive in its capacity to activate N-OH-AAF in this system, and the addition of PAPS had no effect on the mutagenicity (Fig. 3) (43). It has been proposed that the lack of interaction of the sulfate ester of N-OH-AAF in the *Salmonella* system is due to its instability in aqueous solution preventing it from reaching the bacterial DNA.

2. The cytosolic N,O-acyltransferase is capable of activating N-OH-AAF into a mutagen in the *Salmonella* mutagenesis system. However, various investigators have shown that this process is independent of the metabolic activation which results in nucleic acid binding (29,39,40,43). Incubation of equimolar amounts of the primary arylamine AF with N-OH-AAF and partially purified N,O-acyltransferase decreased nucleic acid binding by more than 90%, while it had no effect on the mutation frequency normally observed (39). AF competes with the enzymatically generated N-hydroxy-2-aminofluorene (N-OH-AF) for the acetyl group, thereby inhibiting formation of the reactive N-acetoxy-AF responsible for adduct formation. Similarly, addition of guanosine monophosphate (GMP) had no effect on mutations yet it caused a significant reduction in binding to nucleic acids for the reactive electrophile generated from N-OH-AAF by N,O-acyltransferase (39). Thus the reactive product of this enzyme reaction does not appear to be responsible for mutations generated in the *Salmonella* system. It has been proposed that the mutagenicity is due to the formation of N-OH-AF (29,39,43). Whether this is due to an uncoupling of the acyltransfer process to form the hydroxylamine or to an acyltransferase-independent deacetylation remains to be clarified. However, it is important to note that the N,O-acyltransferase is more proficient in forming N-acetoxy-AF (measured as nucleic acid adducts) than it is in forming the mutagenic derivatives in the *Salmonella* system.

3. The importance of microsomal deacetylation in the mutagenic activation of N-OH-AAF has been clearly demonstrated. Complete inhibition of both mutagenesis and deacetylation was observed in incubation systems containing either liver or

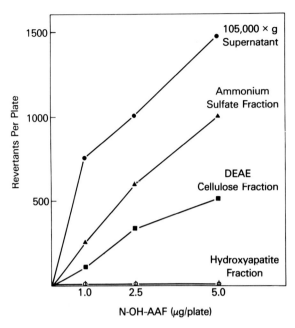

FIG. 3. Mutagenicity of *N*-OH-AAF in *Salmonella* TA 98 mediated by partially purified fractions of rat liver sulfotransferase. Points are the mean number of revertants per plate observed in two experiments and have been corrected for revertants with *N*-OH-AAF in the absence of partially purified sulfotransferase fractions. The protein concentration of each fraction was 1.0 mg/plate. *Solid circle,* experiments utilizing 105,000 x *g* supernatant; *triangle,* fraction obtained after ammonium sulfate precipitation; *square,* fraction obtained after DEAE-cellulose chromatography; *empty circle,* experiments utilizing sulfotransferase activity following hydroxyapatite chromatography. (Data from ref. 43, with permission.)

kidney microsomes and paraoxon (31). Both rat and mouse liver nuclei are also capable of mutagenic activation of *N*-OH-AAF that is readily blocked by paraoxon (29). Furthermore, liver cell nuclei are capable of activating *N*-OH-AAF to derivatives that can interact covalently with intranuclear macromolecules, and this activation is also blocked by paraoxon (29). Paraoxon sensitive deacetylases in liver microsomes from rat, mouse, hamster, and human are also capable of activating other arylhydroxamic acids such as *N*-OH-phenacetin to mutagens (Fig. 4) (42).

Results summarized above from studies over the past few years on the mechanism of *in vitro* mutagenic activation of *N*-OH-AAF and related compounds in both microbial and mammalian mutagenesis systems have demonstrated the importance of deacylation as a key reaction in generating the ultimate mutagen(s). This reaction is catalyzed by both membrane bound deacylase(s) and cytosolic *N,O*-acyltransferase(s), which are found in all target organs for *N*-OH-AAF-induced carcinogenesis. Another metabolic pathway that is intimately associated with AAF and *N*-OH-AAF-induced liver carcinogenesis is sulfation. Although the sulfate ester of *N*-OH-AAF generated *in situ* is not mutagenic in the *Salmonella* system, hepatic sulfotransferase activity is associated with both acute liver toxicity and hepatoma for-

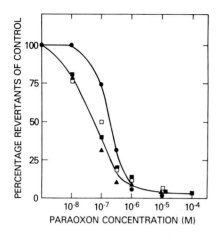

FIG. 4. Effect of paraoxon on the mutagenic activation of *N*-OH-phenacetin in *Salmonella* tester strain TA 100 by B6; *solid square,* mouse liver S-9 fractions; *solid circle,* hamster liver microsomes; *triangles,* human liver microsomes; and *empty square,* rat kidney S-9 fractions. (Data from ref. 42, with permission.)

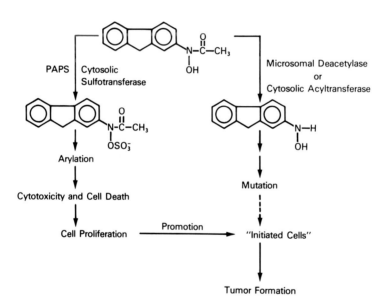

FIG. 5. Proposed roles of sulfotransferase, *N,O*-acyltransferase and deacylase in *N*-OH-AAF-induced hepatocarcinogenesis.

mation after AF or *N*-OH-AAF administration. Moreover, the acute liver toxicity can be prevented by inhibiting sulfotransferase activity. We have therefore proposed, in the context of the multi-stage process involved in chemical hepatocarcinogenesis (28), that the sulfotransferase is primarily involved in the promotional aspect of this process by generating the cytotoxic ester of *N*-OH-AAF. In contrast, *N,O*-acyltransferase and/or deacetylase are responsible for generating the mutagenic species that may initiate the carcinogenic process (Fig. 5).

Although more work is needed to substantiate or refute this proposal, it focuses attention on the possibility that different metabolites generated from procarcinogens, such a N-acetylarylamines, may influence different stages of carcinogenesis. In order to define the precise role of the different metabolites generated from N-OH-AAF and related hydroxamic acids in the carcinogenic process, it is essential to devise experimental model systems both *in vivo* and *in vitro* that clearly separate the initiation and promotional phases of the process. Under these conditions, examination of the formation and removal of nucleic acid and protein adducts, in relation to modulation of the expression of genes that are associated with the transformation process, may provide a powerful approach to the study of carcinogenesis.

REFERENCES

1. Atlas, S. A., Boobis, A. R., Felton, J. S., Thorgeirsson, S. S., and Nebert, D. W. (1977): Oncogenetic expression of polycyclic aromatic compound-inducible monooxygenase activities and forms of cytochrome P-450 in the rabbit. *J. Biol. Chem.*, 252:4712–4721.
2. Atlas, S. A., Thorgeirsson, S. S., Boobis, A. R., Kumaki, K., and Nebert, D. W. (1976): Differential induction of murine Ah locus-associated monooxygenase activities in rabbit liver and kidney. *Biochem. Pharmacol.*, 24:2111–2116.
3. Bahl, O. P., and Gutmann, H. R. (1964): On the binding of the carcinogen N-2-fluorenylacetamide to rat serum albumin *in vivo. Biochim. Biophys. Acta*, 90:391–393.
4. Bartsch, H., and Hecker, E. (1971): On the metabolic activation of the carcinogen N-hydroxy-N-acetylaminofluorene. III. Oxidation with horseradish peroxidase to yield 2-nitrosofluorene and N-acetoxy-N-acetylaminofluorene. *Biochim. Biophys. Acta*, 237:567–578.
5. Benkert, K., Fries, W., Kies, M., and Lenk, W. (1975): N-(9-hydroxy-9H-fluoren-2yl)-acetamide and N-(9-oxo-9H-fluoren-2yl)-acetamide: Metabolites of N-(9H-fluoren-2yl)-acetamide. *Biochem. Pharmacol.*, 24:1365–1380.
6. Cramer, J. W., Miller, E. C., and Miller, J. A. (1960): N-Hydroxylation: A new metabolic reaction observed in the rat with the carcinogen 2-acetylaminofluorene. *J. Biol. Chem.*, 235:885–888.
7. Floyd, R. A. (1981): Free radicals in arylamine carcinogenesis. *Natl. Cancer Inst. Monogr.*, 58:123–131.
8. Gutmann, H. R., and Bell, P. (1977): N-Hydroxylation of arylamides by the rat and guinea pig. Evidence for substrate specificity and participation of cytochrome P_1-450. *Biochim. Biophys. Acta*, 498:229–243.
9. Irving, C. C. (1962): N-Hydroxylation of 2-acetylaminofluorene in the rabbit. *Cancer Res.*, 22:867–873.
10. Irving, C. C., and Russell, L. T. (1970): Synthesis of the O-glucuronide of N-2-fluorenylhydroxylamine. Reaction with nucleic acids and with guanosine monophosphate. *Biochemistry*, 9:2471–2476.
11. Irving, C. C., and Veazey, R. A. (1969): Persistent binding of 2-acetylaminofluorene to rat liver DNA *in vivo* and consideration of the mechanism of binding of N-hydroxy-2-acetylaminofluorene to rat liver nucleic acids. *Cancer Res.*, 29:1799–1804.
12. Irving, C. C., Veazey, R. A., and Hill, J. T. (1969): Reaction of the glucuronide of the carcinogen N-hydroxy-2-acetylaminofluorene with nucleic acids. *Biochim. Biophys. Acta*, 179:189–198.
13. Johnson, E. F. (1979): Multiple forms of cytochrome P-450: Criteria and significance. *Rev. Biochem. Toxicol.*, 1:1–26.
14. Johnson, E. F., Levitt, D. S., Muller-Eberhard, U., and Thorgeirsson, S. S. (1980): Divergent pathways of carcinogen metabolism: Metabolism of 2-acetylaminofluorene by multiple forms of cytochrome P-450. *Cancer Res.*, 40:4456–4460.
15. Kriek, E. (1974): Carcinogenesis by aromatic amines. *Biochim. Biophys. Acta*, 355:177–203.
16. Lotlikar, P. D., Enomoto, M., Miller, J. A., and Miller, E. C. (1967): Species variations in the N- and ring-hydroxylation of 2-acetylaminofluorene and effects of 3-methylcholanthrene pretreatment. *Proc. Soc. Exp. Biol. Med.*, 125:341–346.

17. Lotlikar, P. D., and Zaleski, K. (1974): Inhibitory effect of carbon monoxide on the N- and ring-hydroxylation of 2-acetamidofluorene by hamster hepatic microsomal preparations. *Biochem. J.*, 144:427–430.
18. Lu, A. Y. H., and West, S. B. (1980): Multiplicity of mammalian microsomal cytochromes P-450. *Pharmacol. Rev.*, 31:277–295.
19. Malejka-Giganti, D., McIver, R. C., Glasebrook, A. L., and Gutmann, H. R. (1978): Induction of microsomal N-hydroxylation of N-2-fluorenylacetamide in rat liver. *Biochem. Pharmacol.*, 27:61–69.
20. Marroquin, F., and Farber, E. (1965): The binding of 2-acetylaminofluorene to rat liver ribonucleic acid *in vivo*. *Cancer Res.*, 25:1262–1269.
21. Matsushima, T., Grantham, P. H., Weisburger, E. K., and Weisburger, J. H. (1972): Phenobarbital-mediated increase in ring- and N-hydroxylation of the carcinogen N-2-fluorenyl acetamide and decrease in amounts bound to liver deoxyribonucleic acid. *Biochem. Pharmacol.*, 21:2043–2051.
22. Miller, E. C. (1978): Some current perspectives on chemical carcinogenesis in humans and experimental animals: Presidential address. *Cancer Res.*, 38:1479–1496.
23. Miller, J. A. (1970): Carcinogenesis by chemicals: An overview—G.H.A. Clowes Memorial Lecture. *Cancer Res.*, 30:559–576.
24. Miller, J. A., Wyatt, C. S., Miller, E. C., and Hartmann, H. A. (1961): The N hydroxylation of 4-acetaminobiphenyl by the rat and dog and the strong carcinogenicity of N-hydroxy-4-acetylaminobiphenyl in the rat. *Cancer Res.*, 21:1465–1473.
25. Morris, H. P., Velat, C. A., Wagner, B. P., Dahlgard, M., and Ray, F. E. (1960): Studies on carcinogenicity in the rat of derivatives of aromatic amines related to N-2-fluorenylacetamide. *J. Natl. Cancer Inst.*, 24:149–180.
26. Mulder, G. J., Hinson, J. A., Nelson, W. L., and Thorgeirsson, S. S. (1977): Role of sulfotransferase from rat liver in the mutagenicity of N-hydroxy-2-acetylaminofluorene in *Salmonella typhimurium*. *Biochem. Pharmacol.*, 26:1356–1358.
27. Nebert, D. W. (1979): Multiple forms of inducible drug metabolizing enzymes: A reasonable mechanism by which an organism can cope with adversity. *Mol. Cell. Biochem.*, 27:27–46.
28. Peraino, C. (1981): Initiation and promotion of liver tumorigenesis. *Natl. Cancer Inst. Monogr.*, 58:55–62.
29. Sakai, S., Reinhold, C. E., Wirth, P. J., and Thorgeirsson, S. S. (1978): Mechanism of in vitro mutagenic activation and covalent binding of N-hydroxy-2-acetylaminofluorene in isolated liver cell nuclei from rat and mouse. *Cancer Res.*, 38:2058–2067.
30. Schut, H. A. J., and Thorgeirsson, S. S. (1978): *In vitro* metabolism and mutagenic activation of 2-acetylaminofluorene and N-hydroxy-2-acetylaminofluorene by cotton rat subcellular fractions. *Cancer Res.*, 38:2501–2507.
31. Schut, H. A. J., Wirth, P. J., and Thorgeirsson, S. S. (1978): Mutagenic activation of N-hydroxy-2-acetylaminofluorene in the *Salmonella* test system: The role of deacetylation by liver and kidney fractions from mouse and rat. *Mol. Pharmacol.*, 14:682–692.
32. Seal, U. S., and Gutmann, H. R. (1959): The metabolism of the carcinogen N-(2-fluorenyl)acetamide by liver cell fractions. *J. Biol. Chem.*, 234:648–654.
33. Smith, C. S., and Thorgeirsson, S. S. (1981): An improved high-pressure liquid chromatographic assay for 2-acetylaminofluorene and eight of its metabolites. *Anal. Biochem.*, 113:62–67.
34. Son, O. S., Fouble, J. W., Miller, D. D., and Feller, D. R. (1979): 2-Acetylaminofluorene metabolism in rat liver microsomes: Formation of 9-hydroxy-2-acetylaminofluorene and effects of hepatic enzyme modifiers. *Toxicol. Appl. Pharmacol.*, 51:367–377.
35. Thorgeirsson, S. S., Atlas, S. A., Boobis, A. R., and Felton, J. S. (1979): Species differences in the substrate specificity of hepatic cytochrome P-448 from polycyclic hydrocarbon-treated animals. *Biochem. Pharmacol.*, 28:217–226.
36. Thorgeirsson, S. S., and Nebert, D. W. (1977): The Ah locus and the metabolism of chemical carcinogens and other foreign compounds. *Adv. Cancer Res.*, 25:149–193.
37. Thorgeirsson, S. S., Jollow, D. J., Sasame, H. A., Green, I., and Mitchell, J. R. (1973): The role of cytochrome P-450 in N-hydroxylation of 2-acetylaminofluorene. *Mol. Pharmacol.*, 9:398–404.
38. Thorgeirsson, S. S., Schut, H. A. J., Staiano, N., Wirth, P. J., and Everson, R. B. (1981): Mutagenicity of N-substituted aryl compounds in microbial systems. *Natl. Cancer Inst. Monogr.*, 58:229–236.

39. Weeks, C. E., Allaben, W. T., Louie, S. C., Lazear, E. J., and King, C. M. (1978): Role of arylhydroxamic acid acyltransferase in the mutagenicity of N-hydroxy-N-2-fluorenylacetamide in *Salmonella typhimurium*. *Cancer Res.*, 38:613–618.
40. Weeks, C. E., Allaben, W. T., Tresp, N. M., Louie, S. C., Lazear, E. J., and King, C. M. (1980): Effects of structure of N-hydroxy-N-2-fluorenylacylamides on arylhydroxamic acid acyltransferase, sulfotransferase, and deacetylase activities, and on mutations in *Salmonella typhimurium* TA-1538. *Cancer Res.*, 40:1204–1211.
41. Weisburger, J. H., and Weisburger, E. K. (1973): Biochemical formation and pharmacological, toxicological and pathological properties of hydroxylamines and hydroxamic acids. *Pharmacol. Rev.*, 25:1–66.
42. Wirth, P. J., Dybing, E., von Bahr, C., and Thorgeirsson, S. S. (1980): Mechanism of N-hydroxy-acetylarylamine mutagenicity in the *Salmonella* test system: Metabolic activation of N-hydroxy-phenacetin by liver and kidney fractions from rat, mouse, hamster and man. *Mol. Pharmacol.*, 18:117–127.
43. Wirth, P. J., and Thorgeirsson, S. S. (1981): Mechanism of N-hydroxy-2-acetylaminofluorene mutagenicity in the *Salmonella* test system. *Mol. Pharmacol.*, 19:337–344.

Biochemical Basis of Chemical Carcinogenesis,
edited by H. Greim, R. Jung, M. Kramer,
H. Marquardt, and F. Oesch.
Raven Press, New York © 1984.

Role of Metabolism on the Mutagenicity of Nitroarenes

Elena C. McCoy

*Center for the Environmental Health Sciences and Department of Epidemiology and
Community Health, Case Western Reserve University, School of Medicine,
Cleveland, Ohio 44106*

Since the initial work of Pitts et al. (45), which demonstrated that mutagenic nitrated derivatives of polycyclic aromatic hydrocarbons (nitroarenes) are readily formed in the environment, interest in these chemicals as potential environmental hazards has increased markedly. The presence of nitroarenes in a wide variety of complex mixtures, including the emissions from stationary and mobile combustion sources, is well documented in the literature (9,16,18,20,28,36,40–42,44,45,48,49,53–55). In view of predictions that within the next decade the number of light diesel cars will increase significantly, the biological properties of diesel-emission materials have received considerable scrutiny. A variety of chemical and microbial procedures have revealed that while nitropyrenes are the predominant mutagenic species in diesel emissions, there are in excess of 80 nitroarenes in diesel exhaust (28,37,49,53–55,63).

The mutagenicity and carcinogenicity of nitroarenes depend on their bioconversion to a variety of alternate metabolites. The arylhydroxylamines obtained by reduction appear to be the ultimate or penultimate reactive species (30,51,52). They are capable of reacting at the C-8 position of guanine to form arylamino-DNA adducts (21,25,31). The mutagenic activity of nitroarenes has been most extensively studied in *Salmonella* (2,6,47,50,61). In that species, many nitroarenes are direct-acting, although bacterial enzymes are required to generate mutagenic metabolites. Others require the addition of a mammalian post-mitochondrial fraction (S9) for demonstration of mutagenic activity. Nitroarenes also exhibit significant mutagenic, genotoxic and transforming activities for cultured mammalian cells (Tables 1 and 2). There are obvious differences in the responses of the various cell types which, in turn, may reflect their metabolic capacities. Thus Chinese hamster ovary cells (CHO) require S9 for the expression of the genotoxicity of nitroarenes irrespective of the assay system utilized. On the other hand, neither Chinese hamster fibroblasts nor mouse lymphoma nor rat epithelial liver cells require exogenous metabolic activation.

The requirement for exogenous activation of nitroarenes in human cell lines depends on the origin and passage history. Xeroderma pigmentosum cells were

TABLE 1. *Gene mutations in cultured mammalian cell lines*

Cell line	Chemical	Response	Activation	Reference
Mouse lymphoma	2-Nitrofluorene	+	—	Amacher et al. (1)
(L5178Y)	2,4,7-Trinitro-9-fluorenone	+		Burrell et al. (8)
	1-Nitropyrene	+	Required	Ball et al. (5)
	1,8-Dinitropyrene	+	—	Cole et al. (10)
Chinese hamster ovary	1-Nitropyrene	—	Absent	Ball et al. (5)
Chinese hamster lung	1-Nitropyrene	—	—	Nakayasu et al. (35)
fibroblast	1,3-Dinitropyrene	+	—	Nakayasu et al. (35)
	1,6-Dinitropyrene	+	—	Nakayasu et al. (35)
	1,8-Dinitropyrene	+	—	Nakayasu et al. (35)
	1,3,6-Trinitropyrene	+	—	Nakayasu et al. (35)
	1,3,6,8-Tetranitropyrene	—	—	Nakayasu et al. (35)
(Human) Xeroderma pigmetosum	1,8-Dinitropyrene	—	Absent	Arlett (3)

found to be insensitive to mutation and did not exhibit preferential toxicity. On the other hand, human bronchial explants and HeLa cells were responsive to DNA damages without external metabolic activation. Neoplastic transformation of normal human fibroblasts required either anaerobiosis or the enzymic reduction of the nitroarenes by xanthine oxidase. In addition, nitroarenes are carcinogenic for animals (Table 3).

The specific expression of the mutagenicity, genotoxicity and DNA-adduct formation of nitroarenes may well depend on the enzymic complement of the cell, as evidenced by the catalytic effect of S9 in some systems. However, the contribution of non-enzymatic reaction mechanisms (a notable example could be glutathione conjugation) cannot be ignored (24,32,58). A general scheme for the bioconversions of nitroarenes which is based on analysis of the mutagenicity data in a variety of systems is presented (Fig. 1). The initial step in the reductive activation is catalyzed by flavoprotein enzymes (11,17). Two general types of nitroreductase activities have been described in bacterial cells (4,47). Type I reductase activity is characterized by the transfer of two or more electrons and yields oxygen insensitive products. Type II reductases catalyze the transfer of one electron and generate the nitroradical anion, which in the presence of oxygen, is rapidly reoxidized to the original nitro compound forming superoxide in the process. In hypoxia, nitro and further reduced species are formed (29).

The major microsomal reductase in rat liver is *N*ADPH-cytochrome P-450 reductase (22) which appears to be similar to the bacterial Type II reductase. Nitroreductase activities in the liver cytosol, which have been described, include xanthine oxidase (13,27,33), aldehyde dehydrogenase (62) and DT diaphorase (22). It should be noted that the mechanisms and enzymes described relate to published reports used to explain the genetic activity of 4-nitroquinoline-1-oxide (NQO), and nitrofurans (especially AF$_2$). It has not been ascertained that the same enzyme mechanisms are responsible for the genetic effects of the nitrated polycyclic aromatic

TABLE 2. *Genotoxicity and neoplastic transformation*

Chemical	Assay endpoint	System	Exogenous activation	Result	Reference
2-Nitrofluorene	SCE	CHO	Rat S9	+	Nachtman and Wolf (34)
	Transformation	Hamster BHK21	+S9	+	Styles (57)
	Inhibition of DNA synthesis	HeLa	None	+	Painter and Howard (39)
1-Nitropyrene	SCE	CHO	Rat S9	+	Nachtman and Wolf (34)
	UDS	Human bronchus	None	+	Kawachi (23)
	Cell transformation	Normal human	Anaerobiosis	+	Howard et al. (21)
1,8-Dinitropyrene	SCE	CHO	Rat S9	+	Nachtman and Wolf (34)
	Cell transformation	Mouse Balb 3T3	None		Tu et al. (59)
	Chromosomal aberration	Rat epithelial cell line	None	+	Danford et al. (12)
	Preferential toxicity	Human XP	None	−	Arlett (3)
1,3-Dinitropyrene	UDS	Human bronchus	None	+	Kawachi (23)
	Cell transformation	Mouse Balb 3T3	None	−	Tu et al. (59)
1,6-Dinitropyrene	UDS	Human bronchus	None	+	Kawachi (23)
	Chromosomal aberration	Rat epithelial cell line	None	+	Danford (12)
	Cell transformation	Mouse Balb 3T3	None	−	Tu et al. (59)
2-Nitronaphthalene	Cell transformation	Syrian hamster embryo	None	+	Pienta (43)
Nitrated PAHs[a]	UDS	HeLa	None	+	Campbell et al. (9)
2,4,7-Trinitro-9-fluorene	SCE	CHO	Rat S9	+	Burrell (8)

[a]PAHs used: pyrenes, fluoranthenes, perylenes, chrysenes, anthracenes, benzo(a)pyrenes, benz(a)anthracenes, benz(g,h,i)perylenes. These yield mixtures of nitrated species.
Abbreviations: SCE, sister chromatid exchanges; UDS, unscheduled DNA synthesis; PAH, polyaromatic hydrocarbon.

TABLE 3. *Carcinogenicity of nitroarenes*

Chemical	Carcinogenicity	Reference
1-Nitronaphthalene	—	Griesemer and Cuoto (19)
2-Nitronaphthalene	+	Poirier and Weisburger (46)
5-Nitroacenaphthene	+	Griesemer and Cuoto (19)
2-Nitrofluorene	+	Weisburger and Weisburger (60)
1-Nitropyrene	+	Ohgaki et al. (38)
3-Nitrofluoranthene	+	Ohgaki et al. (38)
6-Nitrochrysene	+ (Tumor initiator)	El-Bayoumi et al. (15)

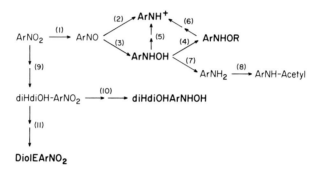

FIG. 1. General scheme for the bioconversion of nitroarenes.

hydrocarbons. However, Quilliam et al. (47) as well as ourselves (50,52) have recently reported that one of the major nitrofurazone reductases can also reduce 1-nitropyrene.

In *Salmonella* the aromatic structure appears to remain intact. Since nitrosoarenes, e.g., 2-nitrosofluorene, do not react with DNA it is proposed that either they dismutate further to form the reactive nitrenium ions (Step 2, Fig. 1) (26) or that they are converted to arylhydroxylamines (Step 3, Fig. 1). Such hydroxylamines are capable of reacting directly with DNA or may also form DNA-reactive nitrenium ion (26,56). The predominant pathway appears to involve the conversion of the arylhydroxylamines to the corresponding hydroxamic acid esters which are potent electrophiles capable of forming DNA adducts (Step 4, Fig. 1).

The mutagenic activities of a variety of nitroarenes in sensitive bacteria as well as strains selected for resistance to the mutagenicity of nitroarenes are presented (Table 4). The data suggest that bacteria possess a family of nitroreductase activities. The strains are still fully sensitive to the mutagenic action of the non-nitrated polycyclic aromatic hydrocarbon 7-bromomethyl-12-methylbromobenzanthracene and quercetin. The NR strain is deficient in the "classical nitroreductase" activity as evidenced by the decreased response to niridazole. It exhibits "wild type" activity with respect to the dinitropyrenes and NQO. Strain TA98/1,8-DNP$_6$ is non-responsive to the mutagenic action of 1,8- and 1,3-dinitropyrene and other nitroarenes, e.g., 2,7-dinitrofluorenone, yet it is sensitive to NQO and to niridazole. The reduced

TABLE 4. *The mutagenic response of* Salmonella *TA98 derivatives*

	Revertants/nmole		
Chemical	TA98	TA98NR	TA98/1,8-DNP$_6$
1-Nitropyrene	453	35	199
1,3-Dinitropyrene	144,760	24,750	2,750
1,6-Dinitropyrene	183,570	190,900	45,890
1,8-Dinitropyrene	254,000	264,160	5,850
1,3,6-Trinitropyrene	40,700	36,300	25,640
1,3,6,8-Tetranitropyrene	15,600	10,400	14,000
Niridazole	390	17	390
4-Nitroquinoline-1-oxide	126	124	106
2,7-Dinitro-9-fluorenone	1,459	184	137
2-Nitrofluorene	84	2	2
5-Nitroacenaphthene	4.6	2.7	0.5

TABLE 5. *Mutagenicity of 2-hydroxylaminofluorene and derivatives*

	Revertants/nmole		
Chemical	TA98	TA98NR	TA98/1,8-DNP$_6$
2-Nitrofluorene	84	2	2
2-Nitrosofluorene	542	504	79
N-Hydroxy-2-aminofluorene[a]	1,175	1,266	31
2-Aminofluorene + S9	154	127	15
N-Hydroxy-2AAF + S9	371	343	20
N-AcAAF	10	9	9
2-Aminoanthracene + S9	494	546	25
DMBA	2	2	2
BMBA	14	15	17
Quercetin	0.9	1.1	1.0
Niridazole	400	17	400

[a]Obtained by the *in situ* reduction of 2-nitrosofluorene by ascorbic acid.
Abbreviations: *N*-AcAAF, *N*-acetoxy-2-acetylaminofluorene; BMBA,7-bromomethyl-12-methylbenz*(a)*anthracene; DMBA, 7,12-dimethyl-benz*(a)*anthracene.

response of strain TA98/1,8-DNP$_6$ observed with 2-nitrofluorene was unexpected, but fortuitous in that it enabled an examination of the proposed reductive pathway leading from 2-nitrofluorene to 2-aminofluorene, as most of the hypothetical intermediates are not only available but have been studied in other contexts, e.g., bioconversion, DNA-adduct formation, carcinogenicity. They include 2-nitrosofluorene, 2-aminofluorene, *N*-hydroxy-2-aminofluorene (*N*-OH-AF), the model ester *N*-acetoxy-2-acetylaminofluorene and the acetylated derivatives: 2-acetylaminofluorene and *N*-hydroxy-2-acetylaminofluorene (Table 5). As would be expected for a strain deficient in nitroreductase, 2-nitrosofluorene and 2-hydroxylaminofluorene bypassed the block in the NR strain. In contrast to the NR strain, reduced intermediates of 2-nitrofluorene did not bypass the block in TA98/1,8-DNP$_6$. These findings suggested that the lesion in that strain was between the arylhydroxylamine and an ultimate mutagenic species. The model electrophilic ester N-acetoxy-2-acetylaminofluorene (AcAAF) was equally active in all strains. These findings are consistent with the hypothesis that the lesion in TA98/1,8-DNP$_6$ is between arylhydroxylamine and an esterified species, and they indicate that a specific gene product, controlling esterification, exists in *Salmonella*. To test this further, 2-aminofluorene (2AF) and 2-acetylaminofluorene (2-AAF), both of which are N-hydroxylated by the microsomal P-450 oxidase to N-OH-AF and N-OH-AAF, prior to showing mutagenicity, were tested in the presence of S9, respectively. The proximate mutagen N-OH-AF may also be generated from N-OH-AAF by liver deacetylase. It is presumed that N-OH-AF is converted to the ultimate mutagen by an esterification mechanism. Bartsch et al. (7) have presented evidence that activation of N-OH-2AAF results from N-O transfer of the acetyl group to yield N-acetoxyaminoarenes which then react with tissue nucleophiles, e.g., DNA.

While all of these manipulations demonstrated the mutagenicity of N-OH-AF for TA98NR, none caused the lesion in TA98/1,8-DNP$_6$ to be bypassed. Similar results were obtained when 2-aminoanthracene and S9 were used, suggesting that a common mechanism (ester formation) may be operative in the mutagenicity of a variety of arylhydroxylamines.

A summary of preliminary results obtained by analyses of HPLC profiles of whole cells incubated for 1 hr in non-growth medium with 2-nitrofluorene, 2-nitrosofluorene, and 2-aminofluorene is presented (Table 6). The tentative identifications are based on co-migration with standards. Although the data are reproducible, definitive chemical identifications have not been performed.

When 2-nitrofluorene was incorporated into the incubation medium, peaks corresponding to 2AF and N-OH-AF, AAF and AcAAF were observed in TA98. As expected these peaks were absent in the NR mutant. TA98/1,8-DNP$_6$ resembled the parental strain with the exception that a peak co-migrating with AcAAF was not observed. An unidentified peak "A" was also present in all.

When 2-nitrosofluorene was used as substrate most of the intermediates were obtained in all strains. However, peaks co-migrating with AAF and AcAAF were markedly reduced in the TA98/1,8-DNP$_6$ mutant. Peak "A" was not observed; however, three additional unidentified peaks—B, C, and D—were noted in all strains.

The results obtained with 2-aminofluorene for TA98 and TA98NR were identical to each other. The strain TA98/1,8-DNP$_6$ did not reveal any material co-migrating with AcAAF, suggesting that the defect in this mutant is at the level of esterification, presumably a transacetylase. None of the unidentified peaks (A,B,C,D) were observed.

In mammalian cells, in addition to reduction, the nitro function may also direct the oxidation of the ring moiety (Step 9, Fig. 1), as evidenced by 6-nitrobenzo(a)pyrene (44). This may be followed by reduction of the nitro function to the hydroxylamino and possibly esterification, as with 5-nitroacenapthene. The

TABLE 6. *Presumed metabolites on HPLC*

	NO$_2$F	NOF	N-OH-F	AF	AAF	AcAAF	A[a]	B[a]	C[a]	D[a]
2-Nitrofluorene										
TA98	+++	?	++	+++	+	+	+	–	–	–
TA98NR	+++	?	–	+/–	–	–	++	–	–	–
TA98/1,8-DNP$_6$	+++	?	+	+++	+?	–	+	–	–	–
2-Nitrosofluorene										
TA98	++	+	+	++	+	++	–	1+	++	++
TA98NR	++	–	–	++	++	+++	–	++	+++	+++
TA98/1,8-DNP$_6$	++	+	+	++	+/–	+/–	–	++	++	++
2-Aminofluorene										
TA98	–	–	?	+++	+++	+++	–	–	–	–
TA98NR	–	–	?	+++	+++	+++	–	–	–	–
TA98/1,8-DNP$_6$	–	–	?	+++	++	–	–	–	–	–

[a]A, B, C, D: unknown metabolites.
NOH AAF: not detected by this chematographic procedure.
Abbreviations: NO$_2$F, 2-nitrofluorene; NOF, 2-nitrosofluorene; AF, 2-aminofluorene; AAF, 2-acetylaminofluorene; AcAAF, N-acetoxyl-2-acetylaminofluorene; N-OH-F, N-hydroxy-2-acetylaminofluorene.

TABLE 7. *Mutagenicity of 5-nitroacenaphthene:*
effect of metabolic activation

S9	TA100	TA100NR	TA98	TA98NR	TA98/1,8-DNP$_6$
None	22.1	4.1	23.0	13.6	2.7
R1	88.9	45.4	96.8	87.4	59.6

R1 = S9 from livers of Araclor-induced rats.
Activities are given as revertants per μg.

results obtained with this chemical are presented (Table 7). Although the parent compound acenaphthene is not mutagenic in any of the *Salmonella* tester strains (TA98, TA100, TA1537, TA1535), the nitro-substituted chemical is mutagenic. Mutagenicity is enhanced by the addition of S9 to the nitroreductase-proficient and -deficient bacteria. The extent of the response in the NR and TA98/1,8-DNP$_6$ strains suggests that S9 bypasses the block in both mutant types. Those data are consistent with the published findings of El-Bayoumi and Hecht (14), who proposed that in the presence of microsomes the 1- and 2-hydroxy and 1- and 2-oxo-5-nitroacenaphthenes are generated which are subsequently reduced to the nitroso and mutagenic hydroxylamino species.

In conclusion, these findings indicate that the activation of nitroarenes to mutagenic species can proceed through a variety of mechanisms and presumably the same applies to their carcinogenicity.

ACKNOWLEDGMENTS

This investigation was supported by the National Institutes of Environmental Health Sciences and the U.S. Environmental Protection Agency.

Portions of this report were the result of a collaborative study with Dr. Robert Mermelstein of Xerox Corporation.

REFERENCES

1. Amacher, D. E., Paillet, S. C., and Turner, G. N. (1979): Utility of the mouse lymphoma L5178Y/ TK assay for the detection of chemical mutagens. In: *Banbury Report No. 2: Mammalian Cell Mutagenesis: The Maturation of Test Systems*, edited by A. W. Hsiu, J. P. O'Neill, and V. K. McElheny, pp. 277–289. Cold Spring Harbor Laboratory, Cold Spring Harbor, L.I., New York.
2. Ames, B. N., McCann, J., and Yamasaki, E. (1975): Methods for detecting carcinogens and mutagens with the *Salmonella*/mammalian-microsome mutagenicity test. *Mutation Res.*, 31:347–364.
3. Arlett, C. (1982): Mutagenicity of 1,8-dinitropyrene in mammalian cells. In: *The Toxicity of Nitroaromatic Compounds*, edited by E. C. Rickert. Hemisphere Publishing Co., New York, (*in press*).
4. Asnis, P. E. (1957): The reduction of furacin by cell-free extracts furacin-resistant and parent-susceptible strains of *Escherichia coli. Arch. Biochem. Biophys.*, 66:208–216.
5. Ball, L. M., Kahan, M. J., Claxton, L., and Lewtas, J. (1982): Mammalian activation and metabolism of 1-nitropyrene. Abstract, Fifth CIIT (Chemical Industry Institute of Toxicology) Conference on Toxicology: Toxicity of Nitroaromatic Compounds, p. 7.

6. Bartsch, H., Malaveille, C., Camus, A.-M., Martel-Planche, G., Brun, G., Hautefeuille, A., Sabadie, N., Barbin, A., Kuroki, T., Drevon, C., Piccoli, C., and Montisano, R. (1980): Validation and comparative studies on 180 chemicals with *Salmonella typhimurium* and V79 Chinese hamster cells in the presence of various metabolizing systems. *Mutation Res.* 76:1–50.

7. Bartsch, H., Dworkin, M., Miller, J. A., and Miller, E. C. (1972): Acetoxyaminoarenes derived from carcinogenic N-hydroxy-N-acetylaminoarenes by enzymatic deacetylation and transacetylation in liver. *Biochem. Biophys. Acta,* 286:272–298.

8. Burrell, A. D., Anderson, J. J., Jotz, J. J., Evans, E. L., and Mitchell, A. D. (1981): Genetic toxicity of 2,4,7-Trinitrofluoren-9-one in the *Salmonella* assay, L5178Y/TK$^{+/-}$ mouse lymphoma mutagenesis assay and sister chromatid exchange assay. *Environ. Mut.,* 3:360.

9. Campbell, J., Crumplin, G. C., Garner, J. V., Garner, R. C., Martin, C. N., and Rutter, A. (1981): Nitrated polycyclic aromatic hydrocarbons: potent bacterial mutagens and stimulators of DNA repair synthesis in cultured human cells. *Carcinogenesis,* 2:559–565.

10. Cole, J., Arlett, C. F., Lowe, J., and Bridges, B. A. (1982): The mutagenic potency of 1,8-dinitropyrene in cultured mouse lymphoma cells. *Mutation Res.,* 93:213–220.

11. Coughlan, M. P. (1980): Aldehyde oxidase, xanthine oxidase and xanthine dehydrogenase: Hydroxylases containing molybdenum, iron-sulfur and flavin. In: *Molybdenum and Molybdenum Containing Enzymes,* edited by M. P. Coughlan, pp. 119–185. Pergamon Press, Oxford.

12. Danford, N., Wilcox, P. and Parry, J. M. (1982): The clastogenic activity of dinitropyrenes in a rat liver epithelial cell line. *Mutation Res.,* 105:349–355.

13. Della Corte, E., Goaaetti, G., Novello, F. and Stupi, F. (1969): Properties of xanthine oxidase from human liver. *Biochim. Biophys. Acta,* 191:164–166.

14. El-Bayoumi, K., and Hecht, S. S. (1982): Identification of mutagenic metabolites formed by C-hydroxylation and nitroreduction of 5-nitroacenaphthene in rat liver. *Cancer Res.,* 42:1245–1248.

15. El-Bayomi, K., Hecht, S. S., and Hoffman, D. (1983): Comparative tumor initiating activity on mouse skin of 6-nitrobenzo(a)pyrene, 6-nitro chrysene, 3-nitroperylene and their parent hydrocarbons. *Cancer Lett.,* 16:333–337.

16. Erickson, M. D., Newton, K. L., Saylor, M. C., Tomer, K. B., Pellizzari, E. D., Zweidinger, T. B., and Tejada, S. (1981): Fractionation and identification of organic components in diesel exhaust particulate. *EPA Diesel Emissions Symposium Abstract.*

17. Feller, D. R., Moura, M., and Gillette, J. R. (1971): Enzymatic reduction of niridazole by rat liver microsomes. *Biochem. Pharmacol.,* 20:203–215.

18. Gibson, T., and Williams, R. (1981): Diesels and other sources of nitro derivatives of polynuclear aromatic hydrocarbons in airborne particulate. *EPA Diesel Emissions Symposium Abstract.*

19. Griesemer, R. A., and Cuoto, C. Jr. (1980): Toward a classification scheme for degrees of experimental evidence for the carcinogenicity of chemicals for animals. In: *Molecular and Cellular Aspects of Carcinogen Screening Tests,* Scientific Publication No. 27. International Agency for Research on Cancer, Lyon.

20. Henderson, T. R., Sun, J. D., Toyer, R. E., Clark, C. R., Harvey, T. M., Hunt, D. F., Fulford, J. E., Lovett, A. M., and Davidson, W. R. (1981): GC/MS and MS/MS studies of direct-acting mutagens in diesel emissions. *EPA Diesel Emissions Symposium Abstract.*

21. Howard, P. C. and Beland, F. A. (1982): Xanthine oxidase catalyzed binding of 1-nitropyrene to DNA. *Biochem. Biophys. Res. Comm.,* 104:727–732.

22. Kato, R., Takadashi, A., and Oshima, T. (1970): Characterizations of nitroreduction of the carcinogenic agent 4-nitroquinoline-N-oxide. *Biochem. Pharmacol.,* 19:45–55.

23. Kawachi, T. (1983): Mutagenicity and carcinogenicity of nitropyrenes. In: *The Toxicity of Nitroaromatic Compounds,* edited by D. E. Rickert. Hemisphere Publishing Co., New York, *(in press).*

24. Ketterer, B. (1981): Xenobiotic metabolism by nonenzymatic reactions of glutathione. *Symposium on the Metabolism and Pharmacokinetics of Environmental Chemicals in Man,* Sarasota, Fla., June 7–12, 1981.

25. King, H. W. S., Thompson, M. H., and Brookes, P. (1975): The benzo(a)pyrene deoxyribonucleoside products isolated from DNA after metabolism of benzo(a)pyrene by rat liver microsomes in the presence of DNA. *Cancer Res.,* 35:1263–1269.

26. Kriek, E. (1965): On the interaction of N-2-fluorenyl-hydroxylamine with nucleic acids *in vitro. Biochem. Biophys. Res. Comm.,* 20:793–799.

27. Krenitsky, T. A., and Tuttle, J. V. (1978): Xanthine oxidase activities: Evidence for two catalytically different types. *Arch. Biochem. Biophys.,* 185:370–375.

28. Lofroth, G. (1981): Comparison of the mutagenic activity in carbon black particulate matter and in diesel gasoline engine exhaust. In: *Application of Short-Term Bioassays in the Analysis of Complex Environmental Mixtures. II.*, edited by M. D. Waters, S. S. Sandhu, J. L. Huisingh, L. Claxton, and S. Nesnow, pp. 319–336. Environmental Science Research, Vol. 22. Plenum Press, New York.

29. Mason, R. P., and Holtzman, J. L. (1975): The mechanism of microsomal and mitochondrial nitroreductase. Electron spin resonance evidence for nitroaromatic free radical intermediates. *Biochemistry*, 14:1626–1632.

30. Mermelstein, R., McCoy, E. C., and Rosenkranz, H. S. (1982): The microbial mutagenicity of nitroarenes. In: *The Genotoxic Effects of Airborne Agents*, edited by R. R. Tice, D. L. Costa, and K. M. Schaich, pp. 369–396. Brookhaven National Laboratory Symposium, Plenum Press, New York.

31. Messier, F., Lu, C., Andrews, P., McCarry, B. E., Quillian, M. A., and McCalla, D. R. (1981): Metabolism of 1-nitropyrene and the formation of DNA adducts in *Salmonella typhimurium*. *Carcinogenesis*, 2:1007–1011.

32. Morita, M., Feller, D. R., and Gillette, J. R. (1971): Reduction of niridazole by rat liver xanthine oxidase. *Biochem. Pharmacol.*, 20:217–226.

33. Muller, G. J., Unruh, L. E., Ketterer, B., and Kadlubar, F. F. (1982): Formation and identification of glutathione conjugates from 2-nitrosofluorene and 2-hydroxy-2-aminofluorene. *Chem.-Biol. Interactions*, 39:111–127.

34. Nachtman, J. P., and Wolff, S. (1982): Activity of nitropolynuclear aromatic hydrocarbons in sister chromatid exchange assay with and without metabolic activation. *Environ. Mut.*, 4:1–5.

35. Nakayasu, M., Sakamoto, H., Wakabayashi, K., Terada, M., Sugimura, T., and Rosenkranz, H. S. (1982): Potent mutagenic activity of nitropyrenes on Chinese hamster lung cells with diphtheria toxin resistance as a selective marker. *Carcinogenesis (London)*, 8:917–922.

36. National Academy of Sciences, U.S. (1981): Health effects of exposure to diesel exhaust, *The Report of the Health Effects Panel of the Diesel Impact Study Committee*, National Research Council-National Academy of Sciences, Washington, D.C.

37. Nishioka, M. G., Petersen, B. A., and Lewtas, J. (1981): Comparison of nitro-PNA content and mutagenicity of diesel emissions. *EPA Diesel Emissions Symposium Abstract.*

38. Ohgaki, H., Matsukara, N., Morino, K., Kawachi, T., Sugimura, T., Morita, K., Tokiwa, H., and Hirota, T. (1982): Carcinogenicity in rats of the mutagenic compounds 1-nitropyrene and 3-nitrofluoranthene. *Cancer Lett.*, 15:1–7.

39. Painter, R. B., and Howard, R. (1982): The HeLa DNA synthesis inhibition test as a rapid screen for mutagenic carcinogens. *Mutation Res.*, 92:427–437.

40. Pederson, T. C., and Siak, J. C. (1981): Dinitropyrenes: Their probable presence in diesel particle extracts and consequent effect on mutagenic activations by NADH-dependent S9 enzymes. *EPA Diesel Emissions Symposium Abstract.*

41. Pederson, T. C., and Siak, J. C. (1981): The role of nitroaromatic compounds in the direct-acting mutagenicity of diesel particle extracts. *J. Appl. Tox.*, 1:54–60.

42. Petersen, B. A., Chuang, C. C., Margard, W. L., and Trayser, D. A. (1981): Identification of mutagenic compounds in extracts of diesel exhaust particulates. *Air Poll. Control Assoc. Abstract, 74th Annual Meeting*, 81–56.1.

43. Pienta, R. J. (1980): Evaluation and relevance of the Syrian hamster embryo cell system. In: *The Predictive Value of Short-Term Screening Tests in Carcinogenicity Evaluation*, edited by G. M. Williams, R. Kroes, H. W. Waaijers and K. W. Van de Poll, pp. 149–169. Elsevier/North Holland, Amsterdam.

44. Pitts, J. N., Jr., Lokensgard, D. M., Harger, W., Fisher, T. S., Mejia, V., Schuler, J. J., Scorziell, G. M., and Katzenstein, Y. A. (1982): Mutagens in diesel exhaust particulate: Identification and direct activites of 6-nitrobenzo(a)pyrene, 9-nitroanthracene, 1-nitropyrene and 5H-phenanthro (4,5-bcd) pyran-5-one. *Mutation Res.*, 103:241–249.

45. Pitts, J. H., Jr., Van Cauwenberghe, K. A., Grosjean, D., Schmid, J. P., Fitz, D. R., Belser, W. L. Jr., Knudson, G. B., and Hunds, P. M. (1979): Atmospheric reactions of polycyclic aromatic hydrocarbons: facile formation of mutagenic nitro derivatives. *Science*, 202:515–519.

46. Poirier, L. A. and Weisburger, E. K. (1979): Selection of carcinogens and related compounds tested for mutagenic activity. *J. Nat. Cancer Inst.*, 62:833–840.

47. Quilliam, M. A., Messier, F., Lu, C., Andrews, P., McCarry, B. E., and McCalla, D. R. (1982): The metabolism of nitro-substituted polycyclic aromatic hydrocarbons in *Salmonella typhimurium*.

In: Polynuclear Aromatic Hydrocarbons: Physical and Biological Chemistry. *Proceedings of the Sixth International Conference on Polycyclic Aromatic Hydrocarbons, Vol. 5*, edited by M. Cooke, A. J. Dennun, and G. Fisher, pp. 667–672. Battelle Laboratories Press, Columbus, Ohio.

48. Rappaport, S. M., Want, Y. Y., Wei, E. T., Sawyer, R., Watkins, B. E., and Rapoport, H. (1980): Isolation of a direct-acting mutagen in diesel-exhaust particulates. *Environ. Sci. and Tech.*, 14:1505–1509.

49. Riley, T., Prater, T., Schuetzle, D., Harvey, T. M., and Hunt, D. (1981): The analysis of nitrated polynuclear hydrocarbons in diesel exhaust particulates by mass spectrometry/mass spectrometry techniques. *EPA Diesel Emissions Symposium Abstract.*

50. Rosenkranz, H. S., and Speck, W. T. (1975): Activation of nitrofurantoin to a mutagen by rat liver nitrorectase. *Biochem. Pharm.*, 24:1555–1556.

51. Rosenkranz, H. S., and Mermelstein, R. (1983): Mutagenicity and genotoxicity of nitroarenes: All nitro-containing chemicals were not created equal. *Mutation Res.*, 114:217–267.

52. Rosenkranz, H. S., Karpinsky, G. E., Anders, M., Rosenkranz, E. J., Petrulla, L. A., McCoy, E. C., and Mermelstein, R. (1982): Adaptability of microbial mutagenicity assays to the study of problems of environmental concern. In: *Induced Mutagenesis: Molecular Mechanisms and their Implications for Environmental Protection*, edited by C. W. Lawrence, L. Prakash and F. Shuman, Plenum Press, New York.

53. Schuetzle, D., Riley, T., Prater, T. J., Harvey, T. M., and Hunt, D. F. (1982): Analysis of nitrated polycyclic aromatic hydrocarbons in diesel particulates. *Anal. Chem.*, 54:265–271.

54. Schuetzle, D., Lee, F. S. C., Prater, T. J., and Tejada, S. B. (1981): The identification of poly-nuclear aromatic hydrocarbon (PAH) derivatives in mutagenic fractions of diesel particulate extracts. *Intern. J. Environ. Anal. Chem.*, 9:1–52.

55. Schuetzle, D., Riley, T., Prater, T. J., Harvey, T. M., and Hunt, D. F. (1981): The identification of nitrated derivatives of PAH in diesel particulates using MS/MS and GC/MS techniques. *28th Congress Inter. Union Pure Appl. Chem. Abstracts (AN 11).*

56. Schut, H. A. J., Wirth, P. J., and Thorgeirsson, S. S. (1978): Mutagenic activation of N-hydroxy-2-acetylaminofluorene in the *Salmonella* test system: The role of deacetylation by liver and kidney fractions from mouse and rat. *Mol. Pharm.*, 14:682–692.

57. Styles, J. A. (1981): Use of the BHK 21/C, 13 cells for chemical screening. In: *Mammalian Cell Transformation by Chemical Carcinogens*, edited by N. Mishra, V. Dunkel, and M. Mehlman, pp. 85–131. Senate Press, Inc., Princeton Junction, New Jersey.

58. Testa, B. (1982): Nonenzymatic contributions to xenobiotic metabolism. *Drug. Metab. Rev.*, 13:25–50.

59. Tu, A. S., Sivak, A., and Mermelstein, R. (1982): Evaluation of *in vitro* transforming ability of nitropyrenes. Abstracts, Fifth CIIT (Chemical Industry Institute of Toxicology) Conference on Toxicology: Toxicity of Nitroaromatic Compounds.

60. Weisburger and Weisburger (1958): Chemistry, carcinogenicity and metabolism of 2-fluorenamine and selected compounds. *Adv. Cancer Res.*, 5:331–341.

61. Wirth, P. J., Dybing, E., von Bahr, C., and Thorgeirsson, S. S. (1980): Mechanism of N-hydroxyacetylamino mutagenicity in *Salmonella* test systems: Metabolic activation of N-hydroxyphenacetin by liver and kidney fractions from rat, mouse, hamster and man. *Mol. Pharmacol.*, 18:117–127.

62. Wolpert, M. K., Althans, J. K., and Johns, D. C. (1973): Nitroreductase activity of mammalian liver aldehyde oxidase. *J. Pharm. Exp. Ther.*, 185:202–213.

63. Xu, X. B., Nachtman, J. P., Jin, A. L., Wei, E. T., Rappaport, S. and Burlingame, A. (1981): Isolation and identification of mutagenic nitroarenes in diesel exhaust particulates. *EPA Diesel Emissions Symposium Abstract.*

Biochemical Basis of Chemical Carcinogenesis,
edited by H. Greim, R. Jung, M. Kramer,
H. Marquardt, and F. Oesch.
Raven Press, New York © 1984.

Diethylstilbestrol: Reactive Metabolites Derived from a Hormonally Active Compound

*Institute of Pharmacology and Toxicology, University of Würzburg,
D-8700 Würzburg, Federal Republic of Germany*

The association of specific tumors in the genital tract of young women with their *in utero* exposure to the synthetic estrogen diethylstilbestrol (DES), first recognized in 1971, is the most dramatic, but certainly not the only, evidence for the carcinogenic potential of this substance (6). In animals, DES has proven carcinogenic in a variety of species (7). The tumors usually arise in tissues considered to be typical estrogen target organs, e.g., uterus and mammary gland. Therefore, it is still widely assumed that the carcinogenic potency of DES is related solely to the hormonal effects of this powerful estrogen.

However, consideration of the chemical structure of DES and data from early metabolic studies led us to propose, in 1975, that metabolic activation of DES may play a role in its tumorigenicity (17). This hypothesis, implying that reactive DES metabolites cause genetic damage in a manner commonly attributed to chemical carcinogens, was subsequently refined and supported by findings from both our laboratory and others. The present communication summarizes most of the available evidence suggesting that a specific metabolic pathway may be critical for DES carcinogenicity.

METABOLISM AND GENETIC TOXICITY OF DES

The DES molecule is not electrophilic per se but requires metabolic alteration in order to become reactive. Hints that DES is metabolically activated came from metabolic studies with radio-labeled DES, where nonextractable binding of radioactivity to cellular macromolecules was observed *in vivo* or under certain metabolic conditions *in vitro* (19). Such investigations with various species, including humans and nonhuman primates, have disclosed an extensive oxidative biotransformation of DES in addition to the previously detected conjugation reactions (18). The major pathways (Fig. 1) comprise aromatic and aliphatic hydroxylation, epoxidation of the stilbene double bond and oxidation of the stilbenediol entity to Z,Z-dienestrol (Z,Z-DIES).

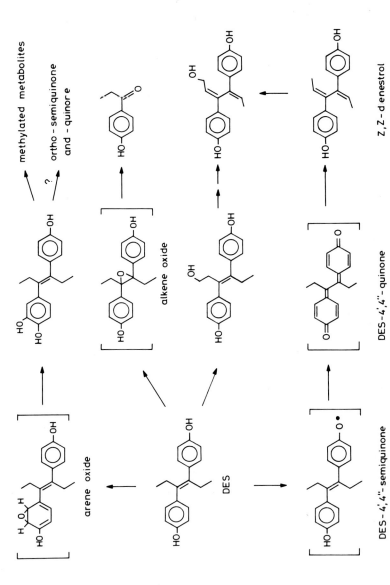

FIG. 1. Major pathways in the metabolism of diethylstilbestrol (DES). (Nomenclature from ref. 20.)

The molecular structures of most of the putative intermediates, such as the arene or alkene oxide and the DES-semiquinone and -quinone, indicate that electrophilic reactivity must be expected. Therefore, it is not surprising that DES produced a positive response in a number of short-term tests used to assay genetic damage (Table 1).

From the results of metabolic studies and short-term tests it may be safely concluded that DES can undergo metabolic activation to electrophiles which are capable of interfering with cellular macromolecules. However, important questions persist: (a) which of the different oxidative pathways is responsible for the genotoxicity of DES? (b) is metabolic activation, even though it is feasible, a *sine qua non* condition for the carcinogenicity of DES? (c) if so, how can one explain the organ specificity of DES carcinogenicity? Although no conclusive answers can be given to any of these questions at the present time, some recent data relevant to them should be considered.

IMPORTANCE OF PEROXIDATIVE METABOLISM OF DES

The formation of Z,Z-DIES (Fig. 1) has been proposed to proceed through the intermediate DES-4', 4"-quinone, which tautomerizes spontaneously to Z,Z-DIES (9,21). As this oxidation of DES is mediated by peroxidases, a semiquinone (phen-oxy radical) is most likely involved as a further intermediate. For several reasons, this pathway in DES metabolism (Fig. 1) appears to be of particular interest for the mechanism of DES carcinogenicity:

1. The intermediates of this pathway are capable of binding covalently to nucleic acids and protein. This has been demonstrated *in vitro* by incubating ^{14}C-DES with DNA and peroxidase (21) and by nonenzymatic reaction of DNA with synthetic DES-quinone (10) or the products of chemical oxidation of DES (3).

2. The intermediates of this pathway are most likely responsible for the mutations in *S. cerevisiae* (Table 1) caused by DES in the presence of iodine or $H_2O_2/FeSO_4$ (16). Under these oxidation conditions, DES has been shown to yield Z,Z-DIES (21).

TABLE 1. *Short-term assays for genetic damage in which DES causes a positive response*

Assay system	Reference no.
Unscheduled DNA synthesis in HeLa cells in the presence of rat liver postmitochondrial supernatant	12
Mutations in a mouse lymphoma cell line	4
Induction of sister chromatid exchange in human fibroblasts	25
Mutations in *S. cerevisiae* in the presence of iodine or hydrogen peroxide/ferrous sulfate	16
Chemical transformation of embryo-derived mouse fibroblasts *in vitro*	24
Chemical transformation of Syrian hamster embryo (SHE) fibroblasts *in vitro*	2,23
Unscheduled DNA synthesis in SHE cells in the presence of rat liver postmitochondrial supernatant	26

3. This pathway is operative in Syrian hamster embryo cells which respond to DES with neoplastic transformation (Table 1). Upon incubation of these cells with ^{14}C-DES, only Z,Z-DIES but none of the other oxidative metabolites was found (5).

4. The peroxidative pathway even appears to be a prerequisite for the capability of DES to transform Syrian hamster embryo cells. Of several DES analogs (Table 2), only those compounds which had retained the stilbenediol structure were able to transform (with the exception of Z,Z-DIES) (15). Most interestingly, there was

TABLE 2. *Comparison of estrogenicity, ability to transform Syrian hamster embryo (SHE) cells, and peroxidase-mediated DNA binding for DES and related compounds*

		Estrogenicity	Transformation of SHE cells	Peroxidase-mediated DNA-binding
E - DES	HO—⟨O⟩—C(=)—⟨O⟩—OH	+	+	1
E-TF-DES	HO—⟨O⟩—C(=)—⟨O⟩—OH (F,F,F,F)	+	+	n.d.
E - DMS	HO—⟨O⟩—C(=)—⟨O⟩—OH	–	+	n.d.
meso - HES	HO—⟨O⟩—CH-CH—⟨O⟩—OH	+	–	3.5
Z,Z - DIES	HO—⟨O⟩—C(=)—⟨O⟩—OH	–	+	1.1
E,E- DIES	HO—⟨O⟩—C(=)—⟨O⟩—OH	+	–	2.9
4'-O-CH₃- DES	CH₃O—⟨O⟩—C(=)—⟨O⟩—OH	–	+	1.0
4;4"-O-di- CH₃-DES	CH₃O—⟨O⟩—C(=)—⟨O⟩—OCH₃	–	–	<0.02

Data on cell transformation are from ref. 15. DNA binding of the DES analogs (Metzler, unpublished data) is expressed relative to DNA binding of DES. n.d. = not determined. Nomenclature of compounds according to ref. 20.

no correlation between transforming activity and estrogenicity in this series of DES analogs (Table 2). For a detailed discussion see ref. 15.

5. This pathway is also operative in a target organ for the transplacental carcinogenicity of DES. When fetal mouse genital tracts were incubated with DES in organ culture, Z,Z-DIES was found. None of the other oxidative metabolites shown in Fig. 1, however, were present (13). DES causes tumors in the genital tract of female mice after prenatal exposure (14).

6. Peroxidatic enzyme activity is particularly high in estrogen target organs such as uterus and mammary gland (11), and can be induced by estrogens (1). This could, in part, explain the organ specificity of the carcinogenic effect of DES.

ROLE OF SEMIQUINONE IN DNA BINDING

Because of the apparent importance of the peroxidase-mediated pathway in DES metabolism for the genetic toxicity and carcinogenicity of this substance, efforts were recently made to clarify whether DNA binding is solely caused by the quinone intermediate or also by the semiquinone (phenoxy radical). This question cannot be solved with DES, because both intermediates are formed simultaneously upon peroxidation. Therefore, analogs of DES were used which could only form a phenoxy radical but no quinone (Metzler, *unpublished data*). When ^{14}C-labelled meso-hexestrol (HES) or the dienestrol (DIES) isomers (Table 2) were incubated *in vitro* with either horseradish peroxidase or mouse uterus peroxidase in the presence of DNA, nonextractable binding similar to or even higher than that for DES was observed (Table 2). This indicates that the phenoxy radical binds DNA very well. The binding of the mono methyl ether of DES (4' -O-CH$_3$-DES), where only a phenoxy radical but no quinone formation is conceivable, also followed this pattern; its binding was as good as that of DES. Blocking of the second hydroxy group (in 4' ,4"-O-diCH$_3$-DES) prevented radical formation and DNA binding (Table 2).

RELEVANCE OF PEROXIDASE-MEDIATED ACTIVATION FOR STEROIDAL ESTROGENS

Steroidal estrogens such as estradiol-17β show the same carcinogenic effect as DES in some animal models (7). Because steroid estrogens and, in particular, their catechol metabolites have structural elements prone to peroxidative metabolism, metabolic activation via phenoxy radicals, semiquinones, and quinones may also be involved in their mechanism of carcinogenicity. In fact, when radioactively labeled estradiol, 17α-ethinylestradiol, and their 2-hydroxy derivatives were incubated *in vitro* with mouse uterus peroxidase and hydrogen peroxide in the presence of DNA, nonextractable binding to DNA was found for all four compounds (22). However, binding was about 20-fold higher for the catechols as compared to the phenols in this case. Covalent binding to DNA of estrone and ethinylestradiol was also reported to occur in rat liver *in vivo* (8). It should prove interesting to test steroid estrogens and their catechol metabolites for genetic damage in the same short-term assays which gave a positive response for DES.

CONCLUSIONS

There is increasing evidence supporting the hypothesis that the carcinogenic activity of the estrogenic compound DES is, at least in part, due to metabolic activation. Most of the available data point to a peroxidatic activation of DES. Thus, DES appears to share characteristic features of chemical carcinogens. The hormonal activity, however, may still be a very important factor in the overall mechanism of DES carcinogenicity, because (a) it determines the distribution within the organism and the cell by binding to transport proteins (such as sex hormone binding globulin and α-fetoprotein) and to intracellular estrogen receptors; (b) it regulates the enzyme activity required for metabolic activation, e.g., by inducing peroxidase; and (c) it stimulates the growth of transformed cells. Thus, by virtue of its metabolic activation and stimulation of cell proliferation, DES may be considered a "complete" carcinogen.

As steroidal estrogens and, particularly, their catechol metabolites can also be metabolically activated, e.g., by peroxidase, the formation of reactive metabolites is not limited to DES but may be a general mechanism in estrogen carcinogenicity.

ACKNOWLEDGMENT

The studies carried out in our laboratory and cited in this paper have been supported by the Deutsche Forschungsgemeinschaft (grant Me 574).

REFERENCES

1. Anderson, W. A., Kang, Y.-H., and DeSombre, E. R. (1975): Endogenous peroxidase: Specific marker enzyme for tissues displaying growth dependency on estrogen. *J. Cell Biol.*, 64:668–681.
2. Barrett, J. C., Wong, A., and McLachlan, J. A. (1981): Diethylstilbestrol induces neoplastic transformation without measurable gene mutation at two loci. *Science*, 212:1402–1404.
3. Blackburn, G. M., Flavell, A. J., and Thompson, M. H. (1974): Oxidative and photochemical linkage of diethylstilbestrol to DNA in vitro. *Cancer Res.*, 34:2015–2019.
4. Clive, D., Johnson, K. O., Spector, J. F. S., Batson, A. G., and Brown, M. M. M. (1979): Validation and characterization of the L5178Y/TK$^{+/-}$ mouse lymphoma mutagen assay system. *Mutation Res.*, 59:61–108.
5. Degen, G. H., Wong, A., and McLachlan, J. A. (1981): Metabolism of diethylstilbestrol (DES) in a model cell culture system for the study of carcinogenicity. *Proc. Am. Assoc. Cancer Res.*, 22:123.
6. Herbst, A. L., Ulfelder, H., and Poskanzer, D. C. (1971): Adenocarcinoma of the vagina: Association of maternal stilbestrol therapy with tumor appearance in young women. *New Engl. J. Med.*, 284:878–881.
7. IARC Working Group (1979): *IARC Monographs on the evaluation of the carcinogenic risk of chemicals to humans, Vol. 21: Sex hormones (II)*. International Agency for Research on Cancer, Lyon.
8. Jaggi, W., Lutz, W. K., and Schlatter, C. (1978): Covalent binding of ethinylestradiol and estrone to rat liver DNA in vivo. *Chem. Biol. Interact.*, 23:13–18.
9. Liao, S., and Williams-Ashman, H. G. (1962): Peroxidase-catalyzed oxidation of diethylstilbestrol. *Biochim. Biophys. Acta*, 59:705–707.
10. Liehr, J. G., Ballatore, A. M., DaGue, B. B., and Henkin, J. (1982): DES quinone—a reactive intermediate in diethylstilbestrol (DES) metabolism. *Fed. Proc.*, 41:1505.
11. Lyttle, C. R., and DeSombre, E. R. (1977): Uterine peroxidase as a marker for estrogen action. *Proc. Natl. Acad. Sci. USA*, 74:3162–3166.
12. Martin, C. N., McDermid, A. C., and Garner, R. C. (1978): Testing of known carcinogens and

noncarcinogens for their ability to induce unscheduled DNA synthesis in HeLa cells. *Cancer Res.,* 38:2621–2627.

13. Maydl, R., Newbold, R. R., Metzler, M., and McLachlan, J. A. (1981): Organ cultures of the fetal mouse genital tract metabolize diethylstilbestrol (DES). *Proc. Am. Ass. Cancer Res.,* 22:104.

14. McLachlan, J. A., Newbold, R. R., and Bullock, B. C. (1980): Long-term effects on the female mouse genital tract associated with prenatal exposure to diethylstilbestrol. *Cancer Res.,* 40:3988–3999.

15. McLachlan, J. A., Wong, A., Degen, G. H., and Barrett, J. C. (1982): Morphological and neoplastic transformation of Syrian hamster embryo fibroblasts by diethylstilbestrol and its analogs. *Cancer Res.,* 42:3040–3045.

16. Mehta, R. D., and Borstel, R. C. (1982): Genetic activity of diethylstilbestrol in Saccharomyces cerevisiae. Enhancement of mutagenicity by oxidizing agents. *Mutation Res.,* 92:49–61.

17. Metzler, M. (1975): Metabolic activation of diethylstilbestrol: Indirect evidence for the formation of a stilbene oxide intermediate in hamster and rat. *Biochem. Pharmac.,* 24:1449–1453.

18. Metzler, M. (1981): The metabolism of diethylstilbestrol. *CRC Crit. Rev. Biochem.,* 10:171–212.

19. Metzler, M., Gottschlich, R., and McLachlan, J. A. (1980): Oxidative metabolism of stilbene estrogens. In: *Estrogens in the Environment,* edited by J. A. McLachlan, pp. 293–303. Elsevier/North-Holland Biomedical Press, New York.

20. Metzler, M., and McLachlan, J. A. (1978): Proposed nomenclature for diethylstilbestrol metabolites. *J. Environ. Pathol. Toxicol.,* 2:579–582.

21. Metzler, M., and McLachlan, J. A. (1978): Peroxidase-mediated oxidation, a possible pathway for metabolic activation of diethylstilbestrol. *Biochem. Biophys. Res. Commun.,* 85:874–884.

22. Metzler, M., and McLachlan, J. A. (1978): Oxidative metabolism of diethylstilbestrol and steroidal estrogens as a potential factor in their fetotoxicity. In: *Role of Pharmakokinetics in Prenatal and Perinatal Toxicology,* edited by D. Neubert, H.-J Merker, H. Nau, and J. Langman, pp. 157–164. Georg Thieme Publishers, Stuttgart.

23. Pienta, R. J. (1980): Transformation of Syrian hamster embryo cells by diverse chemicals and correlation with their reported carcinogenic and mutagenic activities. In: *Chemical Mutagens,* edited by F. J. de Serres, and A. Hollaender, pp. 175–202. Plenum Publishing Corp., New York.

24. Purdy, R. H., Meltz, M. L., Goldzieher, J. W., Goodwin, T. J., and Williams, M. J. (1980): Chemical transformation by estrogens in a mammalian cell culture system. *Proc. 62nd Annual Meeting of the Endocrine Society,* p. 27.

25. Rüdiger, H. W., Haenisch, F., Metzler, M., Oesch, F., and Glatt, H. R. (1979): Metabolites of diethylstilbestrol induce sister chromatid exchange in human cultured fibroblasts. *Nature (Lond.),* 281:392–394.

26. Schiffmann, D., Wong, A., Tsutsui, T., Barrett, J. C., and McLachlan, J. A. (1982): Induction of unscheduled DNA synthesis by some structural analogs of diethylstilbestrol in Syrian hamster embryo fibroblasts. *Proc. 13th Intern. Cancer Congress,* p. 117.

Biochemical Basis of Chemical Carcinogenesis,
edited by H. Greim, R. Jung, M. Kramer,
H. Marquardt, and F. Oesch.
Raven Press, New York © 1984.

Expression of Carcinogen-Metabolizing Enzymes in Continuous Cultures of Mammalian Cells

*Friedrich J. Wiebel, **Maurice Lambiotte, †Jaswant Singh,
*Karl-Heinz Summer, and *Thomas Wolff

*Institute of Biochemistry and Toxicology, Department of Toxicology, Gesellschaft für
Strahlen- und Umweltforschung, D-8042 Neuherberg-München,
Federal Republic of Germany; **Département Unité de Génétique Cellulaire, Institute de
Recherches en Biologie Moléculaire du C.N.R.S., Université Paris VII, Paris, France;
and †Regional Research Laboratory, CSIR, Jammu Tawi, India

Mammalian cells in culture are of increasing interest for the detection of genotoxic chemicals and the analysis of their mechanism of action. They are the models of choice to follow up the sequence of events leading from the metabolic activation of a genotoxic compound to the initial interaction with tissue constituents and the final expression of permanent damage to the genome. The applicability of the cellular systems in such studies largely depends on their competence in the activation and inactivation of the chemical carcinogens. The enzymes involved in the metabolism of xenobiotics including carcinogens constitute a large and heterogeneous group of proteins which are defined only by their common function and differ in every other respect, e.g., their substrate specificity, subcellular, cellular and tissue localization, regulation, ontogeny, etc.

The expression of the xenobiotic-metabolizing enzymes in cells in continuous culture is not well understood. In the present context it is of particular interest to know whether and to what degree they have the status of "differentiated" functions of their cells or tissues of origin. This is important because the acquisition of unlimited growth potential by cells in culture is usually associated with the loss of their differentiated functions. On the other hand, functions of the xenobiotic-metabolizing enzymes which possess some value for the survival of cells are likely to be retained under the conditions of long-term culture.

The following will discuss some of the carcinogen activating and inactivating enzymes under this aspect. In the first part we will be concerned with the general prospects of finding or developing continuous cell lines which express the various carcinogen-metabolizing enzymes. The second part will more specifically explore the expression of differentiated functions of the carcinogen metabolism in these cell systems.

TABLE 1. *Aryl hydrocarbon hydroxylase activity in mammalian cell cultures*

Cell line[b]	AHH-activity (pmoles/ mg protein/30 min)	
	Untreated	BA-treated[a]
From normal tissue		
1. BRL 3C4, epithelial, liver, rat	5	80
2. 3T3-4C2, fibroblastoid, Swiss mouse	10	75
3. 3T3-A31, fibroblastoid, BALB/C mouse	3	20
4. BHK-21, newborn, Syrian hamster	3	48
5. BHK-422E, newborn, Syrian hamster	0.6	6
6. C81, fibroblastoid, cat	1	24
7. Don-C, fibroblastoid, Chinese hamster	4	20
8. XP-2, fibroblastoid, skin, human	<0.5	14
9. FIII, fibroblastoid, rat	<0.5	12
10. HaK, kidney, Syrian hamster	<0.05	6
11. Chang, liver, human	<0.5	1
12. V 79, lung, Chinese hamster	<0.5	<0.5
From tumors		
13. H-4-II-E, hepatoma, rat	13	1,030
14. JEG-3, choriocarcinoma, human	4	150
15. MH_1C_1, hepatoma, mouse	9	25
16. WRC, Walker carcinoma, rat	<0.1	31
17. A-549, adenocarcinoma, lung, human	2	24
18. HEp2, carcinoma, larynx, human	<0.05	3
19. RAG, carcinoma, kidney, BALB/C mouse	<0.5	<0.5
20. L-A9, fibroblastoid, C3H/An mouse	<0.5	<0.5
21. HTC, hepatoma, rat	<0.5	<0.5
In vitro transformed		
22. OBP, newborn, Syrian hamster	2	110
23. JLSV-5, spleen-thymus, mouse	5	50
24. VA-2, fibroblastoid, lung, human	<0.5	2
25. NC37 BaEV, lymphoblastoid, human	<0.5	<0.5

[a]Cultures were kept for 18 hrs in growth medium containing 1 μg/ml benz(*a*)anthracene (BA). AHH-activity was determined as described in ref. 27.

[b]The origin of cells listed under numbers 1–3, 5, 7–9, 14, 17, 19, 20, 22–24 are given in ref. 27; those under 4, 12, 13, 25 in ref. 32. The cell lines under 10, 11, 15, 16, 18, 21 were obtained from the American Type Tissue Culture Collection via Seromed (München, Federal Republic of Germany) or Flow Laboratories (Meckenheim, FRG). C81-cells (Nr. 6) were kindly supplied by Dr. V. Erfle, GSF-Neuherberg, FRG.

EXPRESSION OF CARCINOGEN-METABOLIZING ENZYMES

Monooxygenases

The microsomal monooxygenases are the enzymes of greatest interest since they are responsible for the activation of the majority of chemical procarcinogens. For the purpose of this discussion the various monooxygenases are divided into two groups. The first group, the "cytochrome(s) P-448", is distinguished by the inducibility by polycyclic aromatic hydrocarbons (PAH), the inhibition by modulators such as 7,8-benzoflavone, and the preferential affinity for highly lipophilic, planar substrates. Monooxygenases of the second group, the "cytochrome(s) P-450", are not inducible by PAH and accept as their substrates also nonplanar and hydrophilic compounds. They are preferentially localized in the liver.

Table 1 shows the basal and PAH-induced activity of aryl hydrocarbon (benzo-*[a]*pyrene) hydroxylase (AHH), a typical cytochrome P-448 function, in a large variety of continuous cell lines. Three major conclusions can be drawn from these data: (a) the majority of continuous cell lines express AHH-activity; (b) the levels of monooxygenase activity greatly differ between the various cell lines; and (c) the enzyme is highly inducible by PAH. Similar observations have been made by others on a large variety of rodent and human cell lines (1,12,19). Only very few of the cell lines have been found to express cytochrome P-450-dependent monooxygenases (see below). The lack of this group of monooxygenases has been a major obstacle in the use of continuous cell lines for the detection of genotoxic chemicals.

UDP-Glucuronosyltransferase (EC 2.4.1.17)

The UDP-glucuronosyltransferase form most thoroughly investigated in continuous cell cultures is characterized by its close functional and regulatory relationship to cytochrome P-448, its specificity for substrates such as 1-naphthol or 3-hydroxybenzo-*(a)*pyrene (2,3), and its prenatal development to adult or near-adult levels (35). The

TABLE 2. *UDP-Glucuronosyltransferase activity in continuous cell lines[a]*

Cell line	Glucuronosyltransferase (nmoles/min/mg protein)	Monooxygenase activity
Faza 967	2.17	(+)
MH_1C_1	1.79	+ +
H-4-II-E	0.85	+ + +
RAG	0.83	−
BHK-21	0.36	+ +
3T3/BALB	0.18	+ +
LA9	0.17	−
A549	0.10	+
CHO	0.10	−
WRC	0.04	+
V79	<0.005	−
C81	<0.005	+
NC37BaEV	<0.005	−

Data from ref. 32.
[a]UDP-Glucuronosyltransferase activity directed towards the substrate 3-hydroxybenzo*(a)*pyrene was determined as previously described (23). For the monooxygenase (AHH) activities cf. Table 1.

majority of the continuous cell lines express the glucuronosyltranferase as observed for the cytochrome P-448-dependent AHH-activity (Table 2). Also, the constitutive levels of the transferase widely vary in the cell lines tested. However, no strict correlation exists in individual cell lines between the expression of the monooxygenase and transferase (Table 2). For example, RAG and HTC cells contain high glucuronosyltransferase but no monooxygenase activities. We observed monooxygenase activity in the absence of the glucuronosyltransferase in only one case, the B81 cat cells. The transferase was also found to differ from the monooxygenase by its poor inducibility by PAH (33).

Phenol-Sulfotransferase (EC 2.8.2.1)

The soluble phenol-sulfotransferase competes with the glucuronosyltransferase for many of their phenolic substrates. The majority of the cell lines tested did not express detectable amounts of the sulfotransferase directed toward 3-hydroxy-benzo-(a)pyrene (33). Appreciable activities were only observed in a few cell lines of hepatic origin and their descendents. The sulfotransferase activity in hepatoma cells did not respond to PAH (Wiebel, *unpublished*) but was inducible by dexamethasone (Table 3).

NADPH-Cytochrome c (P-450) Reductase (EC 1.6.2.4) and Glutathione S-Transferase (EC 2.5.1.18)

The NADPH-cytochrome c (P-450) reductase, which is an essential component of the monooxygenase complex, was expressed in all cell lines tested so far independently of the presence or absence of the monooxygenase (Table 4). Furthermore, in contrast to the enzymes shown before, the levels differed only by factor of 4 to 6 between the various cell lines. Similarly to the NADPH-cytochrome c reductase, the glutathione S-transferase activities directed toward 1,2-dichloro-p-nitrobenzene and 1,2-epoxy-3-(p-nitrophenoxy)propane were found in all cell lines which were studied by us (26) and others (24).

TABLE 3. *Induction of phenol-sulfotransferase by dexamethasone*

Cell line	Factor of induction	(n)
H-4-II-E	11.8 ± 2.6	(5)
H_5	11.1 ± 5.7	(4)
HF_{1-4}	21.0 ± 14.0	(2)
Faza 967	5.5 ± 0.7	(2)
WRC	22.4 ± 13.9	(4)

Cells were exposed to dexamethasone (2 μg/ml) for 24 hrs. Enzyme activity was determined as previously described (33). The numbers represent the mean ± S.D. of separate (n) experiments.

TABLE 4. *Cytochrom c reductase activity in various cell lines*

Cell line	Cytochrom c reductase activity (nmoles/min/mg protein)[a]	Monooxygenase activity[b]
HF$_{1-4}$	32.8 ± 5.3[c]	+ +
H-4-II-E	10.7 ± 1.5	+ +
BHK-C21	9.0 ± 2.1	+
HEp2	10.7 ± 0.9	+
Chang	9.9 ± 0.5	+
RAG	28.9 ± 3.1	−
A9	18.8 ± 0.8	−
V79	5.3 ± 0.2	−

[a]The concentration of cellular protein in the reaction mixture was 0.1–0.3 mg/ml. The other conditions are described in ref. 20.

[b]Relative monooxygenase activities. Specific activities are listed in Tables 1 and 6.

[c]Mean ± S.D. of 3 cultures.

CARCINOGEN-METABOLIZING ENZYMES: HOUSEHOLD OR LUXURY PROTEINS?

The data presented show that the expression and inducibility of the carcinogen-metabolizing enzymes differ greatly in the various continuous cell lines. The enzymes may be placed along a scale which reaches from "ubiquitous" to "rare" according to their frequency of expression (Fig. 1). It is reasonable to assume that those on the top of the scale are essential for the survival of the cells in continuous culture, i.e., "household" proteins (9), whereas those on the bottom are obviously nonessential or "luxury" functions.

"Household" proteins in permanent culture grown under constant conditions are likely to exhibit two features: their constitutive activities should only vary within a fairly narrow range between different cell lines, and they should less readily respond to the challenge with exogenous inducing compounds than the "luxury" functions. Both expectations are met by the overall findings in continuous cell lines.

The levels of the presumed essential enzymes, glutathione S-transferase and NADPH-cytochrome c reductase, only vary by a factor of 4 to 6 (Table 4) (26), whereas the levels of the UDP-glucuronosyltransferase differ by more than one order of magnitude (Table 2) and those of the cytochrome P-448 by two orders of magnitude (Table 1). Thus, the variability in the levels of these enzymes appears to decrease with their increased frequency of expression.

Table 5 gives an overview of the differences in the inducibility of these enzymes by two major types of inducers, benz(a)anthracene and dexamethasone in H-4-II-E hepatoma cells. The nonessential functions, cytochrome P-450 or phenol-sulfo-transferase, are highly induced by the glucocorticoid. Cytochrome P-448-dependent monooxygenase shows a moderate response to the glucocorticoid but is highly

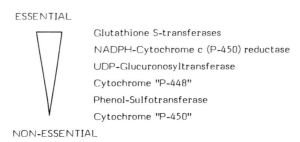

ESSENTIAL

Glutathione S-transferases

NADPH-Cytochrome c (P-450) reductase

UDP-Glucuronosyltransferase

Cytochrome "P-448"

Phenol-Sulfotransferase

Cytochrome "P-450"

NON-ESSENTIAL

FIG. 1. Function of various drug-metabolizing enzymes in the long-term survival of cultured cells.

TABLE 5. *Inducibility of carcinogen-metabolizing enzymes in H-4-II-E-hepatoma cells*

Enzyme	Factor of induction		Reference
	Benz[a]anthracene	Dexamethasone	
Glutathione S-transferase	1.0	1.0	(22, 26)
NADPH-Cytochrome c reductase	1.3	1.0	cf. Text
Glucuronosyltransferase	2.0	1.5	(23, 33)
Cytochrome "P-448"	20–70	2–3	cf. Table 1
Phenol-sulfotransferase	1.0	10–15	cf. Table 3
Cytochrome "P-450"	1.0	5–10	cf. Table 6

inducible by PAH. In contrast, the near ubiquitous UDP-glucuronosyltransferase is only weakly induced by PAH. Finally, the apparent household proteins glutathione S-transferase and NADPH-cytochrome c reductase are not significantly increased either by PAH or by dexamethasone. Aminophylline, another modulator of monooxygenase activity in certain cell lines (27), had no effect on either glutathione S-transferase (26) or NADPH-cytochrome c reductase (Wiebel, *unpublished*) under conditions where the cytochrome P-448 is strongly induced (32).

The survival value of the glutathione S-transferases can be deduced from their role in the trapping of reactive electrophilic species which might arise either from endogenous compounds, such as steroid hormones (8), prostaglandins (4), and α,β-unsaturated acyl-CoA thioesters (25), or from the activation of exogenous chemicals contained in the growth medium. The need for retaining the NADPH-cytochrome c reductase is less apparent. Obviously, the activity of the reductase is not related to the monooxygenase but to some other vital function. It has been postulated that the enzyme is involved in such diverse functions as the reduction of cytochrome b_5 (10), the degradation of heme (17,39) or the fatty acid chain elongation (11). The importance of these functions for the survival of cells in culture remains to be determined. It is also unclear how cells in culture profit from retaining the activity of the cytochrome(s) P-448 and the functionally related glucuronosyltransferase.

EXTINCTION AND REEXPRESSION OF MONOOXYGENASE ACTIVITIES IN HEPATOMA CELLS

As pointed out above, the lack of expression of major functions of the carcinogen-metabolizing enzymes has seriously limited the applicability of continuous cell lines in studies related to chemical carcinogenesis. Are the prospects as poor as they appear from the previous observations? Do cells in continuous culture invariably lose the differentiated functions of their tissue of origin? We attempted to answer this question by using the cytochrome P-450-dependent monooxygenases as a probe. Our efforts were concentrated on hepatoma cells as the most likely candidates for the expression of these virtually liver-specific enzymes. For a model we choose the H-4-II-E cells, derivatives of the H35 Reuber rat hepatoma (21), and their descendents (Fig. 2) which were established and extensively characterized for their status of differentiation by Weiss et al. (5,6,7).

The H-4-II-E cells were previously examined by us (31,32) and by others (20) and were found to contain only PAH-inducible cytochrome P-448-dependent monooxygenase. From these cells two major lines had been selected mainly by morphological criteria (7): The H_5 cells which are poorly differentiated and the Faza 967 and Fao cells which express a large number of differentiated functions such as liver-specific aldolase B and alcohol dehydrogenase, secretion of albumin, glucocorticoid-inducible tyrosine aminotransferase, the key enzymes of the gluconeogenesis pathway (7), or the metabolism of bile acids (14).

Table 6 shows the AHH-activities in these lines and their response to benzo(*a*)anthracene or dexamethasone. The differentiated lines Faza 967, Fao, and C2Rev7 contained only low AHH-activities which were not inducible by the PAH. In contrast, the dedifferentiated H_5 cells responded strongly to the PAH. Dexa-

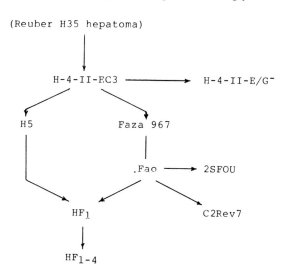

FIG. 2. Filiation of hepatoma clones in the text.

TABLE 6. *AHH- and aldrin epoxidase activity in hepatoma cells: induction by dexamethasone or benz[a]anthracene*

Cell line	AHH (pmoles/min/mg protein)			Aldrin Epoxidase (pmoles/min/mg protein)		
	Control	DEX	BA	Control	DEX	BA
H-4-II-E	0.53	1.83	36.70	0.7	2.6	0.6
Faza 967	0.06	0.24	0.15	14.1	22.6	13.3
Fao	0.19	0.94	0.14	23.0	17.5	18.3
C2Rev7	0.15	1.14	0.18	6.5	29.0	8.1
2SFOU	0.21	0.76	9.80	6.8	9.3	4.2
H_5	0.50	0.75	18.00	<1.0	<1.0	<0,7
HF_1	0.70	1.40	48.00	<1.0	<1.0	<0.7
HF_{1-4}	2.80	21.00	81.90	26.1	69.3	26.3
H-4-II-E/G⁻	1.83	4.30	39.70	16.8	23.9	20.2

Data are partially taken from ref. 28.
Cultures were kept for 20 hrs in medium containing 1 μg/ml dexamethasone (DEX) or 5 μg/ml benz*[a]*anthracene (BA). Experimental conditions are given in ref. 28.

methasone had a stronger effect on the differentiated than on the dedifferentiated cell line. AHH is known to be a function of both cytochrome P-450- and cytochrome P-448-dependent monooxygenases. These two forms may be distinguished by the differential effect of 7,8-benzoflavone (30). As shown elsewhere (34), the flavonoid stimulates the AHH activity in the differentiated cells and inhibits the enzyme in the dedifferentiated line in agreement with the effects on the constitutive and PAH-induced AHH in rat liver microsomes (30).

Previously, Wolff et al. (37,38) established that aldrin is a specific substrate for the cytochrome P-450-dependent monooxygenase(s). As shown in Table 6, the differentiated cells contain appreciable levels of the aldrin epoxidase in contrast to the H_5 cells in which this monooxygenase function was not detectable. The enzyme was not inducible by PAH. Observations in rat liver microsomes (37) and in hepatoma cells (Wiebel, *unpublished*) showed that 7,8-benzoflavone does not affect aldrin epoxidase activity. Thus, aldrin epoxidase and 7,8-benzoflavone-stimulated AHH are indicators for two different cytochrome P-450 forms which are both expressed in the differentiated cells.

The results on the H_5, Faza 967, and Fao cells suggested that the expression of the two monooxygenase forms is mutually exclusive. Recent studies on other descendants of H-4-II-E cells disproved this notion. HF_1, a hybrid line which had been formed from the H_5 and Fao cells, (Fig. 1) exhibited all the characteristics of the dedifferentiated H_5 cells (6) including the expression of PAH-inducible AHH and the lack of aldrin epoxidase activity (Table 6). However the subclone HF_{1-4} (Fig. 1), which was selected by growth in glucose-free medium from the HF_1 cells (6), expressed both cytochrome P-450 and P-448, i.e., PAH-inducible AHH as well as dexamethasone-inducible aldrin epoxidase. Recent observations have shown that HF_{1-4} but not H_5 cells have the capacity to activate the typical cytochrome P-450 substrates, dimethyl- and diethylnitrosamine, to cytotoxic and genotoxic species (16). Similarly to the HF_{1-4} hybrid cells, H-4-II-E/G$^-$, a line directly derived from the H-4-II-E cells, contained both cytochrome P-448 and cytochrome P-450 (Table 6). Finally, closer examination also revealed low aldrin epoxidase activities in the "parental" H-4-II-E cells.

The activity of the PAH-inducible cytochrome P-448, which was not detectable in the differentiated Fao and C2Rev7 cells, may also be reexpressed. Thus, the near-tetraploid line 2SFOU which arose by spontaneous ploidisation of the Fao cells (Fig. 2) expressed not only the cytochrome P-450 but also the PAH-inducible cytochrome P-448 (Table 6).

These observations shed some light on the mode of extinction of the monooxygenase activities in hepatoma cells, i.e., on the general question whether the extinction of differentiated functions in continuous cell lines is due to a loss of genetic material or to epigenetic changes. In the first case, the functions would almost irretrievably be lost; in the second case, they may be recovered, for example, by the resetting of some elements of control either by the removal of suppressing factors or by supplying essential stimulatory factors. Obviously, this is of great practical importance for the prospects of developing continuous cell lines expressing differentiated functions of carcinogen metabolism. Observations on a number of differentiated functions in continuous cell lines have shown that both mechanisms play a role in the extinction process (5). The data presented indicate that the extinction of the functions under consideration, i.e., the induction of cytochrome P-448 and the expression of cytochrome P-450 is not necessarily due to a permanent modification of the genome. The lack of monooxygenase activity in the hepatoma cells more likely is attributable to some form of repression. This is in agreement with previous observations in intraspecific hybrid cells which suggested the existence of a negative control in the regulation of cytochrome P-448 activity (28).

COORDINATE EXPRESSION OF
CARCINOGEN-METABOLIZING ENZYMES

The presence of cytochrome P-450, a "differentiated" monooxygenases form, was closely associated with the overall expression of liver-specific functions in the majority of hepatoma lines tested (Table 6) (5,6,7). Similarly, the "hepatic" form of the UDP-glucuronosyltransferase with 4-hydroxybiphenyl as marker substrate (2) was more strongly expressed in the differentiated than in the dedifferentiated hepatoma lines (Wiebel, *unpublished*). Generally, the observations in the hepatoma cells indicate that the functions of the carcinogen metabolism are handled as part of a larger program of specialized functions of the liver. If cells express whole programs of differentiated functions, including those of the carcinogen metabolism, the question has to be asked whether these programs have a correlate *in vivo*. Specifically, it would be of interest to know whether the set of functions expressed in the hepatoma cells reflects a particular stage of the ontogenesis of the liver.

As noted by Cassio and Weiss (5), many of the liver-specific functions expressed by the differentiated lines derived from the H-4-II-E cells appear *in vivo* only near or after birth. In keeping with these observations, the properties of the monooxygenases in the hepatoma cells strikingly resemble those in the perinatal liver. Firstly, the levels of the monooxygenases, i.e., of AHH and aldrin epoxidase, in differentiated hepatoma cells are comparable to the levels of hepatocytes which were freshly isolated from "fetal" rats near term (13). Generally, the monooxygenase activities ranged between the very low fetal and the high adult activities. Secondly, the 7,8-benzoflavone-stimulated cytochrome P-450-dependent monooxygenase found in the differentiated hepatoma cells appears near the time of birth (13). Thirdly, cytochrome P-450 and cytochrome P-448 are induced by dexamethasone in the hepatoma cells (Table 6) and in freshly isolated "perinatal" cells to a similar degree (13). The inducibility of the monooxygenases by dexamethasone is greatly reduced at a later age (15).

The list of similarities can also be extended to the transferases. Thus, the "neonatal" form of the UDP-glucuronosyltransferase (35) directed toward 4-hydroxybiphenyl exhibits relatively high activities in the hepatoma cells (Wiebel, *unpublished*). The weak response of the glucuronosyltransferase directed toward 3-hydroxybenzo(*a*)pyrene [the "late-fetal" form, (3)] to dexamethasone is compatible with the conditions *in vivo* where a high inducibility by the glucocorticoid during the fetal period is greatly reduced around the time of birth (36). It is also fitting that phenol-sulfotransferase activities which are low during the perinatal period and develop only at later times to adult levels (18) are poorly expressed in the hepatoma cells (33).

CONCLUSIONS

Although only a limited number of the enzymes metabolizing xenobiotics have been studied in sufficient detail in continuous cell cultures, a general pattern emerges of their expression in these cell systems. From these one may derive some broad rules that govern the prospects for retaining or losing specific enzymes or enzyme combinations and for manipulating their activities by induction. Persistent enzymes such as the glutathione S-transferases which presumably serve some household function will strongly resist extraneous modulation. This is particularly true if they play a role in the endogenous metabolism and are not only functions of the cellular adaptation to the culture conditions which can be subject to change. Presently little is known on the nature of the function of these enzymes for the survival of long-term cultures.

The nonessential enzymes present a different problem. It would be of interest to either prevent their extinction or, once they are extinguished, bring them to reappearance. Our observations have shown that differentiated functions thought to be lost in continuous cell cultures may be reexpressed, for example, upon selective pressure or change in gene dosage. Furthermore, cells in continuous culture appear to be capable of expressing not only single differentiated functions of the carcinogen metabolism but also ordered programs which may have a correlate *in vivo*.

In conclusion, the prospects are promising that with the improvements of culture techniques cell lines will be established which will express specific functions or whole sets of functions of the carcinogen-metabolizing enzymes and provide versatile tools to probe for the potential and potency of genotoxic chemicals.

ACKNOWLEDGMENT

We thank Dr. M. C. Weiss (Centre de Génétique Moléculaire, Centre National pour la Recherche Scientifique, Gif-sur-Yvette, France) for generously providing us with the H-4-II-E cells and their derivatives.

REFERENCES

1. Aust, A. E., Antczack, M. R., Maher, V. M., and McCormick, J. J. (1981): Identifying human cells capable of metabolizing various classes of carcinogens. *J. Supramolec. Struct. Cell. Biochem.*, 16:269–279.
2. Bock, K. W., v. Clausbruch, U. C., Kaufmann, R., Lilienblum, W., Oesch, F., Pfeil, H., and Platt, K. L. (1980): Functional heterogeneity of UDP-glucuronyltransferase in rat tissues. *Biochem. Pharmacol.*, 29:495–500.
3. Bock, K. W., Lilienblum, W., and Pfeil, H. (1982): Functional heterogenicity of UDP-glucuronosyltransferase activities in C57BL/6 and DBA/2 mice. *Biochem. Pharmacol.*, 31:1273–1277.
4. Cagen, L. M., Fales, H. M., and Pisano, J. J. (1976): Formation of glutathione conjugates of prostaglandin A_1 in human red blood cells. *J. Biol. Chem.*, 251:6550–6554.
5. Cassio, D., and Weiss, M. C. (1979): Expression of fetal and neonatal hepatic functions by mouse hepatoma-rat hepatoma hybrids. *Somat. Cell Gen.*, 5:719–738.
6. Deschatrette, J., Moore, E. E., Dubois, M., Cassio, D., and Weiss, M. C. (1979): Dedifferentiated variants of a rat hepatoma: analysis by cell hybridization. *Somatic Cell Gen.*, 5:697–718.
7. Deschatrette, J., and Weiss, M. C. (1974): Characterization of differentiated and dedifferentiated clones from a rat hepatoma. *Biochimie*, 56:1603–1611.
8. Elce, J. S., and Harris, J. (1971): Conjugation of 2-hydroxyestradiol-17β (1,3,5,(10)-estratriene-2,3,-17β-triol) with glutathione in the rat. *Steroids* 18:585–591.
9. Ephrussi, B. (1972): *Hybridization of Somatic Cells.* Princeton University Press, Princeton, New Jersey.
10. Estabrook, R. W., Werringloer, J., Capdevila, J., and Prough, R. A. (1978): The role of cytochrome P-450 and the microsomal electron transport system: The oxidative metabolism of benzo[a]pyrene. In: *Polycyclic Hydrocarbons and Cancer, Vol. 1*, edited by Gelboin, H. V., and Ts'o, P. O. P., pp. 285–319. Academic Press, New York.
11. Ilan, Z., Ilan, R., and Cinti, D. L. (1981): Evidence for a new physiological role of hepatic NADPH:ferricytochrome (P-450) oxidoreductase. Direct electron input to the microsomal fatty acid chain elongation system. *J. Biol. Chem.*, 256:10066–10072.
12. Kouri, R. E., Kiefer, R., and Zimmerman, E. M. (1974): Hydrocarbon-metabolizing activity of various mammalian cells in culture. *In Vitro*, 10:18–25.
13. Kremers, P., Goujon, F., De Graeve, J., Van Cantfort, J., and Gielen, J. E. (1981): Multiplicity of cytochrome P-450 in primary fetal hepatocytes in culture. *Eur. J. Biochem.*, 116:67–72.
14. Lambiotte, M., and Thierry, N. (1980): Hydroxylation, sulfation, and conjugation of bile acids in rat hepatoma and hepatocyte cultures under the influence of glucocorticoids. *J. Biol. Chem.*, 255:11324–11331.
15. Leakey, J. E. A., and Fouts, J. R. (1979): Precocious development of cytochrome P-450 in neonatal rat liver after glucocorticoid treatment. *Biochem. J.*, 182:233–235.
16. Loquet, C., and Wiebel, F. J. (1982): Geno- and cytotoxicity of nitrosamines, aflatoxin B_1, and benzo[a]pyrene in continuous cultures of rat hepatoma cells. *Carcinogenesis*, 3:1213–1218.
17. Masters, B. S. S., and Schacter, B. A. (1976): The catalysis of heme degradation by purified NADPH-cytochrome c reductase in the absence of other microsomal proteins. *Ann. Clin. Res. (Suppl.)*, 8:18–27.
18. Matsui, M., and Watanabe, H. (1982): Developmental alteration of hepatic UDP-glucuronosyltransferase and sulphotransferase towards androsterone and 4-nitrophenol in Wistar rats. *Biochem. J.*, 204:441–447.
19. Niwa, A., Kumaki, K., and Nebert, D. W. (1975): Induction of aryl hydrocarbon hydroxylase activity in various cell cultures by 2,3,7,8-tetrachlorodibenzo-p-dioxin. *Molec. Pharmacol.*, 11:399–408.
20. Owens, I. S., and Nebert, D. W. (1975): Aryl hydrocarbon hydroxylase induction in mammalian liver-derived cell cultures. Stimulation of "cytochrome P_1-450-associated" enzyme activity by many inducing drugs. *Molec. Pharmacol.*, 11:94–104.

21. Pitot, H. C., Peraino, C., Morse, P. A., and Potter, V. R. (1964): Hepatomas in tissue culture compared with adapting liver in vivo. *Nat. Cancer Inst. Monogr.*, 13:229–245.
22. Raphael, D., Glatt, H. R., Protić-Sabljić, M., and Oesch, F. (1982): Effects of various enzyme inducers on monooxygenase, glutathione S-transferase and epoxide hydrolase activities in cultured hepatoma cells. *Chem.-Biol. Interactions*, 42:27–43.
23. Singh, J., and Wiebel, F. J. (1979): A highly sensitive and rapid fluorometric assay for UDP-glucuronyltransferase using 3-hydroxybenzo[a]pyrene as substrate. *Analyt. Biochem.*, 98:394–401.
24. Smith, G. J., Huebner, K., and Litwack, G. (1977): Expression of ligandin and glutathione S-transferase activities by cells in tissue culture. *Biochem. Biophys. Res. Commun.*, 76:1174–1180.
25. Speir, T. W., and Barnsley, E. A. (1971): The conjugation of glutathione with unsaturated acyl thiol esters and the metabolic formation of S-carboxyalkylcysteines. *Biochem. J.*, 125:267–273.
26. Summer, K.-H., and Wiebel, F. J. (1981): Glutathione and glutathione S-transferase activities of mammalian cells in culture. *Toxicol. Letters*, 9:409–413.
27. Wiebel, F. J., Brown, S., Waters, H. L., and Selkirk, J. K. (1977): Activation of xenobiotics by monooxygenases: cultures of mammalian cells as analytical tool. *Arch. Toxicol.*, 39:133–148.
28. Wiebel, F. J., Gelboin, H. V. and Coon, H. G. (1972): Regulation of aryl hydrocarbon hydroxylase in intraspecific hybrids of human, mouse and hamster cells. *Proc. Natl. Acad. Sci. USA* 69:3580–3584.
29. Wiebel, F. J., Hlavica, P. and Grzeschik, K. H. (1981): Expression of aromatic polycyclic hydrocarbon-induced monooxygenase (aryl hydrocarbon hydroxylase) in man x mouse hybrids is associated with human chromosome 2. *Hum. Genet.*, 59:277–280.
30. Wiebel, F. J., Leutz, J., Diamond, L., and Gelboin, H. V. (1971): Aryl hydrocarbon (benzo[a]pyrene) hydroxylase in microsomes from rat tissues: Differential inhibition and stimulation by benzoflavones and organic solvents. *Arch. Biochem. Biophys.* 144:78–86.
31. Wiebel, F. J., Schwarz, L. R., and Goto, T. (1980): In: *Short-Term Mutagenicity Test Systems in Detecting Carcinogens*, edited by K. Norpoth, and R. C. Garner, pp. 209–225. Springer Verlag, Berlin, Heidelberg, New York.
32. Wiebel, F. J., and Singh, J. (1980): Monooxygenase and UDP-glucuronyltransferase activities in established cell cultures. *Arch. Toxicol.* 44:85–97.
33. Wiebel, F. J., Singh, J., Schindler, E., and Summer, K.-H. (1980): UDP-Glucuronosyl-, phenol sulfo-, and glutathione S-transferase activities of mammalian cells in permanent culture. *Toxicology*, 17:123–126.
34. Wiebel, F. J., Wolff, T., and Lambiotte, M. (1980): Presence of cytochrome P-450- and cytochrome P-448-dependent monooxygenase functions in hepatoma cell lines. *Biochem. Biophys. Res. Commun.*, 94:466–472.
35. Wishart, G. J. (1978): Functional heterogenicity of UDP-glucuronosyltransferase as indicated by its differential development and inducibility by glucocorticoids. Demonstration of two groups within the enzyme's activity towards twelve substrates. *Biochem. J.*, 174:485–489.
36. Wishart, G. J., and Dutton, G. J. (1977): Regulation on onset of development of UDP-glucuronosyltransferase activity towards *o*-aminophenol by glucocorticoids in late-foetal rat liver *in utero*. *Biochem. J.*, 168:507–511.
37. Wolff, T., Deml, W., and Wanders, H. (1979): Aldrin epoxidation, a highly sensitive indicator specific for cytochrome P-450-dependent mono-oxygenase activities. *Drug Metab. Dispos.*, 7:301–305.
38. Wolff, T., Greim, H., Huang, M.-T., Miwa, G. T., and Lu, A. Y. H. (1980): Aldrin epoxidation catalyzed by purified rat-liver cytochromes P-450 and P-448. High selectivity for cytochrome P-450. *Eur. J. Biochem.* 111:545–551.
39. Yoshida, T., and Kikuchi, G. (1978): Features of the reaction of heme degradation catalyzed by the reconstituted microsomal heme oxygenase system. *J. Biol. Chem.*, 253:4230–4236.

Biochemical Basis of Chemical Carcinogenesis,
edited by H. Greim, R. Jung, M. Kramer,
H. Marquardt, and F. Oesch.
Raven Press, New York © 1984.

Cloning Genes that Encode Enzymes which Metabolize Drugs and Chemical Carcinogens

Daniel W. Nebert, Michitoshi Nakamura, Robert H. Tukey, and
Masahiko Negishi

*Developmental Pharmacology Branch, National Institute of Child Health and Human
Development, National Institutes of Health, Bethesda, Maryland 20205*

The *Ah* locus (Fig. 1) governs the induction of numerous drug-metabolizing enzymes and other proteins by polycyclic aromatic compounds such as 3-methylcholanthrene and 2,3,7,8-tetrachlorodibenzo-*p*-dioxin (TCDD). The cytosolic *Ah* receptor is the gene product of the *Ah* regulatory gene (8,28). In addition to the multiple forms of P-450 induced by 3-methylcholanthrene or TCDD, the induced

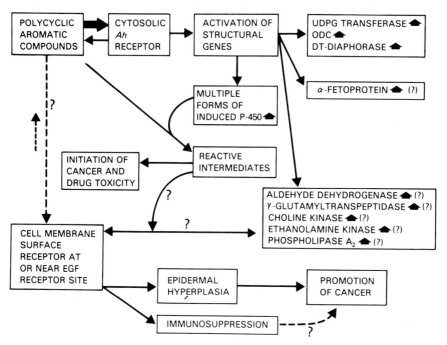

FIG. 1. Heuristic diagram showing possible interrelationship between the *Ah* receptor and the multiple responses. *Question marks* denote that no rigid correlation (among offspring from the B6D2F₁ × D2 backcross) has been determined yet. (Data from ref. 37, with permission.)

activities of UDP glucuronosyltransferase, DT diaphorase, and ornithine decarboxylase have been shown to be closely associated with the Ah^b allele and therefore with the presence of detectable levels of cytosolic *Ah* receptor. These studies were carried out with individual 3-methylcholanthrene-treated progeny from the (C57BL/6N)(DBA/2N)F_1 × DBA/2N (B6D2F_1 × D2) backcross. Inducers known to bind to the *Ah* receptor also enhance α-fetoprotein levels (2), aldehyde dehydrogenase (7), γ-glutamyl-transpeptidase (12), choline kinase (15), ethanolamine kinase (15), and phospholipase A_2 (4) activities; most of these studies were performed in rats, however, and therefore no strict association with the murine *Ah* locus has yet been demonstrated.

It has been proposed (16,17) that these polycyclic aromatic inducers compete with epidermal growth factor (EGF) for the EGF cell-surface receptor in the same order as that seen for compounds competing with [³H]TCDD for the cytosolic *Ah* receptor. In fact, it appears that metabolites of polycyclic hydrocarbons, rather than *Ah* receptor binding *per se*, are important in blocking EGF receptor replenishment (18). These inducers also cause epidermal keratinization (19), birth defects (32,34), immunosuppression (28), and "promoter" effects of chemical carcinogenesis (31,33). The *Ah* receptor and the P_1-450 induction process occur very early in gestation—even before implantation of the mouse embryo (9,11). All these data (Fig. 1) therefore suggest that the *Ah* locus may be involved in certain growth processes such as differentiation and cancer

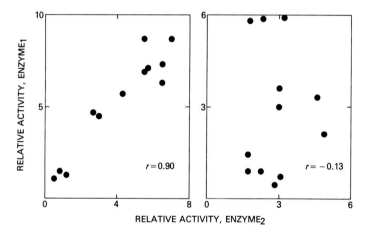

FIG. 2. Experimental attempts to correlate two liver drug-metabolizing enzyme activities among 12 inbred C57BL/6N mice *(left)* and 12 heterogeneous stock (HS) mice *(right)*. Both types of mice were divided into four groups of three each; relative enzyme activities were determined 0, 12, 24, and 48 hr after intraperitoneal treatment with 3-methylcholanthrene, an inducer of certain forms of P-450. The two enzyme activities—believed to represent the same form of P-450 until about 8 years ago—are aryl hydrocarbon (benzo[a]pyrene) hydroxylase and 2-acetylaminofluorene N-hydroxylase on the ordinate and abscissa, respectively. (Data from ref. 24, with permission.)

promotion—in addition to the previously discovered phenomenon of induction of drug-metabolizing enzymes.

In this chapter we will first illustrate some of the difficulties involved in the study of the P-450 proteins. We believe these problems should be solvable with studies at the DNA level. Next, isolation and characterization of the P_1-450 cDNA clone are described. Lastly we show the steps taken for isolating and characterizing the P_1-450 chromosomal gene. P_1-450 is defined as that form of polycyclic-aromatic-inducible P-450 most closely associated with enhanced metabolism of polycyclic aromatic hydrocarbons to their ultimate diol-epoxide carcinogenic intermediates (26). Elucidating the mechanism of P_1-450 gene expression thus may be important to our understanding the reasons for increased genetic risk of environmentally-induced cancers among certain individuals.

PROBLEMS WITH THE P-450 PROTEINS

Data from inbred strain of laboratory animals probably helped to lull all of us into the naive thinking of the 1960s that the P-450 system was simple and straight-forward. An example of this is illustrated in Fig. 2. These two particular drug-metabolizing enzyme activities were chosen for illustration here because of the popular tenet that they represent the same form of P-450, most commonly referred to in pharmacology publications as "3-methylcholanthrene-induced cytochrome P-448." As it turns out, neither activity is "most closely associated" with P-448 (20,21). For example, if one examines 12 inbred mice (Fig. 2, *left*) the correlation coefficient between the two enzyme activities is excellent ($r = 0.90$). Compared with wild mice or randombred strains of mice, any particular strain of inbred laboratory animal is very homogeneous. In fact, colonies of wild mice are not believed to be as diverse as mice of heterogeneous stock (HS).*

HS mice are at least as heterogeneous as any outbred or randombred laboratory animal and, in fact, might approach the degree of variability found in man. With 12 HS mice (Fig. 2, *right*), the two enzyme activities clearly are not correlated ($r = -0.13$). We have similarly studied over 20 drug-metabolizing enzyme activities (20,21) and find that practically no activity correlates well with any other activity. Although such a study cannot determine the exact number of P-450s, we can conclude that almost every "drug-metabolizing enzyme activity" appears to be unique and represents the contribution from multiple forms of P-450.

---

*HS mice originated from an eight-way cross-population developed at the University of California at Berkeley by Dr. Gerald E. McClearn in collaboraton with Dr. W. Meredith. The eight original strains (22) included: C57BL, A, C3H/2, BALB/c, DBA/2, AKR, RIII, and Is/Bi; all were sublines at the Berkeley Cancer Research Genetic Laboratory at the time. The mice were later imported to the Institute of Behavioral Genetics, University of Colorado at Boulder, where they are being maintained as a base stock with 40 mated pairs in each generation. Mates are assigned randomly with the restriction that mates cannot have a common grandparent. With such a large sample of matings used in each generation, this arrangement will maximize outbreeding and prevent many genes from segregation even after 10 or 20 years.

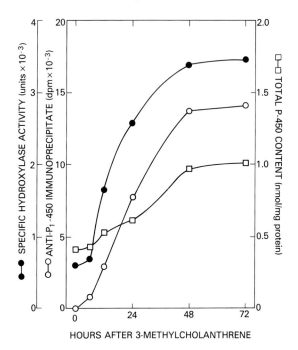

FIG. 3. Kinetics of induction in B6 mouse liver microsomes by 3-methylcholanthrene. At the indicated times, five livers were combined and microsomes were prepared. Aryl hydrocarbon hydroxylase specific activity *(solid circles)*, anti-P₁-450-immunoprecipitable radioactivity *(empty circles)*, and total cytochrome P-450 content *(empty squares)* were determined. (Data from ref. 29.)

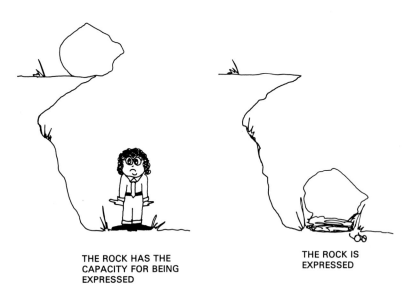

THE ROCK HAS THE
CAPACITY FOR BEING
EXPRESSED

THE ROCK IS
EXPRESSED

FIG. 4. Illustration of the definition of "capacity for expression."

CHARACTERIZATION OF ANTIBODY TO P₁-450

P_1-450 was highly purified from 3-methylcholanthrene-treated B6 liver and an antibody was raised (29). Figure 3 shows the kinetics of P_1-450 induction following a single dose of 3-methylcholanthrene to B6 mice. In the untreated naive control, there is no detectable anti-(P_1-450)-precipitable protein; 6 hrs later measurable amounts are found, and these levels plateau between 48 and 72 hrs after 3-methylcholanthrene administration. In the untreated control there is control aryl hydrocarbon hydroxylase activity, which had been presumed from previous studies (25) to represent some form(s) of P-450 other than P_1-450. The rise in the hydroxylase activity at 6 hrs, and plateauing between 48 and 72 hrs, reflects the rise in newly synthesized P_1-450 protein that is highly specific for benzo[*a*]pyrene metabolism. Figure 4 demonstrates the fact that an individual can have the *capacity* for P-450 gene expression, while the gene product (in this case, P_1-450) is in fact not expressed in the untreated naive control. An example of this point is emphasized in Fig. 4,

FUNDAMENTAL PRINCIPLES OF RECOMBINANT DNA TECHNOLOGY AND ISOLATION OF A P₁-450 cDNA CLONE

Figure 5 illustrates the passage of genetic information from DNA to protein. The positive DNA sense strand is complementary to the negative strand. During transcription, mRNA is synthesized complementary to the negative DNA strand. Triplets of base pairs in the RNA are translated into specific amino acids on polyribosomes. The NH_2-terminal portion of the polypeptide thus corresponds to the 5′ end of the DNA sense strand.

The remainder of this report deals with our success in isolating and characterizing a P_1-450 cDNA clone and ultimately the genomic gene (Fig. 6). We used the *Ah* receptor difference between B6 and D2 mice to our advantage. P_1-450 (23 S) mRNA from 3-methylcholanthrene-treated B6 mice is known (29) to be at least 40 times greater than P_1-450 mRNA from 3-methylcholanthrene-treated D2 mice. [^{32}P]cDNA [reverse-transcribed from total liver poly(A^+)-enriched 23 S RNA from B6 and from D2 mice] was thus used as a probe for colony hybridization (30). Clone 46 (Fig. 7) represents our successfully isolated P_1-450 cDNA clone. Its 1100-bp size represents about one-third of the complete P_1-450 mRNA length.

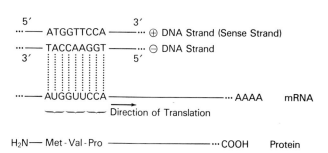

FIG. 5. Diagram of how the genetic message is transmitted from DNA to RNA to protein.

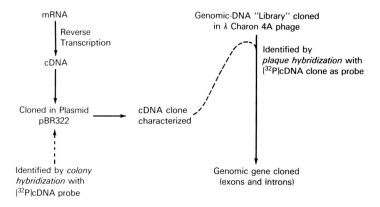

FIG. 6. Scheme by which our laboratory has proceeded from enriched poly(A⁺)-containing total liver RNA to a characterized cDNA clone to a characterized genomic DNA clone.

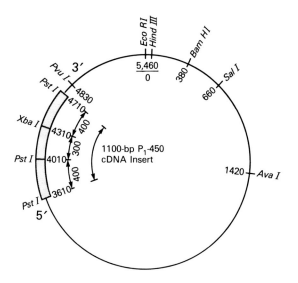

FIG. 7. Restriction map of pBR322 containing clone 46, P₁-450 cDNA. (Data from ref. 30.)

POTENTIAL PITFALLS IN "TRANSLATION ARREST" EXPERIMENTS FOR GENES ENCODING MEMBRANE-BOUND PROTEINS

"Positive" and "negative" translation arrest (Fig. 8) is the usual means for proving that one's cDNA clone is associated with a particular protein. Clone 46 DNA was fixed on a nitrocellulose filter, and 23 S RNA was hybridized to the filter (Fig. 8). When the pass-through mRNA was translated, there was no anti-(P₁-450)-precipitable translation product. Next, the specifically hybridized mRNA was eluted by formamide from the filter and translated; an anti-(P₁-450)-precipitable band at 55 kDa can be seen. These experiments are called "positive" and "negative" translation

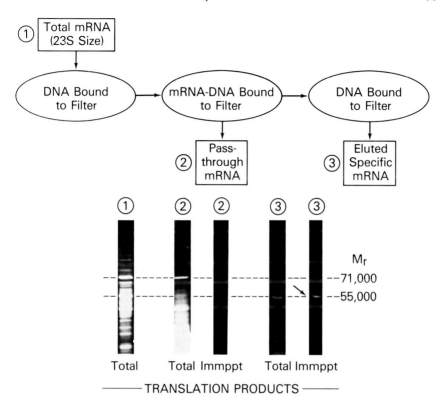

FIG. 8. Demonstration of "positive" and "negative" translation arrest, involving the mouse cDNA clone 46 and anti-(P₁-450). (Data from ref. 30.)

arrest. These data provide immunologic proof that the cDNA clone isolated is associated with one's antibody. The antibody precipitates the protein that has been translated from the mRNA, and this mRNA hybridizes most specifically to the cloned cDNA.

There exist two potential problems with translation arrest experiments. First, mRNAs having 90% or more nucleotide homology with a cDNA clone may hybridize during such an experiment. Figure 9 shows examples of 95% and 40% homology between two DNA sense strands. Although only 20 base pairs are shown in Fig. 9, 95% homology between two 2,000-bp genes derived from a common ancestral gene means that the positions of 1,900 nucleotides are identical and can be matched up; hence, the two genes will hybridize under highly stringent conditions. Second, antibodies to different forms of P-450 (Fig. 10) are notoriously not monospecific. Even monoclonal antibodies have been reported (35) to recognize two distinctly different forms of P-450. We have evidence (manuscript in preparation) for example, that several antibodies—each of which blocks one catalytic activity and not other activities and therefore appear to be relatively specific for distinct forms of P-450—all precipitate protein translated from mRNA that hybrid-

¹⁰   ²⁰
ATGGTTCCAC   TGCTAAATCC

ATGGTTCCAC   TGCTAAATCC
ATGGTTCCAC   TGCTAATTCC

95% Nucleotide sequence homology

ATGGTTCCAC   TGCTAAATCC
ATGGTAGGTC   TGTAGTTCGT

40% Nucleotide sequence homology

FIG. 9. Demonstration, between two DNA sense strands, of 95% nucleotide sequence homology *(top)* and 40% homology *(bottom)*. *Bold letters* in the second and fourth lines represent bases of the second sense strand that differ from bases of the first sense strand.

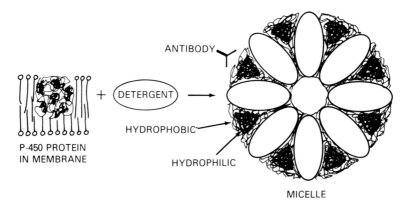

FIG. 10. Diagram of detergent solubilization of a membrane-bound protein such as P-450. Thick-lined portions of the P-450 peptide denote hydrophilic domains, thin-lined portions hydrophobic domains. The detergent-solubilized micelle may comprise 30% or 60% detergent. The solubilized protein will fold with its highly antigenic hydrophilic portions inside and its hydrophobic domains on the outside of the micelle. Antibody formation to such micelles thus will be directed at antigenic determinants of the hydrophobic moieties of all detergent-solubilized P-450 proteins.

izes specifically to a single cloned "P₁-450-like" cDNA in the translation arrest experiments. Therefore, for reasons at both the cDNA-mRNA and the protein levels, translation arrest experiments involving solubilized membrane-bound proteins may lead to difficulties in the interpretation of data. Confusion about which cDNA clone represents P-450*b*, the major rat phenobarbital-inducible form of P-450, is an example of such problems with translation arrest data (1,10,27).

GENETIC PROOF FOR THE P₁-450 cDNA CLONE

With the mouse P₁-450 gene we have the additional criterion of *genetic differences* that have been well characterized over the past decade. Hence, when the *Ah*-responsive F₁ heterozygote (*Ah^b^/Ah^d^*) is crossed with the *Ah*-nonresponsive D2 parent (Ah^d/Ah^d), among the progeny one finds a 50:50 distribution of Ah-responsive heterozygotes and Ah-nonresponsive homozygotes (28).

Figure 11 shows an RNA-DNA hybridization. mRNA was isolated from individual mouse livers; samples 2 through 10 represent individual 3-methylcholanthrene-treated offspring from the B6D2F$_1$ × D2 backcross. With a small piece of liver, their Ah phenotype was previously determined, and we know that numbers 2, 4, 5, 7, and 9 are Ah-responsive heterozygotes; numbers 3, 6, 8, and 10 represent Ah-nonresponsive homozygotes. The mRNA was electrophoresed and probed with labeled clone 46 DNA. There is a perfect correlation between Ah-responsiveness, i.e., induction of aryl hydrocarbon hydroxylase activity and therefore P_1-450 protein, and the presence of induced P_1-450 (23 S) mRNA that hybridizes to clone 46. This experiment, therefore, constitutes genetic proof that clone 46 is highly likely to be associated with the P_1-450 cDNA.

ISOLATION OF THE P_1-450 GENOMIC GENE

With clone 46 as the probe, a mouse plasmacytoma MOPC 41 genomic-DNA library was screened by the Benton-Davis plaque-hybridization procedure (3). Mouse tumor DNA had been digested by *EcoRI* and inserted into λ phage Charon 4A, and 50,000 plaques had been fixed to each filter (generous gift of Dr. Jon Seidman, National Institute of Child Health and Human Development, Bethesda). The entire library consisted of 20 filters, so that we have screened a total of about one million pieces of genomic DNA. A promising "tailed" plaque was found (Fig. 12) and purified to 100%. This positive genomic clone was named λ3NT12 and was found to be 19 kilobase pairs in length (37).

By hybridization between subclones of λ3NT12 and clone 46, we found that clone 46 hybridized to one extreme end of the mouse DNA insert and to an *EcoRI*-digested subclone pMJE12. There are two possible orientations. One is that clone 46 and subclone pMJE12 are located at the 5′ end of λ3NT12; if this were the case, most of the P_1-450 genomic gene would be located 5′-ward of this insert and therefore not contained in λ3NT12. The other possible orientation is that clone 46 and subclone pMJE12 are located at the 3′ end of λ3NT12; if this were the case, the entire P_1-450 chromosomal gene most likely would be contained within λ3NT12. Unfortunately, the former possibility was found to be the case (13,14,23). We therefore returned to the mouse MOPC 41 genomic-DNA library to find another recombinant phage. This time we used as the ^{32}P-labeled probe subclone pMJE12, which is 3 kilobase pairs in length.

By repeating the Benton-Davis plaque-hybridization technique, and characterizing three more genomic clones, we essentially have "walked up" the chromosome with clones λ3NT12, λ3NT13, λ3NT14, and finally λAhP-1. By R-loop analysis, the P_1-450 structural gene is believed to reside in the center of λAhP-1, spanning about 5 kbp (Fig. 13). The chromosomal gene of mouse P_1-450 is in the middle of λAhP-1, a clone which has a total length of 15.5 kbp. The P_1-450 genomic gene has at least 5 exons and 4 intervening sequences. The first and last exon are

Lane   1 2 3 4 5 6 7 8 9 10 11 12 13

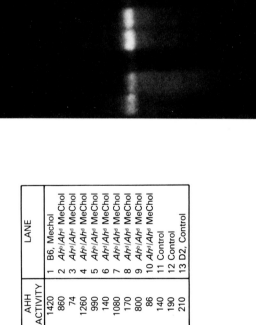

−23 S

AHH ACTIVITY	LANE	
1420	1	B6, Mechol
860	2	Ah^b/Ah^d MeChol
74	3	Ah^b/Ah^d MeChol
1260	4	Ah^b/Ah^d MeChol
990	5	Ah^b/Ah^d MeChol
140	6	Ah^b/Ah^d MeChol
1080	7	Ah^b/Ah^d MeChol
170	8	Ah^b/Ah^d MeChol
800	9	Ah^b/Ah^d MeChol
86	10	Ah^b/Ah^d MeChol
140	11	Control
190	12	Control
210	13	D2, Control

FIG. 11. Northern blot of mRNA from individual mice probed with clone 46 [^{32}P]DNA. AHH, aryl hydrocarbon (benzo[*a*]pyrene) hydroxylase, in units per mg of liver microsomal protein. (Data from ref. 38.)

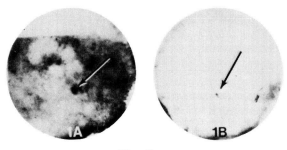

First Step

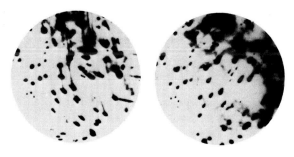

2nd Step Purification

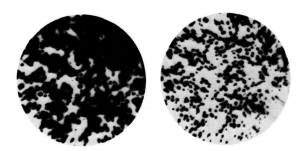

Purified λ Phage

FIG. 12. Autoradiographs of cloned mouse MOPC 41 genomic-DNA library screened with clone 46 [^{32}P]DNA. The plate in duplicate with the positive plaque *(arrow)* is shown at *top* after the initial screening, at *middle* after the first enrichment following the initial screening, and at *bottom* in a purified state (23).

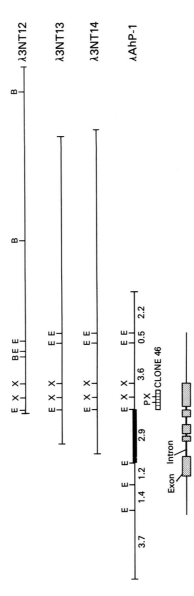

FIG. 13. Restriction maps of four recombinant phage isolated from the mouse genomic-DNA library containing overlapping DNA regions of the P$_1$-450 chromosomal structural gene. The linear DNA maps of individual phage were constructed on the basis of *EcoRI* (E), *XbaI* (X), *BamHI* (B), *PstI* (P), *SstI*, *HindIII*, and *XhoI* digests alone and, in several cases, double digests. The distances in kbp between the *EcoRI* sites of clone λAhP-1 are indicated, and the relative positions of the overlapping *EcoRI* and *XbaI* sites and clone 46 amongst the four phage are shown. By R-loop analysis between λAhP-1 and the P$_1$-450 (23 S) mRNA from 3-methylcholanthrene-treated B6 liver (23), the position of the P$_1$-450 exons and introns was determined and is depicted at *bottom*.

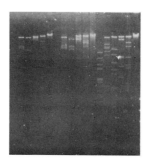

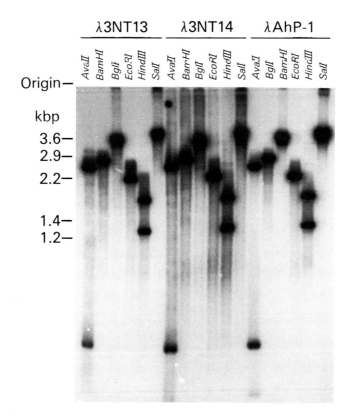

FIG. 14. Hybridization analysis of three recombinant phage digested with each of six restriction endonucleases with the [^{32}P]DNA probe of pAhP-3.6. The ethidium bromide-stained gel *(right)* and the autoradiogram of the Southern hybridization *(left)* are shown. Each well contains 1 μg of DNA. *EcoRI*-digested λAhP-1 DNA fragments were used as standard markers, given in kbp at *left* (23).

remarkably large, being about 1,000 and 1,300 bp, respectively. Total length of all exons together is about 2,700 bp.

Clone 46 is believed to be a unique 3′ sequence and probably exists in the 3′-nontranslating region of the P_1-450 gene. With the clone 46 3′ probe, it should be emphasized that we are unable to hybridize this probe to any other P-450 gene in mouse genomic DNA (30).

The relative position of each genomic clone along the chromosome is shown in Fig. 13. With the four recombinant phages from the mouse genomic-DNA library we have walked up the chromosome to the point where we are certain to have isolated all of the P_1-450 structural gene, including more than 5 kbp 5′-ward of the start of the gene.

EcoRI digestion of recombinant phage λAhP-1 yielded seven fragments of lengths ranging from 0.5 kbp to 3.7 kbp (Fig. 13). Most of these have been subcloned in pBR322 for use as ^{32}P-labeled probes and for nucleotide sequencing presently underway. Clone 46 hybridizes exclusively to the 3.6-kbp fragment, the clone of which we have named pAhP-3.6. Following digestion with each of six restriction endonucleases (Fig. 14), the DNA from genomic clones λ3NT13, λNT14, and λAhP-1 was compared, with use of pAhP-3.6 [^{32}P]DNA as probe. The three genomic clones and genomic DNA prepared from B6 mouse liver (23) exhibited identical patterns. These data are further evidence that λ3NT13, λ3NT14, and λAhP-1 are identical to each other and are truly representative of mouse genomic DNA.

CONCLUSIONS

This laboratory has uncovered several important points of information with the use of the P_1-450 cDNA clone (Table 1). An association of clone 46 with the P_1-450 protein has been demonstrated by both immunologic and genetic criteria (30,38). We believe that P_1-450 induction is under transcriptional control, because increased

TABLE 1. *Our findings with clone 46 (cDNA clone; 1100 bp; 3′-unique sequence)*

Association with P₁-450 protein
  Negative and positive translation arrest with anti-(P₁-450)
  Correlation with *Ahᵇ* allele in offspring from B6D2F₁ × D2 backcross
P₁-450 induction under transcriptional control
  Association with increased mRNA (23 S) levels
  Correlation with intranuclear large molecular weight mRNA precursor
No evidence for gene amplification or gross form of genomic rearrangement
P₁-450 mRNA translation occurs on membrane-bound polysomes
Cross-hybridization with rat and rabbit DNA; rat (23 S) mRNA
P₁-450 gene hypomethylated in adult B6, when compared with that in adult D2, or sperm
  or embryonic B6; no difference in methylation between control and
  3-methycholanthrene-treated B6 mice
Other inducers (such as isosafrole) increase P₁-450 mRNA to small extent
P₁-450 genomic gene characterized by R-loop analysis (~5 kbp; at least 5 exons and 4
  introns)
Excellent correlation (*r* = 0.99) between appearance of inducer-receptor complex in
  nucleus and P₁-450 mRNA induction

---

23 S mRNA and an intranuclear large-molecular-weight mRNA precursor occur concomitantly during the induction process (38). No evidence for gene duplication or gross form of genomic rearrangement has been found, either during induction or during development (6,38). P$_1$-450 mRNA appears to be translated exclusively on membrane-bound polysomes (5). Clone 46 hybridizes with rat and rabbit DNA and with rat but not rabbit mRNA; these data suggest that clone 46 hybridizes to a segment of the rabbit P$_1$-450 gene that is not transcribed into the messenger (6). We found that the P$_1$-450 gene in adult B6 is *hypo*methylated, compared with the gene in B6 sperm, B6 embryo, or adult D2 mice; this hypomethylation pattern could be related to the increased expressivity of the P$_1$-450 gene in B6, compared with that in D2 mice (6). Other P-450 inducers, such as benzo[*a*]anthracene and isosafrole, have been found to induce P$_1$-450 mRNA, as measured by the clone 46 probe (39). With the cDNA probe, we have isolated the chromosomal P$_1$-450 gene from a mouse genomic-DNA library (23). By R-loop analysis, the gene spans about 5 kilobase pairs and has at least 5 exons and 4 introns. Lastly, we have found an excellent correlation between the intranuclear appearance of the inducer-receptor complex and the induction of P$_1$-450 mRNA as measured by the clone 46 probe (36). With clone λAhP-1 and the surrounding regions of this mouse chromosome, we hope to understand much more about the regulation of P-450 induction, the evolution of the P-450 system, and perhaps the ultimate number of P-450 forms that an individual organism is genetically *capable* of expressing. With this knowledge, we hope to gain insight into the mechanism of chemical carcinogenesis, especially since P$_1$-450 is directly responsible for the metabolic activation of polycyclic hydrocarbons, such as benzo[*a*]pyrene, to the ultimate carcinogenic intermediate, which interacts covalently with DNA. Finally, it may be possible to develop an assay, based on recombinant DNA technology, in order to assess the human *Ah* phenotype; such an assay may predict who is at increased risk for certain types of environmentally caused cancers.

REFERENCES

1. Adesnick, M., Bar-Nun, S., Maschio, F., Zunich, M., Lippman, A., and Bard, E. (1981): Mechanism of induction of cytochrome p-450 by phenobarbital. *J. Biol. Chem.*, 256:10340–10345.
2. Becker, F. F., and Sell, S. (1979): α-Fetoprotein levels and hepatic alterations during chemical carcinogenesis in C57BL/6N mice. *Cancer Res.*, 39:3491–3494.
3. Benton, W. D., and Davis, R. W. (1977): Screening λgt recombinant clones by hybridization to single plaques in situ. *Science*, 196:180–182.
4. Bresnick, E., Bailey, G., Bonney, R. J., and Wightman, P. (1981): Phospholipase activity in skin after application of phorbol esters and 3-methylcholanthrene. *Carcinogenesis*, 2:1119–1122.
5. Chen, Y.-T., and Negishi, M. (1982): Expression and subcellular distribution of mouse cytochrome P$_1$-450 mRNA as determined by molecular hybridization with cloned P$_1$-450 DNA. *Biochem. Biophys. Res. Commun.*, 104:641–648.
6. Chen, Y.-T., Negishi, M., and Nebert, D. W. (1982): Cytochrome P$_1$-450 structural gene in mouse, rat and rabbit. Differences in DNA methylation and developmental expression of mRNA. *DNA*, 1:231–238.
7. Deitrich, R. A., Bludeau, P., Roper, M., and Schmuck, J. (1978): Induction of aldehyde dehydrogenases. *Biochem. Pharmacol.*, 27:2343–2347.
8. Eisen, H. J., Hannah, R. R., Legraverend, C., Okey, A. B., and Nebert, D. W. (1983): The *Ah*

receptor: Controlling factor in the induction of drug-metabolizing enzymes by certain chemical carcinogens and other environmental pollutants. In: *Biochemical Actions of Hormones*, edited by G. Litwack, pp. 227-258. Academic Press, New York.

9. Filler, R., and Lew, K. J. (1981): Developmental onset of mixed-function oxidase activity in preimplantation mouse embryos. *Proc. Natl. Acad. Sci. U.S.A.*, 78:6991–6995.

10. Fujii-Kuriyama, Y., Mizukami, Y., Kawajiri, K., Sogawa, K., and Muramatsu, M. (1982): Primary structure of a cytochrome P-450: Coding nucleotide sequence of phenobarbital-inducible cytochrome P-450 cDNA from rat liver. *Proc. Natl. Acad. Sci. U.S.A.*, 79:2793–2797.

11. Galloway, S. M., Perry, P. E., Meneses, J., Nebert, D. W., and Pedersen, R. A (1980): Cultured mouse embryos metabolize benzo[a]pyrene during early gestation: Genetic differences detectable by sister chromatid exchange. *Proc. Natl. Acad. Sci. U.S.A.*, 77:3524–3528.

12. Gupta, B. N., McConnell, E. E., Harris, M. W., and Moore, J. A. (1981): Polybrominated biphenyl toxicosis in the rat and mouse. *Toxicol. Appl. Pharmacol.*, 57:99–118.

13. Ikeda, T , Altieri, M., Nakamura, M., Nebert, D. W., and Negishi, M. (1982): Induction by 3-methylcholanthrene (MC) or isosafrole (ISF) of two P-450 mRNA's which share sequence homology. In: *Cytochrome P-450: Biochemistry, Biophysics and Environmental Implications*, edited by E. Hietanen, pp. 181–184. Elsevier/North-Holland Biomedical Press, Amsterdam.

14. Ikeda, T., Altieri, M., Chen, Y.-T., Nakamura, M., Tukey, R. H., Nebert, D. W., and Negishi, M. (1983): Characterization of P₂-450 (20 S) mRNA. Association with the P₁-450 genomic gene and differential response to the inducers 3-methylcholanthrene and isosafrole. *Eur. J. Biochem.*, 134:13–18.

15. Ishidate, K., Tsuruoka, M., and Nakazawa, Y. (1980): Alteration in enzyme activities *de novo* phosphatidylcholine biosynthesis in rat liver by treatment with typical inducers of microsomal drug-metabolizing system. *Biochim. Biophys. Acta*, 620:49–58.

16. Ivanovic, V., and Weinstein, I. B. (1981): Benz[a]pyrene and other inducers of cytochrome P₁-450 inhibit binding of epidermal growth factor (EGF) to cell surface receptors. *J. Supramol. Struct. Cell. Biochem.*, [Suppl.] 5:232 *(Abstract)*.

17. Ivanovic, V., and Weinstein, I. B. (1982): Benzo[a]pyrene and other inducers of cytochrome P₁-450 inhibit binding of epidermal growth factor to cell surface receptors. *Carcinogenesis*, 3:505–510.

18. Kärenlampi, S. O., Eisen, H. J., Hankinson, O., and Nebert, D. W. (1983): Effects of cytochrome P₁-450 inducers on the cell-surface receptors for epidermal growth factor, phorbo 112, 13-dibutyrate, or insulin of cultured mouse hepatoma cells. *J. Biol. Chem., (in press)*.

19. Knutson, J. C., and Poland, A. (1980): Keratinization of mouse teratoma cell line XB produced by 2,3,7,8-tetrachlorodibenzo-p-dioxin: An *in vitro* model of toxicity. *Cell*, 22:27–36.

20. Lang, M. A., Gielen, J. E., and Nebert, D. W. (1981): Genetic evidence for many unique liver microsomal P-450-mediated monooxygenase activities in heterogeneic stock mice. *J. Biol. Chem.*, 256:12068–12075.

21. Lang, M. A., and Nebert, D. W. (1981): Structural gene products of the *Ah* locus. Evidence for many unique P-450-mediated monooxygenase activities reconstituted from 3-methylcholanthrene-treated C57BL/6N mouse liver microsomes. *J. Biol. Chem.*, 256:12058–12067.

22. McClearn, G. E., Wilson, J. R., and Meredith, W. (1970): The use of isogenic and heterogenic mouse stocks in behavioral research. In: *Contributions to Behavior-Genetic Analysis—The Mouse as a Prototype*, edited by G. Lindzey, and D. D. Thiessen, pp. 3–22. Appleton-Century-Crofts, New York.

23. Nakamura, M., Negishi, M., Altieri, M., Chen, Y.-T., Ikeda, T., Tukey, R. H., and Nebert, D. W. (1983): Structure of the mouse cytochrome P₁-450 genomic gene. *Eur. J. Biochem.*, 134:19–25.

24. Nebert, D. W. (1981): Possible clinical importance of genetic differences in drug metabolism. *Br. Med. J.*, 283:537–542.

25. Nebert, D. W., and Jensen, N. M. (1979): The *Ah* locus: Genetic regulation of the metabolism of carcinogens, drugs, and other environmental chemicals by cytochrome P-450-mediated monooxygenases. In: *CRC Critical Reviews in Biochemistry*, edited by G. D. Fasman, pp. 401–437. CRC Press, Inc., Cleveland, Ohio.

26. Nebert, D. W., Levitt, R. C., and Pelkonen, O. (1979): Genetic variation in metabolism of chemical carcinogens associated with susceptibility to tumorigenesis. In: *Carcinogens: Identification and Mechanisms of Action*, edited by A. C. Griffin, and C. R. Shaw, pp. 157–185. Raven Press, New York.

27. Nebert, D. W., and Negishi, M. (1982): Multiple forms of cytochrome P-450 and the importance of molecular biology and evolution. *Biochem. Pharmacol.*, 31:2311–2317.
28. Nebert, D. W., Negishi, M., Lang, M. A., Hjelmeland, L. M., and Eisen, H. J. (1982): The *Ah* locus, a multigene family necessary for survival in a chemically adverse environment: Comparison with the immune system. *Advanc. Genet.*, 21:1–52.
29. Negishi, M., and Nebert, D. W. (1979): Structural gene products of the *Ah* locus. Genetic and immunochemical evidence for two forms of mouse liver cytochrome P-450 induced by 3-methylcholanthrene. *J. Biol. Chem.*, 254:11015–11023.
30. Negishi, M., Swan, D. C., Enquist, L. W., and Nebert, D. W. (1981): Isolation and characterization of a cloned DNA sequence associated with the murine *Ah* locus and a 3-methylcholanthrene-induced form of cytochrome P-450. *Proc. Natl. Acad. Sci. U.S.A.*, 78:800–804.
31. Pitot, H. C., Goldsworthy, T., Campbell, H. A., and Poland, A. (1980): Quantitative evaluation of the promotion by 2,3,7,8-tetrachlorodibenzo-*p*-dioxin of nepatocarcinogenesis from diethylnitrosamine. *Cancer Res.*, 40:3616–3620.
32. Poland, A., and Glover, E. (1980): 2,3,7,8-Tetrachlorodibenzo-*p*-dioxin: Segregation of toxicity with the *Ah* locus. *Mol. Pharmacol.*, 17:86–94.
33. Poland, A., Palen, D., and Glover, E. (1982): Tumour promotion by TCDD in skin of HRS/J hairless mice. *Nature*, 300:271–273.
34. Shum, S., Jensen, N. M., and Nebert, D. W. (1979): The *Ah* locus: *In utero* toxicity and teratogenesis associated with genetic differences in benzo[a]pyrene metabolism. *Teratology*, 20:365–376.
35. Thomas, P. E., Reik, L. M., Ryan, D. E., and Levin, W. (1982): Some hybridoma antibodies against rat liver cytochrome P-450c cross-react with cytochrome P-450d. *Fed. Proc.*, 41:297 *(Abstract)*.
36. Tukey, R. H., Hannah, R. R., Negishi, M., Nebert, D. W., and Eisen, H. J. (1982): The *Ah* locus. Correlation of intranuclear appearance of inducer-receptor complex with induction of cytochrome P₁-450 mRNA. *Cell*, 31:275–284.
37. Tukey, R. H., Nakamura, M., Chen, Y.-T., Negishi, M., and Nebert, D. W. (1982): Genetic regulation of P-450 induction in the mouse. Studies with a cloned DNA sequence. In: *Microsomes, Drug Oxidations, and Drug Toxicity*, edited by R. Sato, and R. Kato, pp. 353–360. Japan Scientific Societies Press, Tokyo.
38. Tukey, R. H., Nebert, D. W., and Negishi, M. (1981): Structural gene product of the [*Ah*] complex. Evidence for transcriptional control of cytochrome P₁-450 induction by use of a cloned DNA sequence. *J. Biol. Chem.*, 256:6969–6974.
39. Tukey, R. H., Negishi, M., and Nebert, D. W. (1982): Quantitation of hepatic cytochrome P₁-450 mRNA with the use of a cloned DNA probe. Effects of various P-450 inducers in C57BL/6N and DBA/2N mice. *Mol. Pharmacol.*, 22:779–786.

Biochemical Basis of Chemical Carcinogenesis,
edited by H. Greim, R. Jung, M. Kramer,
H. Marquardt, and F. Oesch.
Raven Press, New York © 1984.

Epoxide Hydrolases in Laboratory Animals and in Man

H. R. Glatt, I. Mertes, T. Wölfel and F. Oesch

*Institute of Pharmacology, University of Mainz,
D-6500 Mainz, Federal Republic of Germany*

Many olefinic and aromatic xenobiotics, and also some endogenous compounds, are metabolized by mammalian monooxygenases to epoxes (8,41). In general, epoxides are electrophilically reactive (although their reactivity greatly varies). By covalent binding to tissue components they can elicit mutagenic, carcinogenic and other toxic effects. Therefore, enzymes which metabolize epoxides are of substantial toxicological interest. Two systems are known: conjugation with glutathione and hydrolysis to dihydrodiols by epoxide hydrolases (EHs). Whereas the former metabolic pathway is also operative with other electrophiles, epoxides are the only known substrates for the latter enzymes. Despite functions usually protective, both systems are involved in toxication in rare cases. By conversion of some arene oxides derived from polycyclic aromatic hydrocarbons to less reactive dihydrodiols, EHs provide the metabolic precursors for highly reactive vicinal dihydrodiol-epoxides, the major ultimate carcinogens of various polycyclic hydrocarbons (27,58). Hence, EHs do not always have a purely protective function, but also are involved in the formation of some reactive metabolites. In mammalian enzyme-mediated bacterial tests it was demonstrated that the levels of EH activities strongly affect the effect of various proximate and ultimate mutagens (4,11,16,17,44).

Various aspects of EHs have been reviewed in detail (25,35,41,48). Here we report on EHs in man and, in so far as is relevant for extrapolation from toxicological studies to man, in laboratory animals. The first paragraphs will deal with EHs in the liver, the organ where these enzymes, due to their high levels and the general importance of the liver in drug metabolism, have been studied most thoroughly.

EHs IN THE LIVER

Multiplicity of EHs

Hepatic microsomes from the investigated mammalian species including rat and man hydrolyze numerous epoxides of widely different chemical structures (3,26,29,40,43,63). With minor exceptions (5), induction led to parallel increases in activity towards different substrates (26,56,63). Studying interindividual variation in man, Kapitulnik et al. (29) observed an excellent correlation among the activities towards 11 substrates. Enzymes which were purified to apparent homogeneity according to several criteria possessed broad substrate specificities which were similar to those in microsomes (3,20,36). However, differences in purification factors have been observed (3,36). They may be the result of the presence of multiple enzymes, but alternatively trivial technical reasons might also explain their occurrence, e.g., differential accessibilities of different (often highly lipophilic) substrates to the membrane-bound and purified enzyme. Antibodies raised against the purified enzyme precipitated the activity towards different substrates (styrene 7,8-oxide, benzo(*a*)pyrene 4,5-oxide, estroxide, androstene oxide) from solubilized microsomes completely and with non-distinguishable dose-response curves (63). Together, these experiments demonstrate that various epoxides are hydrolyzed by a single enzyme or, alternatively, that several enzymes exist that possess very similar structures and are under very similar biosynthetic control. The latter interpretation may be true since Guengerich et al. (20,21) reported on a separation and purification of several EH_m of slightly different amino acid composition and immunochemical properties from inbred rats as well as from a single human liver. As these preparations did not greatly differ in their substrate specificities and were similarly affected by enzyme activators and inhibitors, a biological significance of this heterogeneity is not yet known.

Using bovine liver microsomes, Watabe et al. (66) could differentially inhibit the hydrolysis of cholesterol $5\alpha,6\alpha$-oxide and cholesterol $5\beta,6\beta$-oxide as opposed to styrene oxide and safrole oxide. We found cholesterol oxide hydrolase activity also in rat liver and could separate it physically from other EH_m activities (Timms et al., unpublished results). Whether other epoxides are also metabolized by cholesterol 5,6-oxide hydrolase and whether further EH_m with special substrate specificities exist is unknown.

However, it is clear that liver cytosol contains EH which differ(s) from the microsomal enzyme not only by its subcellular localization, but also immunochemically, in its pH-optimum, in its molecular weight and in that it is not inhibited by 1,1,1-trichloropropene oxide (23,25,50,54,64). The most important difference is that cytosol metabolizes various epoxides, such as *trans*-β-methyl styrene oxide and *trans*-stilbene oxide (25,50,54), that are very poor substrates for microsomal enzymes. On the other hand, benzo(*a*)pyrene 4,5-oxide is readily metabolized by mouse liver microsomes, but not by cytosol (50). Other arene oxides, which are good substrates for microsomal enzymes, are metabolized at very low rates by cytosol (50). Hammock et al. (25) noticed a similar purification factor towards different substrates in a partially purified preparation from mouse liver cytosol. Otherwise little is known about whether the cytosolic activities result from a single enzyme or several enzymes.

EH activities have also been found in all other investigated subcellular fractions. Plasma membrane, Golgi apparatus and nuclear membranes from rat liver metabolize benzo(*a*)pyrene 4,5-oxide with about one quarter of the specific activities in microsomes (59). Mouse liver mitochondria contain a soluble EH which is very similar to or structurally identical with EH_c (14,25).

Species Differences in Hepatic EHs

Liver of all investigated vertebrate species have EH_m activities. The substrate specificities vary greatly between species which are phylogenetically far apart from each other (Table 1). Within the class of mammals qualitative differences also occur (albeit to a smaller extent) and, hence, do not allow a simple quantitative comparison among species. With all substrates used so far, mouse has a particularly low hepatic EH_m activity (Table 1). The substrate specificity appears to be very similar to rat EH_m. Kapitulnik et al. (29), using styrene oxide, octene 1,2-oxide and 9 arene oxides found very similar specificities in rat and human microsomes. From rat, human, rabbit and mouse liver, EH_m has been purified to apparent homogeneity (2,20,24,30,36,37). Species differences in substrate specificity and the effect of enzyme inhibitors and activators have been demonstrated, but were of minor extent (20,36,43,65). Immunochemical studies indicated great structural similarities (or identity) of mouse and rat EH_m (30,33,37), whereas only few antibody preparations showed cross-reactivity between human and rat enzyme (33,37). N-terminal amino acid sequences and peptide maps showed marked similarities, but no identity between purified human and rat EH_m (10).

EH_c has been studied in relatively few species; mouse, rat, guinea pig, rabbit and man (13,25). The interspecies variations in activity and substrate specificity appear greater than for EH_m. As an example, rabbit cytosol readily hydrolyzes styrene 7,8-oxide (64), whereas no activity was found in rat, mouse and guinea pig (54). With all investigated substrates, rat cytosol had very low EH activities,

TABLE 1. *Epoxide hydrolase activity in liver microsomes from various species with three substrates*

Species	Sex	Activity (nmoles diol/mg protein/min)		
		HEOM[a]	Styrene oxide	Benzo(a)pyrene 4,5-oxide
Mouse (various strains)	Male	0.87-1.1	0.73-1.3	1.5-2.1
Rat (Sprague-Dawley)	Male	3.0	6.4	6.1
Guinea pig	Male	15	12	18
Rabbit (New Zealand White)	Male	82	10	16
Cat (single specimen)	Female	1.7	1.5	4.8
Pig (single specimen)	Female	30	6.8	6.9
Japanese quail (Coturnix japonica)	Male	0.40	8.9	0.2
Feral pigeon (Columba livia)	Male	0.31	3.0	0.94
Toad (Xenopus laevis)	Mixed	0.3	0.98	0.97
Rainbow trout (Salmo gairdnerii)	Mixed	0.08	2.7	0.6

Data from ref. 54, with permission.
Except for the cat and pig each assay was performed using a pooled sample of microsomes from 4 to 6 animals.
[a]1,2,3,4,9,9-Hexachloro-6,7-epoxy-1,4,4a,5,6,7,8,8a-octahydro-1,4-methanonaphthalene.

whereas with most substrates, the mouse had the highest activity among the investigated species (25,54).

Strain Differences in Hepatic EHs

Systematic investigations on strain differences were performed in the mouse (13,38,42,65) and rat (53) and were limited to microsomal activities with one exception (13). Mice showed a polymorphism in that the pH-optimum of EH_m in some strains was at 8.7 and in others at 9.5 (38). Genetic analysis demonstrated inheritance on a single locus on chromosome 1 with expression of both alleles in heterozygotes (38). In spite of this polymorphism, activity, when measured at pH≤9.0, varied less than 2-fold among different strains (38,42). These investigations were performed with a single substrate, styrene oxide. In a study using styrene oxide, benzo(*a*)pyrene 4,5-oxide and HEOM (1,2,3,4,9,9-hexachloro-6,7-epoxy-1,4,4a,5,6,7,8,8a-octahydro-1,4-methanonaphthalene), differences in substrate specificity among mouse strains were not observed (65). No polymorphism, but somewhat larger (about 3-fold) variation in EH_m was found in rat strains (53). pH-Optimum and substrate specificity (using styrene oxide, benzo(*a*)pyrene 4,5-oxide and estroxide as substrates) did not differ in strains with low (F344), intermediate (Sprague-Dawley) or high (DA) hepatic EH_m activity. Immunochemical experiments showed quantitative but not qualitative differences in enzyme protein (53). As in mice, the hepatic EH_m activities in rats were inherited in a codominant, autosomal mode (53).

EH_c activity was compared in 4 mouse strains, whereby the specific activity in hepatic cytosol differed maximally 1.4-fold (13).

Sex Differences in Hepatic EHs

The specific EH activities in microsomes from females of various rat strains, measured with styrene oxide, benzo(*a*)pyrene 4,5-oxide, androstene oxide and estroxide as substrates, are about 75% of those in males (31,45,53,63). Adult, but not newborn male mice have higher hepatic EH_c activities than females (13). No other sex differences in hepatic or extrahepatic EH_s are known in any species. Specifically in man, very similar hepatic EH_m and EH_c activities are found in both sexes (31 and below).

Inhibition and activation of EHs

Various epoxides (40,43), ketones (1,12,43,55) and *N*-heterocyclics (43,55,62) activate or inhibit EH_m. It is important to know that the same modulator may have opposite effects towards the enzyme activity when using different substrates (33).

As some compounds, such as 5,6-benzoflavone and 7,8-benzflavone, activate EH_m in intact (human) cells and as this activation even occurs at a concentration of 1 μM (18) it is likely that modulation of EH_m by endogenous or exogenous compounds may be of significance *in vivo*. So far no potent, specific modulators of EH_c have been found (25).

Induction of Hepatic EHs

Various compounds including phenobarbital (5,26,39,61), 3-methylcholanthrene (5,26,39,61), pregnenolone 16α-carbonitrile (61), Aroclor 1254 (45), *trans*-stilbene oxide (56), lindane (52), various antioxidants (6,28), and hepatocarcinogens (9,34,57) induce hepatic EH_m activities in rats and/or mice. In rats, the maximal induction rarely exceeds the 3-fold of the control activity. In mice, which have lower control activities than rats, up to 11-fold increases have been observed (6). There is some evidence that phenobarbital, phenytoin and rifampicin at therapeutic doses induce EH_m activity in man (see below). Rifampicin was inactive in the mouse, the only laboratory animal investigated (A. Zimmer, H. R. Glatt and F. Oesch, unpublished results). EH_c is induced by phenobarbital, but no other inducers are known (25).

Interindividual differences in EH activities in human liver

Biopsies obtained from different human subjects varied greatly in their specific EH_m (63-fold) and EH_c activities (539-fold), using benzo(*a*)pyrene 4,5-oxide and *trans*-stilbene oxide as substrates, respectively (Fig. 1). The two activities varied independently from each other (Spearman's correlation: $r = 0.039$, $p = 0.45$).

One possible reason for the large interindividual variation may be that most biopsies were from patients with liver disease and/or under drug treatment. Table 2 shows the activities in different classes of patients. With one exception, no association between EH activities and diseases, drug treatment, sex, smoking habits and alcohol consumption of the biopsy donors occurred. The exception was that tuberculosis patients treated with rifampicin, isoniazid and ethambutol had increased EH_m activities. We suspect that rifampicin was the inducing agent, because this compound induces other enzymes in human liver and EH activity in cultured human lymphocytes (see below). Other studies (7,29) suggest that hepatic EH_m activity is also increased in patients treated with phenobarbital or phenytoin.

Large interindividual variations in human EH_m activities have also been observed when other substrates were used, such as the pesticide HEOM (7) or the drug metabolite carbamazepine 10,11-oxide (60), styrene oxide (29), octene 1,2-oxide (29) and various arene oxides (29). In the last study (29), the activities towards each substrate correlated highly with the activities towards each other substrate. The enormous interindividual variation in human hepatic EH activities contrasts to the small interindividual (and even interstrain) variations in laboratory animals under uniform conditions used in toxicologic studies. The results underline the importance of performing toxicologic studies in more than one species and, if possible, to complete them with biochemical investigations. Moreover, as in clinical studies on

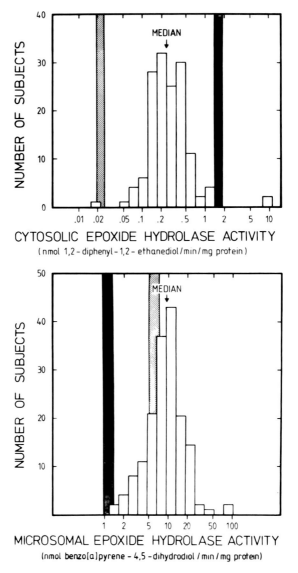

FIG. 1. Microsomal and cytosolic epoxide hydrolase activity in liver biopsis from different human individuals. The activities in C57BL/6 mice *(black bars)* and Sprague-Dawley rats *(hatched bars)* are indicated for comparison (the values are means ± S.D. from 3 to 6 adult male animals). (From F. Oesch, I. Mertes, R. Fleischmann, and H. R. Glatt, manuscript in preparation.)

a limited number of subjects, individuals with extreme enzyme activities not necessarily occur, it may be fruitful to study which genetic, developmental and environmental factors affect the enzymes which are important in the metabolism of a compound.

TABLE 2. *Hepatic epoxide activities in different human groups*

Group	Microsomal epoxide hydrolase[a] (nmoles BP-4,5-diol/min/mg protein)	Cytosolic epoxide hydrolase[a] (nmoles 1,2-diphenyl-1,2-ethanediol/min/mg protein)
Controls[b]	9.81 ± 5.02 (29)	.287 ± .159 (26 + 1*)
Fatty liver disease	9.59 ± 4.86 (31)	.289 ± .122 (30 + 3*)
Cirrhosis	10.23 ± 6.08 (18 + 1*)	.261 ± .098 (16)
Hepatitis	8.95 ± 6.26 (10)	.227 ± .140 (16)
Hodgkin/non-Hodgkin lymphoma	7.54 ± 2.67 (6)	.378 ± .120 (7 + 1*)
Stomach carcinoma	7.93 ± 3.43 (11)	.564 ± .700 (3)
Tuberculosis[c]	16.71 ± 7.63 (11)[e]	.336 ± .190 (5)
Estrogen therapy	9.61 ± 4.24 (6)	.223 ± .061 (5 + 1*)
Cholangiolar diseases	10.35 ± 4.54 (13 + 1*)	.292 ± .130 (9)
Other miscellaneous diseases	9.45 ± 6.98 (28 + 1*)	.232 ± .127 (21)
Males	8.52 ± 3.88 (93 + 10*)	.273 ± .130 (88 + 4*)
Females	10.44 ± 5.79 (62 + 1*)	.274 ± .147 (49 + 2*)
Non-smokers	9.16 ± 4.84 (99 + 4*)	.280 ± .147 (85 + 4*)
Smokers[d]	8.74 ± 3.97 (37 + 4*)	.279 ± .136 (32 + 1*)
Non-alcoholics	9.22 ± 5.03 (99 + 4*)	.239 ± .128 (77 + 6*)
Alcoholics[d]	10.16 ± 4.23 (28)	.218 ± .044 (14 + 4*)

[a]Mean activity ± S.D. from n (first number in brackets) subjects. Some additional subjects, marked with an asterisk, were not used for calculation of means and S.D. because of their strong deviation from the mean activity. (Frequency in normal distribution less than 1% according to the Nalimov-test.)

[b]Subjects not treated with drugs for at least 20 days prior to biopsy, with normal liver histology and normal levels of plasma proteins, and without indications of liver or intestinal diseases except cholelithiasis.

[c]Treated with rifampicin and, in part, isoniazid and ethambutol.

[d]Only smokers and alcoholics who continued this habit during hospitalization were used for the comparison.

[e]Different from controls $p < 0.001$, (Kolmogroff-Smirnov test). All other groups did not differ from the respective controls ($p > 0.1$, independent of whether or not outlying values were included).

EHs IN EXTRAHEPATIC TISSUES

Extrahepatic EHs in Laboratory Animals

In the rat, EH_m activity towards benzo(*a*)pyrene 4,5-oxide could be measured in 26 of 27 investigated tissues (45). The specific activity in microsomal preparations varied from 8 (in triceps muscle) to 6400 pmoles/min/mg protein (in liver). In whole blood, no measurable activity (<5 pmoles/min/mg protein) could be detected [however, various individual human blood components, which have been investigated with more sensitive methods, showed low but clear activity (15, see also below)]. In rat kidney, testis, ovary, adrenal, and lung activities have also been determined with estroxide and androstene oxide (63), in rat and mouse skin with various other arene oxides (46). In all these cases the substrate specificities were very similar to those in the liver. Antibodies raised against purified rat EH_m precipitated >90% of the EH_m activity (with styrene oxide as substrate) from rat kidney, lung or testis (21). Whilst no indications for qualitative differences in EH_m in different tissues exist, the biosynthetic control may vary: whereas hepatic EH_m activities are induced by various compounds, no effects are often observed on EH_m in extrahepatic tissues of the same animals (45,47,61). Extrahepatic tissues, however, do not for the most part lack inducibility, as seen from increased EH_m activity in the kidney of rats treated with *trans*-stilbene oxide (47) or in the lung of mice treated with 2(3)-*tert*-butyl-4-hydroxyanisole (6). Differences in the biosynthetic control in different tissues could account for the finding that strain differences in EH_m activity vary in different tissues (Table 3). A consequence of this finding is that determination of the activity in one tissue is not a reliable measure for the relative activity in other tissues of the same animals (unless a specific correlation between the activities in the two tissues has been established). Differences in organ distribution become more pronounced when different species, instead of strains, are compared. Table 3 shows that mice possess higher specific EH_m activity in testis than in liver, the tissue with the highest activity in most species. Syrian hamsters have a particularly high activity in the lung and a very low activity in the testis.

EH_c activity [with 1-(4'-ethylphenoxy)-3,7-dimethyl-6,7-epoxy-*trans*-2-octene as substrate] has been found in kidney, duodenum, skeletal muscle, colon, lung, and spleen of New Zealand white rabbits and in kidney, lung, testis and spleen of Swiss Webster mice; the specific activities were 1 to 67% of those in hepatic cytosol (13).

EHs in Extrahepatic Tissues of Man

EH activities have been determined in lung and in skin, both tissues of great toxicological significance, as well as in fibroblast and blood components, the latter

TABLE 3. *Species and strain differences in organ distribution of microsomal epoxide hydrolase activity*

	pmoles BP-4,5-diol/min/mg protein			
Species	Liver	Lung	Kidney	Testis
Rat				
Sprague-Dawley	6400 ± 600	360 ± 50	700 ± 120	1470 ± 250
DA	9100 ± 900	300 ± 40	650 ± 140	1180 ± 210
F344	3800 ± 800	240 ± 60	1170 ± 280	1500 ± 260
Mouse (NMRI)	1020 ± 120	370 ± 40	71 ± 11	2540 ± 310
Syrian hamster	11700 ± 1300	3700 ± 200	3500 ± 400	107 ± 8
Rabbit (New Zealand white)	16000	1300	1700	2400

Data from refs. 45, 53, 65 and unpublished results (H.R. Glatt, H.U. Schmassmann, and F. Oesch).

Values are means with S.D. from determinations in 1 to 8 pools of microsomes, whereby each pool was obtained from 1 to 5 animals.

having the advantages that samples can be easily taken at different occasions from the same subject and that the cells can be cultured, i.e. environmental differences can be minimized and enzyme inductions, activations and inhibitions can be studied in a flexible manner. In all studies on extrahepatic human EH the measurements were performed in microsomal fractions, total cell homogenates or intact cells, so that nothing is known specifically about cytosolic activities. Where activities in total homogenates or whole cells were measured, the substrate used, benzo(a)-pyrene 4,5-oxide, and inhibition by 1,1,1-trichloropropene oxide indicate a close relationship to the microsomal, but not to the cytosolic enzyme in the liver.

Most measurements of extrahepatic human EH activity were performed with benzo(a)pyrene 4,5-oxide. Where other substrates were used, such as various other K-region arene oxides with skin (46) and pulmonary preparations (51), no obvious differences from the substrate specificity of hepatic EH_m were noticed.

Table 4 shows that interindividual variations in EH activity were substantially smaller in the investigated extrahepatic tissues than in liver. Nevertheless, persistent differences between individuals could be observed, when lymphocytic EH activity was determined in samples which had been taken from the same subjects on several occasions at approximately monthly intervals (15).

The relatively small interindividual variations in extrahepatic EH activities are in line with animal studies, where EH_m is much more readily induced in the liver than in other tissues (45,47,61). Due to the relatively weak interindividual variations, only a few factors are known which affect (or are associated with) levels of

TABLE 4. *Epoxide hydrolase activity in various human cells and tissues*

Tissue, cells	Preparation	Number of subjects	Range of spec.act.(pmoles BP-4,5-diol/ min/mg protein)	Reference no.
Liver	⎫	166	1,390 − 87,700	a
Lung	⎪	57	410 − 1,890	51[b]
Skin	microsomes	1	447	46
Epidermis	⎪	1	359	46
Subepidermis	⎭	1	112	46
Native lymphocytes	intact cells	2	5.3 − 6.1	18
Native lymphocytes	⎫	88	2.0 − 9.9	15,18,[c]
Cultured lymphocytes	⎪	125	1.8 − 7.0	15,18,[c]
Monocytes	⎪	4	8.6 − 19.0	c
Granulocytes	homogenate	56	7.8 − 19.0	c
Thrombocytes	⎪	53	3.8 − 15.4	c
Erythrocytes	⎪	4	0.11 − 0.24[d]	c
Skin fibroblast cultures	⎭	4	80 − 313	49

[a]F. Oesch, I. Mertes, R. Fleischmann and H.R. Glatt *(manuscript in preparation)*.
[b]Similar activities (610–1600 pmoles BP-4,5-diol/min/mg protein) were found by Greene and Jernström (19) in pulmonary microsomes from 18 subjects.
[c]H.R. Glatt, T. Wölfel, J. Herborn, H. Halfer-Wirgus and F. Oesch *(manuscript in preparation)*.
[d]Incomplete removal of leukocytes cannot be excluded.

extrahepatic EH activities. No differences occur between males and females in the investigated tissues, liver (31, Table 2), lung (51), native and cultured blood components (T. Wölfel, J. Herborn, H. Halfer-Wirgus, H. R. Glatt, and F. Oesch, manuscript in preparation) and in cultured fibroblasts (49). Smokers showed slightly higher activities than nonsmokers in pulmonary microsomes (51), but not in hepatic microsomes (Table 2), lymphocytes (15) nor in cultured fibroblasts (49). Tuberculosis patients treated with rifampicin (and usually with ethambutol and isoniazid) showed not only elevated EH_m activity in the liver, but had also slightly increased EH activities in native lymphocytes and granulocytes, whereas the activities in cultured lymphocytes from treated patients were for unknown reasons even slightly below control (Table 5). Addition of rifampicin to the culture medium of lymphocyte cultures led to an increase in EH activity (Table 6). An increase was also observed with phenobarbital (Table 6), a compound that induces hepatic EH_m activity in man (7). As these increases in activity only occurred after a considerable delay after the addition of rifampicin and phenobarbital, they were probably due to enzyme induction.

Two other compounds, 5,6-benzoflavone and 7,8-benzoflavone, also increased EH activity in lymphocytes (Fig. 2,3). In contrast to phenobarbital and rifampicin, the effects occurred immediately after their addition to the cells. Even addition after homogenization had the same effect, indicating enzyme activation as the mechanism. Figure 3 also demonstrates that EH activities in whole and homogenized lymphocytes were similar. Moreover, the effects of the benzoflavones were practically identical in both systems. This indicates that results obtained in studies on subcellular preparations can provide valid information on the enzyme in its phys-

TABLE 5. *Effect of* in vivo *exposure to rifampicin on epoxide hydrolase activity in liver microsomes and in blood cells*

| | Activity (pmoles BP-4,5-diol/min/mg protein) | | |
Preparation	Control subjects[a]	Treated subjects[b]	(% control)
Liver (microsomes)	9810 ± 5020 (29)	16710 ± 7630 (11)***	(170%)
Lymphocytes (homogenized native cells)	5.70 ± 0.77 (20)	6.89 ± 1.59 (10)**	(121%)
Lymphocytes (homogenized cultured cells)	4.79 ± 0.74 (20)	4.20 ± 0.76 (10)*	(88%)
Granulocytes (homogenized cells)	12.49 ± 2.79 (17)	14.74 ± 2.88 (10)*	(118%)

EH activity was measured as described (15). The conditions used for the culture of lymphocytes were the same as reported (18). For technical reasons, most blood donors were treated for a much shorter time with rifampicin that the subjects from whom liver biopsies were taken. As there was a statistical significant correlation between EH activity in blood cells and treatment period, the data do not allow quantitative comparison between the induction of hepatic and blood EH activities.
[a]Values are means ± S.D. from n (number in brackets) subjects.
[b]Wilcoxon's rank test (two-tailed): * $p < 0.10$; ** $p < 0.05$; *** $p < 0.001$.

TABLE 6. *Induction of epoxide hydrolase activity in cultured lymphocytes*

Subject no.	Activity in control culture (pmoles BP-4,5-diol/ min/mg protein)	Activity compared to control			
		Rifampicin		Phenobarbital	
		4.2 μM	12.5 μM	250 μM	750 μM
		Treatment for 72 hours			
337	4.01 ± .29	157%	197%	113%	142%
302	4.93 ± .38	124%	190%	101%	151%
353	4.39 ± .19	141%	149%	102%	119%
354	5.19 ± .37	153%	166%	140%	166%
355	4.26 ± .17	115%	155%	122%	130%
301	5.51 ± .42	104%	136%	184%	136%
		Treatment for 10 minutes			
301	6.35 ± .23	n.d.[a]	103%	n.d.	95%

EH activity was measured in lymphocyte homogenates as described (15). The conditions used for the lymphocyte cultures were identical with those reported in (18).
[a] n.d., not determined.

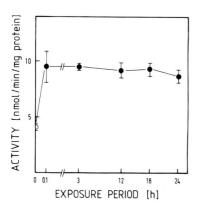

FIG. 2. EH activity in homogenized human lymphocytes after various periods of culturing in the presence of 5,6-benzoflavone (27 μM in medium). The cells of all treatment groups were seeded and harvested at the same time. Different duration of treatment was obtained by addition of 5,6-benzoflavone at different time points. Benzo(*a*)pyrene 4,5-oxide was used as substrate. Values are means with S.D. for 4 determinations. Solvent control *(empty circle)*. (Data from ref. 18, with permission.)

iological environment. These studies with native and cultured lymphocytes show that, in spite of their low specific EH activities with moderate interindividual variation, they are useful for the investigation of various aspects of regulation of human EH.

EPOXIDE HYDROLASES AND TUMOURS

Addition of pure EHs or of EH inhibitors decreases or increases the mutagenicity, DNA-binding and other toxic effects of many compounds in *in vitro* tests (4,11,16,17,22,27). Therefore, it is expected that EH activity levels are partially responsible for determining the susceptibility to such carcinogens. Particularly large differences in EH levels occur between species and tissues, and presumably are of accordingly high significance (albeit in these cases an estimation of this significance is impeded by the occurrence of numerous other differences). A quite different

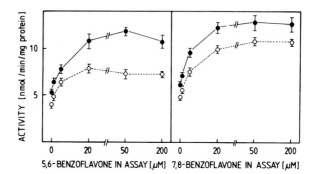

FIG. 3. Effect of 5,6-benzoflavone and 7,8-benzoflavone on EH activity in whole *(solid circle)* or homogenized *(empty circle)* native human lymphocytes. The flavones were added to the cells or cell homogenates immediately before the substrate, benzo(a)pyrene 4,5-oxide. Values are means with S.D. for 4 determinations. (Data from ref. 18, with permission.)

question is whether in man interindividual variations in EH can lead to epidemiologically recognizable differences in carcinogenic risks. So far, the following observations have been made with this respect:

1. Melanoma patients: Normal EH activities (with benzo(a)pyrene 4,5-oxide as substrate) were found in cultures of skin fibroblasts (49).
2. Patients with stomach tumours: Hepatic EH_m (with benzo(a)pyrene 4,5-oxide as substrate) and EH_c activities (with *trans*-stilbene oxide as substrate) did not significantly differ from control subjects (Table 2).
3. Patients with Hodgkin and non-Hodgkin lymphoma: Hepatic EH_m (with benzo(a)pyrene 4,5-oxide as substrate) and EH_c activities (with *trans*-stilbene oxide as substrate) did not significantly differ from control subjects (Table 2).
4. Patients with bronchogenic tumours: Normal levels of EH (with benzo(a)pyrene 4,5-oxide as substrate) were observed in cultures of skin fibroblasts (49). In pulmonary microsomes, specific EH activities (with benzo(a)pyrene 4,5-oxide as substrate) compared to controls (nonsmokers without tumours) were slightly but significantly increased in smokers without cancer (160%, $p<0.0125$) and in bronchogenic carcinoma patients independently of whether they used tobacco products (130%, $p<0.005$) or not (140%, $p<0.05$) (51). On the other hand, smokers with bronchogenic tumours had similar or lower EH_m activities (90%, $p>0.05$) than had smokers without tumours. In two patients with squamous cell carcinoma, EH_m activity was investigated in the tumour and in non-diseased areas of the lung (51). Both tumours only had about one third of the enzyme activity in non-diseased tissue.
5. Patients with hepatocellular carcinoma: So far we have investigated three subjects (I. Mertes, R. Fleischmann, H. R. Glatt, and F. Oesch, unpublished results). Hepatic EH_m (with benzo(a)pyrene 4,5-oxide as substrate) and EH_c activities (with *trans*-stilbene oxide as substrate) in non-diseased tissue did not significantly differ from the activities in control subjects, while in the tumour EH_m activity was markedly decreased.

These data do not yet allow a definite conclusion on the role of EH activities as interindividually varying disposing factors in human carcinogenesis. For instance, if in addition to epoxides other carcinogens also give rise to tumours in the same tissue, even a strong disposition by EHs for epoxide-evoked tumours may be difficult to recognize. Moreover, in all above described studies, EH activities were determined at times long after the initiation of tumours and when treatment and other secondary effects of the tumours may have affected EH activities.

The situation is further complicated by the following interesting, but little understood findings. In animal experiments, many liver carcinogens induce EH_m (9,34,57). This is the case even with carcinogens which are probably not metabolized to epoxides. The induction occurs a few days after application of the compound. After the treatment is ended, EH_m levels in most cells soon return to control levels, but a few foci with increased concentrations of EH_m persist and may develop to hyperplastic nodules (32). Hyperplastic nodules also have a characteristic increase in EH_m levels (32,34,57). It is probable that the liver tumours, which only occur later, develop from some hyperplastic nodules. Various groups have observed increased EH_m levels in these tumours (32,34,57). Kuhlmann et al. (32) interestingly observed increases in EH_m levels in all benign hepatomas, but not in any of the hepatocellular carcinomas investigated. It is not known, whether these changes in EH_m levels during experimental hepatocarcinogenesis are of causal significance or only represent accidental epiphenomena. (In the latter case, they still could serve as markers for more fundamental changes.)

In conclusion, there exist multiple connections between tumour formations and EHs. The changes in EH_m levels during hepatocarcinogenesis suggest that EH_m may be involved in the process of carcinogenesis not only during the metabolism of carcinogens. The limited epidemiological data available on EH characteristics in human subjects developing tumours do not yet allow clear prediction on how strongly individual EH levels affect the probabilities of developing tumours whilst the roles of EHs in the metabolism of several carcinogens are established quite well.

ACKNOWLEDGMENTS

The authors thank C. Timms from our laboratory for critically reading the manuscript. This work was supported by the Bundesministerium für Forschung und Technologie.

REFERENCES

1. Alworth, W. L., Dang, C. C., Ching, L. M., and Viswanathan, T. (1980): *Xenobiotica*, 10:395–400.
2. Bentley, P., and Oesch, F. (1975): *FEBS Lett.*, 59:291–295.
3. Bentley, P., Schmassmann, H. U., Sims, P., and Oesch, F. (1976): *Eur. J. Biochem.*, 69:97–103.
4. Bentley, P., Oesch, F., and Glatt, H. R. (1977): *Arch. Toxicol.*, 39:65–75.
5. Bresnick, E., Mukhtar, H., Stoming, T. A., Dansette, P. M., and Jerina, D. M. (1977): *Biochem. Pharmacol.*, 26:891–892.

6. Cha, Y.-N., Martz, F., and Bueding, E. (1978): *Cancer Res.*, 38:4496–4498.
7. Craven, A. C. C., Walker, C. H., and Murray-Lyon, I. M. (1982): *Biochem. Pharmacol.*, 31:1321–1324.
8. Daly, J. W., Jerina, D. M., and Witkop, B. (1972): *Experientia*, 28:1129–1149.
9. Dent, J. G., and Graichen, M. E. (1982): *Carcinogenesis*, 3:733–738.
10. DuBois, G. C., Appella, E., Ryan, D. E., Jerina, D. M., and Levin, W. (1982): *J. Biol. Chem.*, 257:2708–2712.
11. El-Tantawy, M. E., and Hammock, B. (1980): *Mutat. Res.*, 79:59–71.
12. Ganu, V. S., and Alworth, W. L. (1978): *Biochemistry*, 17:2876–2881.
13. Gill, S. S., and Hammock, B. D. (1980): *Biochem. Pharmacol.*, 29:389–395.
14. Gill, S. S., and Hammock, B. D. (1981): *Nature*, 291:167–168.
15. Glatt, H. R., Kaltenbach, E., and Oesch, F. (1980): *Cancer Res.*, 40:2252–2556.
16. Glatt, H. R., Vogel, K., Bentley, P., Sims, P., and Oesch, F. (1981): *Carcinogenesis*, 2:813–821.
17. Glatt, H. R., Cooper, C. S., Grover, P. L., Bentley, P., Merdes, M., Waechter, F., Vogel, K., Guenthner, T. M., and Oesch, F. (1982): *Science*, 215:1507–1509.
18. Glatt, H. R., Wölfel, T., and Oesch, F. (1983): *Biochem. Biophys. Res. Commun.*, 110:525–529.
19. Greene, F. E., and Jernström, B. (1980): *Cancer Lett.*, 8:235–239.
20. Guengerich, F. P., Wang, P., Mitchell, M. B. and Mason, P. S. (1979): *J. Biol. Chem.*, 254:12248–12254.
21. Guengerich, F. P., Wang, P., Mason, P. S., and Mitchell, M. B. (1979): *J. Biol. Chem.*, 254:12255–12259.
22. Guengerich, F. P., Mason, P. S., Stott, W. T., Fox, T. R., and Watanabe, P. G. (1981): *Cancer Res.*, 41:4391–4398.
23. Guenthner, T. M., Hammock, B. D., Vogel, U., and Oesch, F. (1981): *J. Biol. Chem.*, 256:3163–3166.
24. Halpert, J., Glaumann, H., and Ingelmann-Sundberg, M. (1979): *J. Biol. Chem.*, 254:7434–7441.
25. Hammock, B. D., Gill, S. S., Mumby, S. M., and Ota, K. (1979): In: *Molecular Basis of Environmental Toxicity*, edited by R. S. Bhatnagan, pp. 229–271. Ann Arbor Science, Ann Arbor, Michigan.
26. Jerina, D. M., Dansette, P. M., Lu, A. Y. H., and Levin, W. (1977): *Mol. Pharmacol.*, 13:342–351.
27. Jerina, D. M., Lehr, R., Schaefer-Ridder, M., Yagi, H., Karle, J. M., Thakker, D. R., Wood, A. W., Lu, A. Y. H., Ryan, D., West, S., Levin, W., and Conney, A. H. (1977): In: *Origins of Human Cancer*, edited by H. Hiatt, J. D. Watson, and J. A. Winsten, pp. 639–658. Cold Spring Harbor Laboratory, New York.
28. Kahl, R., and Wulff, U. (1979): *Toxicol. Appl. Pharmacol.*, 47:217–227.
29. Kapitulnik, J., Levin, W., Lu, A. Y. H., Morecki, R., Dansette, P. M., Jerina, D. M., and Conney, A. H. (1977): *Clin. Pharmacol. Ther.*, 21:158–165.
30. Knowles, R. G., and Burchell, B. (1977): *Biochem. Soc. Trans.*, 5:731–732.
31. Kremers, P., Beaune, P., Cresteil, T., de Graeve, J., Columelli, S., Leroux, J.-P., and Gielen, J. E. (1981): *Eur. J. Biochem.*, 118:599–606.
32. Kuhlmann, W. D., Krischan, R., Kunz, W., Guenthner, T. M., and Oesch, F. (1981): *Biochem. Biophys. Res. Commun.*, 98:417–423.
33. Levin, W., Thomas, P. E., Korzeniowski, D., Seifried, H., Jerina, D. M., and Lu, A. Y. H. (1978): *Mol. Pharmacol.*, 14:1107–1120.
34. Levin, W., Lu, A. Y. H., Thomas, P. E., Ryan, D., Kizer, D. E., and Griffin, M. J. (1978): *Proc. Natl. Acad. Sci. USA*, 75:3240–3243.
35. Lu, A. Y. H., and Miwa, G. T. (1981): *Ann. Rev. Pharmacol. Toxicol.*, 20:513–531.
36. Lu, A. Y. H., Jerina, D. M., and Levin, W. (1977): *J. Biol. Chem.*, 252:3715–3723.
37. Lu, A. Y. H., Thomas, P. E., Ryan, D., Jerina, D. M., and Levin, W. (1979): *J. Biol. Chem.*, 254:5878–5881.
38. Lyman, S. D., Poland, A., and Taylor, B. A. (1980): *J. Biol. Chem.*, 255:8650–8654.
39. Oesch, F., Jerina, D. M., and Daly, J. (1971): *Biochim. Biophys. Acta*, 227:685–691.
40. Oesch, F., Kaubisch, N., Jerina, D. M., and Daly, J. W. (1971): *Biochemistry*, 10:4858–4866.
41. Oesch, F. (1973): *Xenobiotica*, 3:305–340.

42. Oesch, F., Morris, N., Daly, J. W., Gielen, J. E., and Nebert, D. W. (1973): *Mol. Pharmacol.*, 9:692–696.
43. Oesch, F. (1974): *Biochem. J.*, 139:77–88.
44. Oesch, F., Bentley, P., and Glatt, H. R. (1976): *Int. J. Cancer*, 18:448–452.
45. Oesch, F., Glatt, H. R., and Schmassmann, H. U. (1977): *Biochem. Pharmacol.*, 26:603–607.
46. Oesch, F., Schmassmann, H. U., and Bentley, P. (1978): *Biochem. Pharmacol.*, 27:17–20.
47. Oesch, F., and Schmassmann, H. U. (1979): *Biochem. Pharmacol.*, 28:171–176.
48. Oesch, F., (1979): In: *Progress in Drug Metabolism, Vol. 3*, edited by J. W. Bridges and L. F. Chasseaud, pp. 253–301. John Witly, Chichester (England).
49. Oesch, F., Tegtmeyer, F., Kohl, F.-V., Rüdiger, H., and Glatt, H. R. (1980): *Carcinogenesis*, 1:305–309.
50. Oesch, F., and Golan, M. (1980): *Cancer Lett.*, 9:169–175.
51. Oesch, F., Schmassmann, H. U., Ohnhaus, E., Althaus, U., and Lorenz, J. (1980): *Carcinogenesis*, 1:827–835.
52. Oesch, F., Friedberg, T., Herbst, M., Paul, W., Wilhelm, N., and Bentley, P. (1982): *Chem.-Biol. Interact.*, 40:1–14.
53. Oesch, F., Zimmer, A., and Glatt, H. R. (1983): *Biochem. Pharmacol.*, 32:1783–1788.
54. Ota, K., and Hammock, B. D. (1980): *Science*, 207:1479–1480.
55. Raphael, D., Glatt, H. R., Protić-Sabljić, M., and Oesch, F. (1982): *Chem.-Biol. Interact.*, 42:27–43.
56. Schmassmann, H. U., Sparrow, A., Platt, K., and Oesch, F. (1978): *Biochem. Pharmacol.*, 27:2237–2245.
57. Sharma, R. N., Gurtoo, H. L., Farber, E., Murray, R. K., and Cameron, R. G. (1981): *Cancer Res.*, 41:3311–3319.
58. Sims, P., Grover, P. L., Swaisland, A., Pal, K., and Hewer, A. (1974): *Nature*, 252:326–328.
59. Stasiecki, P., Oesch, F., Bruder, G., Jarasch, E.-D., and Franke, W. W. (1980): *Eur. J. Cell Biol.*, 21:79–92.
60. Tybring, G., von Bahr, C., Bertilsson, L., Collste, H., Glaumann, H., and Solbrand, M. (1981): *Drug. Metab. Disp.*, 9:561–564.
61. van Cantfort, J., Manil, L., Gielen, J. E., Glatt, H. R., and Oesch, F. (1977): *Biochem. Pharmacol.*, 26:603–607.
62. Vaz, A. D., Fiorica, V. M., and Griffin, M. J. (1981): *Biochem. Pharmacol.*, 30:651–656.
63. Vogel-Bindel, U., Bentley, P., and Oesch, F. (1982): *Eur. J. Biochem.*, 126:425–431.
64. Waechter, F., Merdes, M., Bieri, F., Stäubli, W., and Bentley, P. (1982): *Eur. J. Biochem.*, 125:457–461.
65. Walker, C. H., Bentley, P., and Oesch, F. (1978): *Biochim. Biophys. Acta*, 539:427–434.
66. Watabe, T., Kanai, M., Isobe, M., and Ozawa, N. (1981): *Biochim. Biophys. Acta*, 619:414–419.

Biochemical Basis of Chemical Carcinogenesis,
edited by H. Greim, R. Jung, M. Kramer,
H. Marquardt, and F. Oesch.
Raven Press, New York © 1984.

Carcinogen Metabolism and Carcinogen-DNA Adducts in Human Tissues and Cells

*Curtis C. Harris, *Roland C. Grafstrom,
*†Abulkalam M. Shamsuddin, *Nuntia T. Sinopoli,
†Benjamin F. Trump, and *Herman Autrup

*Laboratory of Human Carcinogenesis, National Cancer Institute, Bethesda, Maryland
20205; †Department of Pathology, University of Maryland School of Medicine,
Baltimore, Maryland 21201

Since many environmental chemical carcinogens require metabolic activation to exert their mutagenic and carcinogenic effects, studies of carcinogen metabolism in human tissues and cells are of obvious importance. Early studies were mostly restricted to measuring enzyme activities in subcellular fractions of human tissues obtained at surgery. Although these studies have provided much useful information, a number of limitations are evident including (a) limited possibility for experimental manipulation of the tissues such as testing the effects of enzyme inducers and (b) so called "fresh" tissues obtained at surgery have frequently undergone various degrees of ischemic injury (6). Peripheral blood cells and amniotic cells have also been utilized (see Chapter 10), but metabolism in these cells may not necessarily quantitatively reflect the metabolism of carcinogens in specific target tissues.

One successful approach for investigating carcinogen metabolism has been to develop the methodology to maintain human tissues in a controlled *in vitro* environment (9,13). Tissues from many of the major sites of human cancer can be maintained *in vitro* for periods of weeks to more than 1 year (15,16). Culture of the tissue prior to exposure to carcinogens has the advantage that tissues collected at surgery or autopsy display morphological and biochemical evidence of ischemic injury which can be readily reversible in the cultured tissues (Fig. 1). Chemically defined media have certain advantages, including less variability when compared to media containing sera, and such media have been developed for explant cultures of human bronchus, colon, pancreatic duct, and esophagus (15,16). In addition, human epithelial cells from either bronchus (23) or skin (28) can be cloned and grown for 20 to 30 cell generations in chemically defined media.

Using these *in vitro* model systems, the metabolism of chemical carcinogens, formation of carcinogen-macromolecular adducts, and DNA repair can now be studied at several levels of biological organization, i.e., cells and tissues. Since we have recently reviewed the published studies concerning carcinogen metabolism

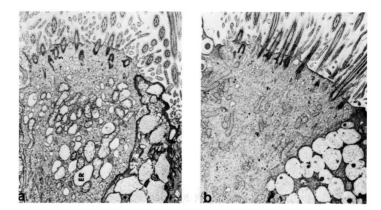

FIG. 1. a, Morphologic changes including swollen endoplasmic reticulum and mitochondrial swelling indicate irreversible ischemic cellular damage in the human bronchial epithelium. **b,** Reversal of the ischemic injury is seen in bronchial explants cultured for 24 hrs. (Data adapted from ref. 6).

and DNA repair in human tissues and cells (1,5,10,17,18), we will focus this report primarily on investigations concerning interspecies and interindividual differences in carcinogen metabolism conducted in our laboratories and present examples of recent results.

CARCINOGEN METABOLISM AND CARCINOGEN DNA ADDUCTS

Our strategy has been to first select representative procarcinogens from several chemical classes that are found in tobacco smoke and/or in the environment and then determine whether or not these procarcinogens are activated to metabolites that bind to DNA. The amount of binding could be considered as a simplistic estimate of the balance between metabolic activation and deactivation of the procarcinogen.

Mean binding values of several chemical carcinogens to DNA in cultured human bronchus are shown in Table 1. Interestingly, cultured human bronchus can activate carcinogens from all the chemical classes tested to date. Several of these procarcinogens have been studied in detail. In collaboration with our coworkers, the major carcinogen-DNA adducts have been identified for aflatoxin B_1, benzo(a)pyrene, 7,12-dimethylbenz(a)anthracene, N-nitrosodimethylamine, and N-nitrosomethylbenzylamine (Fig. 2). In each case, the predominant adducts are identical to those found in experimental animals in which these chemicals have been shown to be carcinogenic.

As a representative polycyclic aromatic hydrocarbon, benzo(a)pyrene metabolism has been extensively investigated. The metabolic pathway leading to the major carcinogen-DNA adduct is shown in Fig. 3. Binding of benzo(a)pyrene metabolite to bronchial DNA is dependent on substrate concentration, length of exposure time, and temperature of incubation (11). Aryl hydrocarbon hydroxylase activity is in-

TABLE 1. *Binding of chemical carcinogens to DNA in cultured human bronchus and colon[a]*

	Bronchus	Colon
Polycyclic Aromatic Hydrocarbons (1.5 μM)		
benzo*(a)*pyrene 7,8-diol	471[b] (3)[c]	9 (4)
7,12-dimethylbenz*(a)*anthracene	118 (28)	8 (3)
3-methylcholanthrene	34 (2)	15 (3)
benzo*(a)*pyrene	32 (15)	6 (145)
dibenz*(a,h)*anthracene	28 (4)	nt[d]
Mycotoxin (1.5 μM)		
aflatoxin B$_1$	14 (17)	3 (29)
N-Nitrosamines (100 μM)		
N-nitrosodimethylamine	906 (15)	215 (24)
N-nitrosodiethylamine	264 (4)	4 (6)
N-nitrosopyrrolidine	183 (4)	<1 (4)
Others		
1,2-dimethylhydrazine (100 μM)	675 (4)	904 (120)
2-acetylaminofluorene (1.5 μM)	73 (13)	nt
Trp-P-1 (10 μM)	nt	11 (2)

[a]The explants were cultured for 1 (colon) or 7 (bronchus) days in chemically defined media prior to addition of the radioactively labeled carcinogens. After incubation for 24 hrs, mucosa was removed by scraping and the DNA isolated and purified by either CsCl gradient centrifugation or by hydroxylapatite chromatography.
[b]pmoles carcinogen bound per 10 mg DNA.
[c]number of cases studied.
[d]nt, not tested.

duced by pretreatment of the cultured bronchi with benz(*a*)anthracene and is reduced by cycloheximide, an inhibitor of protein synthesis (12). Benz(*a*)anthracene does not induce epoxide hydrolase. Cultured mean bronchial epithelial cells metabolize benzo(*a*)pyrene and bind its metabolites to DNA three-fold greater than do human bronchial fibroblasts (12,23). When metabolism of benzo(*a*)pyrene is compared at different levels of biological organization, bronchial cells and explants provide similar qualitative profiles of metabolites but qualitative and quantitative differences in organosoluble and water-soluble metabolites are found in a subcellular fraction (5). Binding of benzo(*a*)pyrene metabolite to colonic or bronchial DNA is reduced by inhibitors of aryl hydrocarbon hydroxylase, i.e., 7,8-benzoflavone, disulfiram, and butylated hydroxytoluene, and not affected by either β-retinyl acetate or nicotine (Table 2). When compared to the parent compound, the proximate carcinogenic form of benzo(*a*)pyrene 7,8-diol, is more readily metabolized to diol epoxide which is bound to DNA. In addition, benzo(*a*)pyrene 9,10-diol is activated, possibly by epoxidation of 4-5 positions, to a metabolite that forms an unidentified DNA adduct in cultured human bronchus (29).

INTERSPECIES COMPARISONS

If the metabolism of a carcinogen and the resultant carcinogen-DNA adducts are similar in experimental animals and humans, then the extrapolation of carcinogenesis

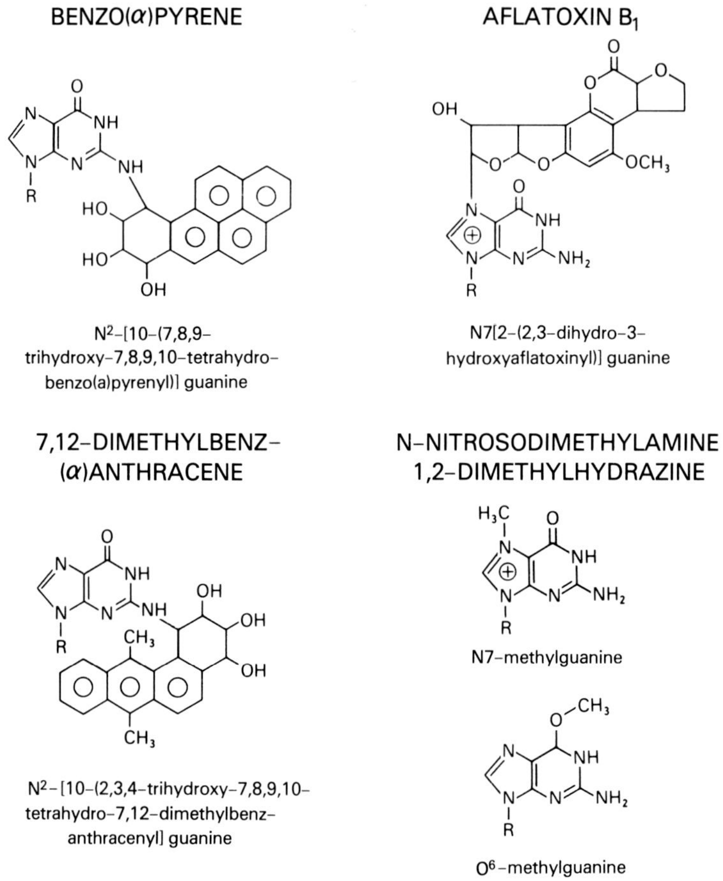

BENZO(α)PYRENE

AFLATOXIN B$_1$

N^2–[10–(7,8,9–
trihydroxy–7,8,9,10–tetrahydro–
benzo(a)pyrenyl)] guanine

N7[2–(2,3–dihydro–3–
hydroxyaflatoxinyl)] guanine

7,12–DIMETHYLBENZ–
(α)ANTHRACENE

N–NITROSODIMETHYLAMINE
1,2–DIMETHYLHYDRAZINE

N7–methylguanine

N^2–[10–(2,3,4–trihydroxy–7,8,9,10–
tetrahydro–7,12–dimethylbenz–
anthracenyl] guanine

O^6–methylguanine

FIG. 2. Major DNA adducts found in cultured human tissues exposed to chemical carcinogens.

data from experimental animals to the human situation is more likely to be valid than if the metabolic pathways differ. The available data are consistent with this hypothesis.

Comparison of xenobiotic metabolism, including metabolism of chemical carcinogens in animal species, has revealed qualitative differences (7). Examples of defective reactions include (a) *N*-hydroxylation of aromatic amines in guinea pigs, (b) *N*-hydroxylation of aliphatic amines in rats, (c) acetylation of many primary amino groups in dogs, and (d) glucuronidation of small phenols and aromatic acids in cats. The deficiency in *N*-hydroxylation of carcinogenic aromatic amines may be responsible for the resistance of guinea pigs to these carcinogens. Although humans have defective metabolism of specific chemicals, none of the pathways important in the activation of chemical carcinogens are defective in all humans. As will be discussed in the next section of this brief review, quantitative differences

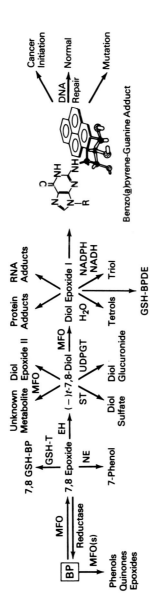

FIG. 3. Alternative pathways to diol epoxide I formation and DNA binding. Metabolic pathways of benzo(a)pyrene leading to its major DNA adduct that can either be removed with good fidelity by DNA repair enzymes or, if not, lead to mutagenic and carcinogenic events. *MFO*, mixed function oxidase; *EH*, epoxide hydrolase; *GSH*, glutathione; *GSH-T*, glutathione transferase.

TABLE 2. *Effect of exogenous chemicals on the binding of benzo*(a)*pyrene to DNA by cultured human bronchus and colon[a]*

Compound	Concentration (μM)	Percentage of control	Number of cases
Bronchus			
7,8-Benzoflavone	20	33 $\pm$ 7[c]	4
Disulfiram	10	80 $\pm$ 21	4
	100	69 $\pm$ 19	6
DL-α-Tocopherol	10	106 $\pm$ 16	4
	100	63 $\pm$ 13	4
β-Retinyl acetate	3	128 $\pm$ 38	5
	30	101 $\pm$ 27	5
Aminophylline[b]	100	121 $\pm$ 33	4
	1000	198 $\pm$ 96	5
Colon			
Butylated hydroxytoluene	100	49 $\pm$ 10	3
Bisacodyl	10	76 $\pm$ 75	5
Disulfiram	100	89 $\pm$ 20	4
Lithocholic acid	1	142 $\pm$ 51	15
Taurodeoxycholic acid	5	178 $\pm$ 129	12
Phenobarbital[b]	100	315 $\pm$ 153	3

[a]Data adapted from ref. 1.
[b]Preincubation of the explants with the compounds for 24 hrs prior to addition of [^{3}H]-benzo*(a)*pyrene. The other compounds dissolved in DMSO (0.05%) were added concomitantly with [^{3}H]-benzo*(a)*pyrene.
[c]The results represent the mean $\pm$ S.D.

are found among individuals in outbred populations, including humans, and among inbred strains of experimental animals.

The subject of interspecies differences in metabolism of chemical carcinogens has been recently reviewed (5). In our studies, benzo(a)pyrene has been used as a prototype to investigate differences in metabolism in tracheobronchial tissues (3). The distributions of organosoluble and water-soluble metabolites are qualitatively similar in the experimental animals tested and humans (Table 3). Quantitative differences are evident including the total amount of metabolites and ratio of organosoluble to water-soluble metabolites. A ratio of less than one is found in CD rats and C57 black mice which are relatively less susceptible to benzo(a)pyrene carcinogenicity when compared to Syrian golden hamsters and the C3H mice. The mean binding values of benzo(a)pyrene metabolite to DNA in the cultured tracheobronchial tissues are within one order of magnitude. As will be discussed later, interindividual differences are narrow in the inbred animals and wide in outbred animals, including cows and humans. The major DNA adduct has been shown to be formed by the reaction of (+)-(7β, 8α)-dihydroxy(9α, 10α)-epoxy-7,8,9,10-tetrahydrobenzo(a)pyrene with the 2-amino group of guanine in both animal species. Similar results have been observed in a comparative study of benzo(a)pyrene metabolism in tracheobronchial and bladder tissues of monkey, dog, hamster, rat, and human (8).

TABLE 3. *Metabolism of benzo(a)pyrene by cultured tracheobronchial tissues[a]*

	Bovine bronchus	Syrian hamster trachea	Rat trachea	Mouse trachea		Human bronchus
				C57B1/6N	DBA/2N	
Total metabolites[b]	0.93 ± 0.12	1.34 ± 0.13	0.65 ± 0.10	1.00 ± 0.25	0.40 ± 0.13	1.33 ± 0.72
Total water-soluble[b]	0.83 ± 0.06	0.61 ± 0.03	0.43 ± 0.01	0.42 ± 0.11	0.27 ± 0.07	0.50 ± 0.28
% of water-soluble metabolites						
Sulphate esters	24	20	31	31	28	44
Glucuronides	29	17	13	30	27	7
Glutathione-conjugates	38	63	56	39	44	51
Total organic extractable metabolites[b]	0.10 ± 0.04	0.73 ± 0.08	0.21 ± 0.07	0.58 ± 0.08	0.13 ± 0.03	0.83 ± 0.46
% of organosoluble metabolites						
(7,10/8,9)-Tetrol	26	28	2	4	7	10
(7,9,10/8)-Tetrol	10	10	6	7	17	10
(7,9,10/8)-Tetrol	4	ND[c]	5	1	5	1
(7/8,9)-Triol and trans-9,10-diol	8	22	12	9	12	28
trans-4,5-diol	16	1	8	1	4	4
trans-7,8-diol	5	6	6	16	4	5
3-hydroxy	3	3	8	3	6	2
9-hydroxy	2	3	8	6	3	4
Quinones	17	3	27	6	28	26
Unidentified	21	2	8	29	13	3

[a]Data adapted from ref. 3.
[b]Expressed as pmoles metabolites per 1 μg DNA. The results are mean ± S.D. of at least three experiments.
[c]Not detectable.

Metabolism of benzo(a)pyrene, aflatoxin B_1, and 1,2-dimethylhydrazine has been studied using cultured rat or human colon (2). Both rat and human colon activate these carcinogens into metabolites that react with cellular macromolecules. The major DNA adducts and metabolic profiles of 1,2-dimethylhydrazine and aflatoxin B_1 are qualitatively similar as in both rats and humans. However, the mean binding values to DNA of 1,2-dimethylhydrazine and aflatoxin B_1 are higher in rats than in humans. Although benzo(a)pyrene-guanine adducts were the major ones in both species, benzo(a)pyrene-adenine adducts are detectable only in the cultured rat colon.

When compared to polycyclic aromatic hydrocarbons (benzo(a)pyrene), a mycotoxin (aflatoxin B_1), and a methylhydrazine (1,2-dimethylhydrazine), marked differences in the metabolism of N-nitrosamines have been found in rat and human esophagi (4). Metabolism of both acyclic (N-nitrosodimethylamine, N-nitrosoethylmethylamine, N-nitrosodiethylamine) and cyclic (N-nitrosopyrrolidine) N-nitrosamines has been investigated by measuring CO_2 production, metabolites with an oxo group, and metabolites bound to DNA. N-Nitrosobenzylmethylamine, a potent organotropic carcinogen for the rat esophagus, is oxidized to metabolites that are bound to rat esophageal DNA in at least 100-fold higher amounts when compared to cultured human esophagus. Rat esophageal DNA is methylated at positions 7 and 0^6 of guanine by N-nitrosobenzylmethylamine. The level of benzylation in rat is one-tenth the level of methylation. Since formation of benzaldehyde exceeded that of formaldehyde plus CO_2, the methylene group of N-nitrosobenzylmethylamine is preferentially oxidized. N-Nitrosopyrrolidine is oxidized by both rat and human esophagus in the position as measured by the formation of 2,4-dinitrophenylhydrazone derivative of 4-hydroxybutanal. Although binding of metabolites of N-nitrosopyrrolidine to DNA is detected only in rat esophagus, N-nitrosodimethylamine is metabolized as measured by the formation of both CO_2 and formaldehyde, by both human and rat esophagus. Again, methylation of the guanine positions 7 and 0^6 is detected by chromatography of the hydrolyzed rat DNA. The results indicate significant quantitative and perhaps qualitative differences between cultured rat and human esophagus in their ability to activate N-nitrosamines.

INTERINDIVIDUAL DIFFERENCES

One would predict that metabolism of chemical carcinogens among individual humans would be quantitatively different by one or more orders of magnitude based on predictions from clinical investigations of drug metabolism (22) and from studies of carcinogen metabolism among inbred strains of experimental animals (25).

Wide interindividual differences in the activities of enzymes important in the metabolism of polycyclic aromatic hydrocarbons have been reported. Using primarily subcellular fractions of human tissues and cells obtained at surgery, more than a 10-fold difference in activity of aryl hydrocarbon hydroxylase has been found in human skin, bronchus, liver, and placenta (Table 4). Differences in epoxide

TABLE 4. *Interindividual variation in aryl hydrocarbon hydroxlase and epoxide hydrolase activities in human tissues[a]*

Specimen	Aryl hydrocarbon hydroxylase activity		Epoxide hydrolase activity	
	Interindividual variation in activity	Number of cases in each study	Interindividual variation in activity	Number of cases in each study
Liver	3	6	2	6
	4	26	8	8
	7	6	17	71
	14	20		
	30	27		
	60	15		
	76	32		
Lung	5	14	4	57
	13	13		
	20	76		
Bronchus	10	13	3	4
	20	10		
Placenta	156	97	8	21
	275	21		
	300	24		
	350	24		
Skin	3	13	3	6
	3	6		
	7	27		
	7	13		
Kidney	3	10		
	12	23		

[a]Data adapted from ref. 18.

hydrolase and enzymes important in detoxification pathways are less than those observed in activity of aryl hydrocarbon hydroxylase (see Chapter 12). The relative importance of genetic versus environmental factors in determining these differences is as yet unknown.

As mentioned earlier, binding values of carcinogens to DNA vary among individuals in outbred populations. Wide interindividual differences in binding of activated chemical carcinogen to DNA in cultured human tissues have been observed (17). The magnitude (50- to 150-fold) of these differences among individuals is wider than differences found among either tissues (bronchus, esophagus, colon, and duodenum) from the same individual (5) or anatomic segments of each tissue type (3,14). These inter- and intra-tissue differences are generally within one order of magnitude.

Interindividual differences have also been investigated using tissue- or cell-mediated mutagenesis assays (19,20). Human tissue explants or cells serve as a procarcinogen activating system, and the frequencies of either mutations or sister chromatid exchanges are measured in cocultivated Chinese hamster V-79 cells. A very significant statistical correlation exists between binding values of benzo(*a*)pyrene metabolite to DNA in cultured human bronchi and the frequency of ouabain-resistant mutations in the V-79 cells. The variation in tissue-mediated mutation frequency among bronchi from different donors is approximately 50-fold. In addition, human pulmonary alveolar macrophages also have the capability to activate benzo(*a*)pyrene and to mediate mutagenesis in V-79 cells.

Investigations in biochemical epidemiology are providing us with intriguing albeit preliminary results. In our ongoing study, benzo(*a*)pyrene metabolism and DNA adduct formation is being investigated in cultured, nontumorous bronchi from patients either with or without lung cancer. Binding values are similar in nontumorous bronchi from patients without cancer or with lung carcinomas displaying primarily features of well-differentiated adenocarcinomas. In contrast, significantly higher values are found in bronchi from individuals with primarily epidermoid differentiated cancers. In each category, a family history of cancer is associated with higher binding values which is most significant in the epidermoid group. The contribution of possible confounding factors is being studied.

DETECTION OF CARCINOGEN-DNA ADDUCTS IN HUMAN POPULATIONS

Knowing that several chemical carcinogens found in the environment and/or tobacco smoke are both metabolically activated into electrophilic metabolites and form specific DNA adducts in cultured human tissues and cells, the next logical step is to determine if such adducts can be detected in people who are exposed to these carcinogens due to either occupation or personal habits, e.g., tobacco smoking. Advances in biotechnology have made this search for adducts feasible. Both immunologic and biophysical approaches are now available. The initial investigations have utilized specific antibodies to carcinogen-DNA adducts, e.g., benzo(*a*)pyrene-modified DNA (26) and highly sensitive enzyme radioimmunoassays (21). Perera et al. and Harris et al. have recently reported at an international meeting ("The Development and Possible Use of Immunological Techniques to Detect Individual Exposure to Carcinogen," Essen, November 30, 1981) the finding of benzo(*a*)pyrene-DNA antigenicity in lung and samples of white blood cells obtained from individuals suspected to be exposed to this carcinogenic polycyclic aromatic hydrocarbon. For example, 7 of 20 samples from foundry workers and 7 of 28 samples from roofers were positive for benzo(*a*)pyrene-DNA antigenicity (range 0.04 to 2.5 femtomoles per μg DNA) in white blood cells (unpublished data). Similar levels of antigenicity have also been found in nontumorous lung tissues obtained at either surgery or autopsy (unpublished data). These results were confirmed by an independent biophysical approach, i.e., photon-counting fluorimetry.

Another promising biophysical approach has been recently described by Randerath et al. (27). They have developed an enzymatic ^{32}P post-labeling method in which the nucleotides, including carcinogen modified ones, are labeled with ^{32}P, resolved by anion-exchange thin-layer chromatography on polyethyleneimine-cellulose, and detected by autoradiography.

Therefore, by using these complementary immunologic and biophysical approaches, it will be possible to investigate the relationship between environmental exposure to chemical carcinogens and amount of DNA damage in various cells and tissues. The rate of removal of these DNA adducts can also be studied. Eventually, the association between these DNA lesions and cancer risk can be determined.

CONCLUSIONS

Recent progress in the development of conditions to culture epithelial tissues and cells from adult humans has provided cancer researchers an opportunity to investigate various facets of carcinogenesis directly in human cells. Studies of activation and deactivation of several chemical classes of carcinogens have revealed that the metabolic pathways and the predominant adducts formed with DNA are generally similar in humans and experimental animals; however, wide interindividual differences are found in humans and other outbred animal species. When the metabolic capabilities of specimens from different levels of biological organization are compared, the profiles of benzo(*a*)pyrene metabolites are similar in cultured tissues and cells, but subcellular fractions, e.g., microsomes, produce a qualitative and quantitative aberrant pattern. To test the interactive effects of cell types in individual differences among people, human tissue- and cell-mediated mutagenesis assays have been developed. The fact that terminally differentiated cells such as pulmonary alveolar macrophages can activate benzo(*a*)pyrene and mediate an increase in frequencies of both mutations and sister chromatid exchanges in cocultivated "detector" cell populations, i.e., Chinese hamster V-79 cells, suggests that nontarget cells of chemical carcinogens may play an important role in the activation of environmental carcinogens. Interindividual differences in carcinogen-DNA adducts are also being found in studies of biochemical epidemiology. Using specific antibodies and highly sensitive enzyme radioimmunoassays, benzo(*a*)pyrene-DNA antigenicity have been detected in lung specimens and white blood cells. The relationship between environmental exposure and tissue levels of benzo(*a*)pyrene is being studied.

Carcinogenesis studies using cultured human tissues and cells are providing new insights into the mechanisms of human carcinogenesis and are aiding efforts to identify host factors that influence individual risk to environmental and endogenous carcinogens.

ACKNOWLEDGMENTS

We are indebted to our coworkers, A. Apostolides, J. Essigmann, I.-C. Hsu, A. Jeffreys, J. Lechner, P. Schafer, T. Sugimura, I. B. Weinstein, and G. N. Wogan who have contributed to our investigations. We appreciate the secretarial aid of N. Paige.

REFERENCES

1. Autrup, H. (1982): Metabolism of chemical carcinogen by cultured human tissues and cells. *Drug. Metab. Rev.*, 13:603–648.

2. Autrup, H., Schwartz, R. D., Essigmann, J. M., Smith, L., Trump, B. F., and Harris, C. C. (1980): Metabolism of aflatoxin B_1, benoz(a)pyrene, and 1,2 dimethylhydrazine by cultured rat and human colon. *Teratogenesis, Mutagenesis and Carcinogenesis*, 1:3–13.
3. Autrup, H., Wefald, F., Jeffrey, A., Tate, H., Schwartz, R. D., Trump, B. F., and Harris, C. C. (1980): Metabolism of benzo(a)pyrene by cultured tracheobronchial tissues from mice, rats, hamsters, bovines, and humans. *Int. J. Cancer*, 25:293–300.
4. Autrup, H., and Stoner, G. D. (1982): Metabolism of N-nitrosamines by cultured human and rat esophagus. *Cancer Res.*, 42:1307–1311.
5. Autrup, H., Grafstrom, R. C., and Harris, C. C.: Metabolism of chemical carcinogens by tracheobronchial tissues. In: *Organ and Species Specificity in Chemical Carcinogenesis*, edited by J. Rice, R. Langenbach, and S. Nesnow. Plenum Press, New York (*in press*).
6. Barrett, L., McDowell, E., Harris, C., and Trump, B. (1977): Studies on the pathogenesis of ischemic cell injury. XV. Reversal of ischemic cell injury in hamster trachea and human bronchus by explant culture. *Beitrage zur Pathologie*, 161:109–122.
7. Caldwell, J. (1981): The current status of attempts to predict species differences in drug metabolism. *Drug. Metab. Rev.*, 12:221–237.
8. Daniels, F. B., Stoner, G. D., Sandwisch, D. W., Schenck, K. M., Hoffman, C. A., Schut, H. A. J., and Patrick, J. R.: Interspecies comparisons of benzo(a)pyrene metabolism and DNA-adduct formation in cultured human and animal bladder and tracheobronchial tissues. *Cancer Res.* (*in press*).
9. Harris, C. (1976): Chemical carcinogenesis and experimental models using human tissues. *Beitrage zur Pathologie*, 158:389–404.
10. Harris, C. C.: Role of carcinogens, cocarcinogens, and host factors in human cancer risk. In: *Human Carcinogenesis*, edited by C. C. Harris and H. Autrup. Academic Press, New York (*in press*).
11. Harris, C., Frank, A., van Haaften, C., Kaufman, D., Connor, R., Jackson, F., Barrett, L., McDowell, E., and Trump, B. (1976): Binding of [³H] benzo(a)pyrene to DNA in cultured human bronchus. *Cancer Res.*, 36:1011–1018.
12. Harris, C., Autrup, H., Stoner, G., Yang, S., Leutz, J., Gelboin, H., Selkirk, J., Connor, R., Barrett, L., Jones, R., McDowell, E., and Trump, B. F. (1977): Metabolism of benzo(a)pyrene and 7,12-dimethylbenz(a)anthracene in cultured human bronchus and pancreatic duct. *Cancer Res.*, 37:3349–3355.
13. Harris, C., Autrup, H., Stoner, G., and Trump, B. (1978): Carcinogenesis studies in human respiratory epithelium: An experimental model system. In: *Pathogenesis and Therapy of Lung Cancer*, edited by C. Harris, pp. 559–608. M. Dekker, Inc., New York.
14. Harris, C. C., Autrup, H., Stoner, G. D., Trump, B. F., Hillman, E., Schafer, P., and Jeffrey, A. (1979): Metabolism of benzo(a)pyrene, N-nitrosodimethylamine, and N-nitrosopyrrolidine and identification of the major carcinogen-DNA adducts formed in cultured human esophagus. *Cancer Res.*, 39:4401–4407.
15. Harris, C. C., Trump, B. F., and Stoner, G. D., editors (1980): *Cultured Normal Human Tissues and Cells, Vol. 21A*. Academic Press, New York.
16. Harris, C. C., Trump, B. F., and Stoner, G. D., editors (1980): *Cultured Normal Human Tissues and Cells, Vol. 21B*. Academic Press, New York.
17. Harris, C. C., Trump, B. F., Grafstrom, R., and Autrup, H. (1982): Differences in metabolism of chemical carcinogens in cultured human epithelial tissues and cells. *J. Cell Biochem.*, 18:285–294.
18. Harris, C. C., Grafstrom, R. C., Lechner, J. F., and Autrup, H.: Metabolism of N-nitrosamines and DNA repair in cultured human tissues and cells. In: *Banbury Reports, Vol. 12*, edited by P. Magee. Cold Spring Harbor Laboratory, Cold Spring Harbor (*in press*).
19. Hsu, I.-C., Autrup, H., Stoner, G. D., Trump, B. F., Selkirk, J. K., and Harris, C. C. (1978): Human bronchus-mediated mutagenesis of mammalian cells by carcinogenic polynuclear aromatic hydrocarbons. *Proc. Natl. Acad. Sci. USA*, 75:2003–2007.
20. Hsu, I.-C., Harris, C. C., Trump, B. F., Schafer, P. W., and Yamaguchi, M. (1979): Induction of ouabain-resistant mutation and sister chromatid exchanges in Chinese hamster cells with chemical carcinogens mediated by human pulmonary macrophages. *J. Clinical Invest.*, 64:1245–1252.
21. Hsu, I.-C., Poirier, M. C., Yuspa, S. H., Grunberger, D., Weinstein, I. B., Yolken, R. H., and Harris, C. C. (1981): Measurement of benzo(a)pyrene-DNA adducts by enzyme immunoassays and radioimmunoassays. *Cancer Res.*, 41:1091–1096.

22. Idle, J. R., and Ritchie, J. C.: Probing genetic variable carcinogen metabolism using drugs. In: *Human Carcinogenesis*, edited by C. C. Harris and H. Autrup. Academic Press, New York (*in press*).
23. Lechner, J. F., Haugen, A., Autrup, H., McClendon, I. A., Trump, B. F., and Harris, C. C. (1981): Clonal growth of epithelial cells from normal adult human bronchus. *Cancer Res.*, 41:2294–2304.
24. Lechner, J. F., Haugen, H. A., McClendon, I. A., and Pettis, E. W. (1982): Clonal growth of normal adult human bronchial epithelial cells in a serum-free medium. *In Vitro*, 18:636–642.
25. Nebert, D. W., Levitt, R. C., and Pelkonen, O. (1979): Genetic variation in metabolism of chemical carcinogens associated with susceptibility to tumorigenesis. In: *Carcinogens: Identification and Mechanisms of Action*, edited by A. C. Griffin and C. R. Shaw, pp. 157–185. Raven Press, New York.
26. Poirier, M. C., Santella, R., Weinstein, I. B., Grunberger, D., and Yuspa, S. H. (1980): Quantitation of benzo(a)pyrene-deoxyguanosine adducts by radioimmunoassay. *Cancer Res.*, 40:412–416.
27. Randerath, K., Reddy, M. W., and Gupta, R. C. (1981): ^{32}P-labeling test for DNA damage. *Proc. Natl. Acad. Sci.*, 78:6126–6129.
28. Tsao, M. C., Walthall, B. J., and Ham, R. G. (1982): Clonal growth of normal human epidermal keratinocytes in a defined medium. *J. Cell Physiol.*, 110:219–229.
29. Yang, S. F., Gelboin, H. V., Trump, B. F., Autrup, H. N., and Harris, A. C. (1977): Metabolic activation of benzo(a)pyrene and DNA binding in cultured human bronchus. *Cancer Res.*, 37:1210–1215.

Biochemical Basis of Chemical Carcinogenesis,
edited by H. Greim, R. Jung, M. Kramer,
H. Marquardt, and F. Oesch.
Raven Press, New York © 1984.

Oncogenes and Chemical Carcinogenesis

Robert A. Weinberg

*Whitehead Institute for Biomedical Research, Center for Cancer Research and
Department of Biology, Massachusetts Institute of Technology,
Cambridge, Massachusetts 02139*

The molecular basis of carcinogenesis is poorly understood. Although a carcin ogen may introduce a large number of lesions in the genomes of target cells, only a few of these are likely to be relevant to subsequent appearance of the malignant phenotype. Moreover, the chemical structure of the lesions that are productive for oncogenesis is unclear; and the identity of critical target sequences in the cellular genome has similarly eluded definition.

One might even question whether alteration of DNA is directly involved in the process of carcinogenesis, since the literature suggests only correlations between mutation and oncogenic transformation rather than proving any causal role on the part of the mutations. It was this last issue that we addressed several years ago by undertaking experiments which analyzed the DNAs of 3-methyl-cholanthrene trans- formed mouse fibroblasts (12). We extracted the DNA from these transformed cells and applied it to untransformed NIH3T3 mouse fibroblast cultures, using the gene transfer technique of Graham and van der Eb (6). As a consequence of these manipulations, foci of transformed cells appeared in the culture that had undergone gene transfer. DNA of untransformed cells was unable to elicit this effect. This indicated directly a structural difference between the two DNAs which was highly relevant to oncogenic phenotype. It showed, moreover, that the phenotype was encoded, at least in part, by sequences of the tumor cell DNA.

The tumor cells from which these DNAs had been prepared were C3H10T1/2 cells transformed by exposure to 3-methyl cholanthrene. One can presume that this carcinogen was able to effect an alteration of the target cell genome in a way that led to creation of the transforming sequences. This work does not resolve the issue of whether this important alteration arose as a direct or indirect consequence of the carcinogen-genome interaction.

Gene transfers (transfections) of this type were subsequently used by several groups to demonstrate the presence of transforming sequences in a number of human tumors. These tumors range from promyelocytic leukemias and Burkitt's lymphomas to a series of carcinomas including those of the colon, breast, and lung (3). These results prove that the oncogenic sequences of these various tumors can transform cells of quite different tissue and species origin. This means that the NIH3T3 transfection-focus assay is potentially useful in analyzing sequences from a wide variety of tumor cells. Unfortunately, only 10 to 15% of any group of tumor cell DNAs is able to yield DNAs that are active in this assay. The explanation of such results is unclear. It may be that only these tumors have dominantly acting oncogenes that are capable of transforming mouse fibroblasts. Alternatively, it remains possible that the transfection assay has not been developed and exploited to its full potential, and the negative results may disappear as refinements are introduced into the gene transfer procedures and the type of recipient cells used.

ISOLATION OF AN ONCOGENE

The isolation of any cellular gene is absolutely dependent upon the recently developed techniques of gene cloning. Such isolation must depend more specifically on the exploitation of lambdaphage vectors into which one can introduce 10 to 20 kb segments of the genome of interest. The resulting cellular-phage chimeric genomes are able to transduce the cellular inserts effectively. Cloning can be achieved by identifying the rare bacteriophage carrying the inserted cellular sequence of interest. In the case of tumor oncogenes, one could introduce the fragmented genome of a tumor cell into lambdaphage vectors and attempt to identify which bacteriophage carries DNA that has oncogenic transforming potencies. Following such a strategy, one might transfect the DNAs of different pools of chimeric bacteriophage until one had identified a group of phage that carried the gene of interest. Further identification could be achieved by sub-dividing the pool of phage, until this narrowing search routine identified the single phage clone carrying the sequence of biological interest.

We reasoned that this strategy was compromised by two factors. First, the oncogene might be too large to be inserted in its entirety into a single bacteriophage. Thus, no single bacteriophage would be able to transduce a biologically active oncogene segment. Second, such a "sib-selection" protocol ignores one of the most powerful aspects of the genomic library procedure: the ability to rapidly identify, by use of sequence-specific probes, those bacteriophage carrying genes of interest. Consequently, we attempted to identify a bacteriophage of interest using sequence-specific hybridization probes. These probes could not be made reactive with the oncogene itself, since we knew nothing of its structure or origin. Instead, we utilized probes that would not identify the oncogene DNA, but instead react with closely linked repetitive sequences present in the cellular genome.

The repetitive sequences, termed "Alu" sequences, are present in the human genome in 300,000–500,000 copies, and located in an interspersed array along the DNA (7). Any human gene is consequently closely linked to one or more copies of these Alu sequences. It should be mentioned that these Alu sequences are widely diverged from homologues present in the mouse genome. This makes possible the generation of a human Alu-specific sequence probe that is not cross-reactive with mouse DNA.

When one introduces, via transfection, a human oncogene into a mouse cell, a large number of human sequences are concomitantly acquired by the recipient cell.

Many of these co-transfected sequences carry Alu blocks. The presence of the oncogene can thus be demonstrated by detection of the concomitantly acquired Alu sequences, using an Alu-specific sequence probe. DNA segments carrying a human oncogene are identifiable not by their biological activity, but by their affiliation with these useful sequence tags.

This strategy was followed to identify a bacteriophage carrying the oncogene of the EJ human bladder carcinoma (11). The oncogene that was isolated is 6.6 kb long, and this segment of DNA appears to contain the entire biological activity previously attributed to the tumor cell as a whole. The cloned oncogene is biologically very potent, since 1 μg of the cloned DNA introduces $>10^4$ foci when applied to NIH3T3 monolayers.

Using the cloned oncogene DNA as sequence probe reveals its close relationship to a DNA sequence present in the genome of normal human cells (11). This proves another, perhaps not unexpected, point: the oncogene arose via alteration of novel human DNA sequences, as an apparent consequence of a somatic mutational event. This bladder carcinoma oncogene is not closely related in sequence to several other human oncogenes elucidated by transfection—those of colon and lung carcinomas and a neuroblastoma. These data support a conclusion drawn from other experiments (8) that there are different human oncogenes present in different types of tumors.

The above-mentioned evidence indicates the derivation of the oncogene from a closely related sequence. This sequence can be termed the "proto-oncogene". Such a relationship of normal cellular gene, the proto-oncogene, with an activated oncogene counterpart is reminiscent of a relationship observed in the study of retroviruses. Many of these viruses carry oncogenes that have been acquired from the genome of an infected host animal. For example, the v-*src* gene of Rous sarcoma virus derives from a closely related c-*src* proto-oncogene present in the chicken genome (14). At least 14 other cellular proto-oncogenes have been elucidated by their association with various retroviruses (2). Two groups of proto-oncogenes are thus implied by these various studies. Gene transfer procedures elucidated the first group, while the second is known from retrovirology.

Experiments were undertaken to determine whether any relationship existed between these two groups of cellular genes. These studies, pursued in three laboratories, revealed that the bladder carcinoma oncogene, whose isolation was described above, is a close homologue of the oncogene acquired by Harvey murine sarcoma virus from the rat genome (4,9,10). This indicates that the same proto-oncogene can become activated by two separate routes. On the one hand, activation can be achieved by a somatic mutational event of the type that led to creation of the bladder carcinoma oncogene. On the other hand, a retrovirus can acquire the proto-oncogene and convert to an active oncogene.

The oncogene of the Harvey sarcoma virus is termed v-Ha-*ras*. The cellular counterpart, that also served as precursor of the bladder carcinoma oncogene, is termed c-Ha-*ras*l. The *ras* genes have been studied by Scolnick et al. for many years (5). Because of this, the structure of these genes and the nature of the gene product is well-established. The viral *ras* genes encode proteins of 21,000 daltons, and this has been shown to pertain to the bladder oncogene as well. The oncogenes of colon and lung tumors are also members of the *ras* family (4) and they also encode these proteins (4; E. M. Scolnick and R. A. Weinberg, in preparation).

The origin of the oncogenes carried by the 3-methyl-cholanthrene-transformed fibroblasts is relevant to chemical carcinogenesis. These oncogenes are homologues of the oncogene of Kirsten murine sarcoma virus, which is also a member of the *ras* gene family. In this case, as a consequence of application of the carcinogen, the c-Ki-*ras* proto-oncogene has become activated (L. Parada and R. A. Weinberg, in preparation). It is possible that this proto-oncogene became activated in a similar manner to the c-Ha-*ras* proto-oncogene, as described below.

The human c-Ha-*ras*l gene has been isolated by Chang et al. (1). It represents the proto-oncogene counterpart of the bladder carcinoma oncogene. In a collaboration with these workers, we initiated a comparison between clones of the bladder oncogene and this proto-oncogene. The differences between the two genes could be explained by two alternative hypotheses. Possibly the two genes are expressed at different levels, e.g., the proto-oncogene might be expressed at a low level and the oncogene at a high level. This over-expression might be responsible for the transformation of the cell. It is also possible that the two genes are expressed at comparable levels, but that the structure of the proteins encoded by them differs.

This work (13) began by examining the levels of expression of the oncogene and proto-oncogene in normal human bladder epithelial cells and in the EJ bladder carcinoma. The levels of RNAs homologous to the oncogene/proto-oncogene were comparable in the two cell types. Additionally, the levels of the 21,000 dalton proteins encoded by the genes, in the normal and malignant cells, were within a factor of 3 in their amounts. This measurement of protein level could be pursued by use of specific monoclonal sera in immunoprecipitations of radiolabeled lysates from these two cell types. Taken together such experiments indicated that the two genes were not expressed at greatly different levels.

Such comparisons of the two genes could be more directly achieved by study of NIH3T3 cells transfected with the oncogene or proto-oncogene clones. Such cells differed greatly in their appearance. Those cells acquiring the oncogene were extremely transformed while their counterparts carrying the proto-oncogene appeared quite normal. Once again, the levels of expression of the two genes, as measured in RNA and protein gels, were comparable. This showed even more persuasively that the differences in cellular phenotype were not due to the over- or under-expression by the oncogene. In fact, close analysis of immunoprecipitates of the 21,000 dalton proteins encoded by the two genes indicated a slight difference in electrophoretic mobility. This provided the beginnings of evidence that the differences between the two genes lay in the structure of the proteins that they encoded.

Experiments were undertaken to definitively resolve the genetic lesion which led to conversion of the proto-oncogene into the oncogene. It was possible to derive total nucleotide sequences of the two genes and compare them. However, we reasoned that this would not be a productive exercise, since many differences in sequence might be seen which were in no way related to the contrasting functional properties of the two genes. We chose, therefore, to construct a series of recombinants between the oncogene and proto-oncogene clones. For example, we cleaved a 1.2 kb segment from the left end of the oncogene clone, prepared this segment, and introduced it into the corresponding position of the proto-oncogene clone. Such a recombinant was actively transforming, thus indicating that this segment of the oncogene could impart activity to the proto-oncogene, and that the biologically important lesion lay within the confines of this segment.

A repeated series of these recombinations finally led to identification of a 350 nucleotide segment of the oncogene that was able to induce activation of the proto-oncogene after being recombined with the latter. This segment was then subjected to sequencing by Ravi Dhar of the National Cancer Institute. The 350 nucleotide proto-oncogene counterpart was sequenced as well. The sequencing indicated that the two segments differed in only one nucleotide. This nucleotide was at a position that encoded the twelfth amino acid residue of the 21,000 dalton protein. This nucleotide alteration causes the glycine residue normally present in this position of the proto-oncogene encoded protein to be replaced by a valine residue. The consequences of this replacement on the functioning of the protein are dramatic. This localization of the lesion confirms the supposition from the earlier work that the critical lesion in the gene affects protein structure and not gene regulatory functions.

It would seem unlikely that such an amino acid replacement could exert such a profound affect. Several arguments confer greater plausibility on the importance of this change. The replacement of glycine by virtually any other amino acid means a drastic change in the local stereochemistry of the protein. This derives from the unique structure of glycine, which lacks a side chain. More persuasive arguments perhaps arise from comparison of the v-Ha-*ras* oncogene of Harvey murine sarcoma virus with its genetic precursor, the rat c-Ha-*ras*l proto-oncogene. The amino acid sequence of the 21,000 protein encoded by the rat proto-oncogene differs in this region from the derived oncogene at one position—residue 12, where the normal glycine residue is replaced by the more bulky arginine. Taken together, these data begin to suggest that alteration of residue 12 of the 21,000 dalton protein is repeated even in different, independent oncogenic activations. This hypothesis clearly needs to be extended by examination of other oncogenes.

It is likely that alterations of the 21,000 dalton *ras* proteins are important in a number of human malignancies. This insight, however, hardly provides anything but a small part of the solution to the problem of molecular carcinogenesis. It remains unclear how carcinogens are able to induce biologically productive lesions in target cell genomes. It is even more obscure how many alterations must occur in order for a normal cell to become converted to a tumor cell. Surely the creation of an active oncogene is an important step in this process, but it is only one step. Perhaps the most complex of problems revolves around the 21,000 dalton oncogene protein. Elucidating its mode of action could consume our energies for the coming decade.

ACKNOWLEDGMENTS

This work was supported by Grants CA26717, CA31649, and CA17537 of the U.S. National Cancer Institute and by a grant from the Whitehead Institute for Biomedical Research.

REFERENCES

1. Chang, E. H., Gonda, M. A., Ellis, R. W., Scolnick, E. M., and Lowy, D. R. (1982): Human genome contains four genes homologous to transforming genes of Harvey and Kirsten murine sarcoma viruses. *Proc. Natl. Acad. Sci. USA*, 79:4848–4852.
2. Coffin, J. M., Varmus, H. E., Bishop, J. M., Essex, M., Hardy, W. D., Martin, G. S., Rosenberg, N. E., Scolnick, E. M., Weinberg, R. A., and Vogt, P. K. (1981): Proposal for naming host cell-derived inserts in retrovirus genomes. *J. Virology*, 40:953–957.
3. Cooper, G. M. (1982): Cellular transforming genes. *Science*, 218:801–806.
4. Der, C., Krontiris, T., and Cooper, G. M. (1982): Transforming genes of human bladder and lung carcinomas are homologous to the *ras* genes of Harvey and Kirsten sarcoma viruses. *Proc. Natl. Acad. Sci. USA*, 79:3637–3640.
5. Ellis, R. W., Lowy, D. R., and Scolnick, E. M. (1982): The viral and cellular p21 (ras) gene family. In: *Advances in Viral Oncology*, edited by G. Klein, pp. 107–126. Raven Press, New York.
6. Graham, F. L., and van der Eb, A. J. (1973): A new technique for the assay of infectivity of human adenovirus 5 DNA. *Virology*, 52:456–471.
7. Jelinek, W. R., Toomey, T. P., Leinward, L., Duncan, C. H., Biro, P. A., Choudary, P. V., Weissman, S. M., Rubin, C. M., Houck, C. M., Deininger, P. L., and Schmid, C. W. (1980): Ubiquitous interspersed repeated sequences in mammalian genomes. *Proc. Natl. Acad. Sci. USA*, 77:1398–1402.
8. Murray, M. J., Shilo, B., Shih, C., Cowing, D., Hsu, H. W., and Weinberg, R. A. (1981): Three Different Human Tumor Cell Lines Contain Different Oncogenes. *Cell*, 25:355–361.
9. Parada, L. F., Tabin, C. J., Shih, C., and Weinberg, R. A. (1982): Human EJ Bladder Carcinoma Oncogene is Homologue of Harvey Sarcoma Virus *ras* Gene. *Nature*, 297:474–478.
10. Santos, E., Tronick, S. R., Aaronson, S. A., Pulciani, S., and Barbacid, M. (1982): T24 human bladder carcinoma oncogene is an activated form of the normal human homologue of BALB- and Harvey-MSV transforming genes. *Nature*, 298:343–347.
11. Shih, C., and Weinberg, R. A. (1982): Isolation of a Transforming Sequence from a Human Bladder Carcinoma Cell Line. *Cell*, 29:161–169.
12. Shih, C., Shilo, B., Goldfarb, M., Dannenberg, A., and Weinberg, R. A. (1979): Passage of Phenotypes of Chemically Transformed Cells via Transfection of DNA and Chromatin. *Proc. Natl. Acad. Sci. USA*, 76:5714–5718.
13. Tabin, C. J., Bradley, S. M., Bargmann, C. I., Weinberg, R. A., Papageorge, A. G., Scolnick, E. M., Dhar, R., Lowy, D. R., and Chang, E. H. (1982): Mechanism of Activation of a Human Oncogene. *Nature*, 300:143–149.
14. Stehelin, D., Varmus, H. E., Bishop, J. M., and Vogt, P. K. (1976): DNA related to the transforming gene(s) of avian sarcoma viruses is present in normal avian DNA. *Nature*, 260:170–173.

Biochemical Basis of Chemical Carcinogenesis,
edited by H. Greim, R. Jung, M. Kramer,
H. Marquardt, and F. Oesch.
Raven Press, New York © 1984.

Role of DNA Lesions and Excision Repair in Carcinogen-Induced Mutagenesis and Transformation in Human Cells

Veronica M. Maher and J. Justin McCormick

Carcinogenesis Laboratory-Fee Hall, Department of Microbiology and Department of Biochemistry, Michigan State University, East Lansing, MI 48824-1316

A wealth of data derived from experimental studies in animals and epidemiologic studies of human cancer incidence indicates that carcinogenesis is a multistepped or multistage process. To quote Peto (40) this implies "that a few distinct changes (each heritable when cells carrying them divide) are necessary to alter a normal cell into a malignant cell and that human cancer usually arises from the proliferation of a clone derived from a single cell that suffered all the necessary changes and then started to proliferate malignantly." Although studies with intact animals are indispensable in analyzing many aspects of carcinogenesis, the use of cells in culture permits a more direct experimental manipulation and quantitation of the individual steps involved and can yield information on the nature of these steps. A further advantage of using cell-culture systems is that they allow experimental studies with *human* cells, which would otherwise be impossible for obvious ethical reasons. In fact, dissection of the steps involved in the neoplastic transformation of human cells in culture represents, perhaps, the only experimental approach for obtaining such information. Therefore, a great deal of effort has gone into the development of assays for "*in vitro* transformation" of mammalian cells in culture by chemical carcinogens or radiation (3).

As part of this effort to dissect the steps in carcinogenesis, we and our coworkers have developed reproducible, quantitative assays for measuring the frequency of mutations induced in diploid human fibroblasts by such carcinogens (1,2,15,20–25,28,29,31,44–46) and, more recently, for determining the frequency of neoplastic transformation of these same cells in culture (28,32–34,42). We have, as our working hypothesis for these studies, the idea that chemical carcinogens and radiation cause cancer by acting as mutagens and that an event leading ultimately to the neoplastic transformation of normal cells into tumor-forming cells results from damage to DNA which is converted into a somatic cell mutation.

It is instructive to recall that less than 15 years ago this idea was not commonly accepted, even though Brookes and Lawley had shown in 1964 that the carcinogenicity of a series of polycyclic aromatic hydrocarbons correlated with their binding to DNA rather than to RNA or proteins (10). Early demonstrations that there was a good correlation between carcinogenicity and mutagenicity of reactive derivatives of chemical carcinogens (26,27) were followed by those of a number of workers (13,17,30) which brought renewed interest in the discarded theory of Boveri (11) that somatic cell mutations were causally involved in the induction of cancer. Indirect support for the involvement of mutations in neoplastic transformation came from the finding by Cleaver (12) that cells derived from xeroderma pigmentosum (XP) patients who are genetically predisposed to sunlight-induced skin cancer (41) were deficient in the rate of excision of ultraviolet induced DNA lesions. This finding predicted that cells from such XP patients would be abnormally susceptible to sunlight-induced mutations.

We proved this was true in studies comparing the sensitivities of a series of XP cells, each with a different capacity for excision repair of UV-induced DNA lesions, and fibroblasts from the skin of normal persons to the cytotoxic and mutagenic effects of UV radiation (254 nm) (20–22,24,29). Cytotoxicity was defined as the inability of a cell to form a colony, i.e., reproductive death; mutagenicity was defined as an increase in 8-azaguanine or 6-thioguanine resistant cells in the population (resulting from the loss of active hypoxanthine(guanine)phosphorybosyltransferase). The results indicated that mutations by these particular agents are not introduced during excision repair, but result from semi-conservative DNA synthesis on a template containing unexcised lesions, e.g., by misreplication or failure to replicate a portion of the DNA. We extended these comparative mutagenicity and/or cytotoxicity studies to include broad spectrum sunlight (36) and several classes of chemical carcinogens which result in DNA lesions which XP cells are unable, or less able, to excise (16,23–25,31,43–45).

The genetic marker used for these mutagenesis studies served only as a model for the kinds of mutational events by which carcinogens were considered to affect cellular processes or structures involved in neoplastic transformation. Therefore, we have concentrated our efforts on developing quantitative methods for selecting, or otherwise identifying, transformed cells induced in populations of these same diploid human cells by exposure to chemical carcinogens and/or radiation (28,32–34,42). For many years, workers had tried without success to induce the neoplastic transformation of human fibroblasts with such agents. Finally, in 1977, Kakunaga (18) demonstrated that human fibroblasts treated with 4NQO or MNNG could give rise to cells which formed foci (small areas, apparently clonal in origin, where cells grow in a three dimensional array) on the top of confluent monolayers. The progeny of these cells proved to be tumorigenic when injected subcutaneously into athymic mice (18). This was a very important accomplishment, but his focus assay for these human cells was not quantitative enough to be of use in determining the number or kinds of steps in carcinogenesis.

The following year, Milo and DiPaolo (35) reported inducing anchorage independence (ability to form large colonies in soft agar) in fibroblasts from neonatal foreskins by chemical carcinogens. The soft-agar colony assay can be much more quantitative. Therefore, we have used it as a basis for developing a reproducible, quantitative assay for dissecting the steps involved in neoplastic transformation of human cells, including XP cells (28,32–34,42). Because of our conviction that the transformation process was likely to involve one or more mutagenic events, we deliberately modeled our human cell transformation assay on our human cell mutagenesis assays (28,42). For example, we expected the process of transformation of human fibroblasts to have in common with the process of mutagenesis: (a) an expression period, i.e., a period of time between carcinogen damage of cells and their ability to express the new (i.e., transformed) phenotype; (b) a linear increase in the frequency of transformants with increase in carcinogen dose; (c) a concentration dependence for the carcinogenic agent which resembled that required for induction of mutations so that strong mutagens would usually be strong transforming agents; (d) a low, but measurable frequency of transformed cells in noncarcinogen treated cell population just as one finds low, but measurable, frequency of mutant cells in such populations; (e) a higher frequency of transformation per dose in DNA repair-deficient cells than in normal cells, as we had shown for the induction of mutants in XP cells; (f) a cell cycle dependence similar to that which occurs for mutation induction, so that populations of cells treated just before S phase would show a higher frequency of transformation than cell populations treated with the same dose of the agent far from S phase. Our results described below confirmed each of these predictions. The cells derived from these anchorage independent colonies produce fibrosarcomas upon injection into appropriate host animals (28,42).

In contrast to our approach to "*in vitro* transformation" and that of several others (6,8,9,37,38), many earlier researchers assumed either explicitly or implicitly that the transformation event(s) was not the result of mutations, and so did not design their transformation assay system to yield information simultaneously on transformation frequencies and mutation frequencies using the same treated cell population. In fact, some of the protocols used, as well as the type of mammalian cell line employed (aneuploid), often precluded recognizing whether a mutation was involved in transformation. Even when early passage diploid cells were used, e.g., derived from Syrian hamster embryos, the earliest end point, morphologic transformation, developed at such a high frequency (0.1 to 1%) as to rule out genetic mutations as the cause (3–5,7,14). The cells in these morphologically transformed colonies are not tumorigenic *per se*, but cells able to cause tumors arise randomly in progeny of the carcinogen-treated cultures after 35 to 70 population doublings posttreatment (3). By that time, control cells from nontreated cultures have senesced and the surviving treated cell population has become aneuploid. This delay, as well as the aneuploid state of the cells after passing through crisis, makes it difficult to associate the ultimate tumorigenicity with the original carcinogen treatment and rules out direct correlation with typical mutagenic events. Nevertheless, these studies with nonhuman mammalian cells in culture, taken together with our own studies and those of many others, have already shed light on the nature of several of the steps in the neoplastic transformation of cells in culture.

EVIDENCE THAT DNA EXCISION REPAIR CAN DECREASE THE POTENTIALLY MUTAGENIC AND CYTOTOXIC EFFECTS OF UV RADIATION

Effect of Varying the Rate of Excision

Our earliest comparative studies with human skin fibroblasts showed that the sensitivity of the cells to the potentially lethal or mutagenic effect of UV (254 nm) paralleled their excision repair capability (21,22,24). Cells from normal persons exhibited a rapid rate of excision repair (20) and were much more resistant to the potentially lethal and mutagenic effect of UV than were repair-deficient XP strains. After exposure to low doses (1 J/m^2), XP12BE cells, with little or no excision repair capacity (39), exhibited approximately 5% survival; XP7BE, which excises very slowly (41), exhibited a survival of about 18%; XP2BE cells, which excise damage more rapidly, had a survival of about 25%; normally repairing cells exhibited 100% survival. This same dose of UV increased the frequency of thioguanine resistant cells in the population of XP12BE cells to 315×10^{-6}, of XP7BE cells to 300×10^{-6}, but did not induce any significant increase over the background frequency (15×10^{-6}) in the normal cells. A 10-fold higher dose of radiation was required to cause comparable cytotoxicity and mutagenicity in the normal cells (20,22,28).

These results are expected if the XP12BE cells, which are virtually devoid of excision repair capacity, exhibit essentially the maximum potential cytotoxicity and mutagenicity of a given dose of UV, whereas XP2BE of XP7BE cells can reduce their load of DNA damage to a level 15 to 30% of that initially received and the normal cells, with rapid excision repair, can reduce their load to an insignificant number of photolesions. Since an essential difference between these strains is their respective rates of excision repair of UV-induced damage, the data are consistent with the hypothesis that there is a finite amount of time for excision repair between the initial radiation and the onset of the critical events responsible for cell killing and/or mutation induction in these cells. We suggested that the loss of ability to form a clone and the frequency of mutations induced in these cells reflected the number of unexcised lesions remaining in DNA at the time of some "critical cellular event" which translated the DNA lesions into their biological manifestations and that this critical event could be semiconservative DNA synthesis on a damaged template (22,25).

Effect of Lengthening the Time Available for Excision Repair Between Irradiation and Onset of DNA Synthesis

If semiconservative DNA synthesis, rather than the excision repair process itself, is involved in these processes, extending the period between the introduction of the lesions in DNA and the onset of DNA replication in cells which have repair capacity should decrease the cytotoxic effect of UV and the frequency of mutant cells induced. To test this, we grew cells to confluence to cause density inhibition of cell replication, irradiated them with doses large enough to cause significant cell killing and mutation induction in exponentially growing populations (e.g. $9J/m^2$), and held them in the nonreplicating state for various lengths of time to allow excision repair of potentially cytotoxic or mutagenic DNA lesions. Normal cells released from confluence immediately exhibited 20% survival and about 60 mutants per 10^6 cells plated. Cells held 8 hrs showed a survival of approximately 45% and about 30 mutants per 10^6 cells; those assayed after 16 hrs showed 100% survival and the frequency of mutants reached the background level of the unirradiated population, i.e., about 15×10^{-6}. In contrast, XP12BE cells irradiated in confluence with 0.5 J/m^2 and released immediately or after 24, 48, or 120 hrs showed a survival of about 20% and about 200 mutants per 10^6 cells. There was no evidence of recovery in these excision-minus cells (22).

We noted that, although the frequency of mutants observed in the UV irradiated XP12BE cells released from confluence was similar to that of such cells irradiated with 0.5 J/m^2 in exponential growth, this was not true for the normal cells. A dose of 9 J/m^2 induced about 200×10^{-6} mutants in normal cells irradiated in exponential growth. but only about 50×10^{-6} were observed in cells irradiated in confluence and released immediately. The survival of the two populations did not differ significantly (about 20%). We investigated and found that confluent cells released from the noncycling state under our experimental conditions are synchronized and do not begin DNA synthesis (S-phase) for approximately 24 hr (20). Therefore, a reasonable explanation for this lower frequency is that mutations are "fixed" during semiconservative DNA replication, and this extended G_1 phase gives the cells more time for excision repair processes to remove the majority of the potentially mutagenic lesions from the DNA than is available to cells irradiated in exponential growth. Such additional time before S phase would not be expected to affect the excision-minus XP12BE cells.

The gradual increase in survival and decrease in mutation frequency in cells capable of excision repair with time held in the nonreplicating state supported our hypothesis that the cellular event responsible for killing and mutation induction was semiconservative DNA replication on a template still containing unexcised lesions. The low doses of UV radiation employed in these comparative studies made it difficult to demonstrate the high correlation between the rate of removal of lesions and the rate of recovery from the potentially harmful effects of UV (19). To get around this difficulty, we used a series of labeled chemical carcinogens of high specific radioactivity which we had found caused lesions in DNA (covalently-bound adducts) which the XP12BE cells were unable to excise, i.e., aromatic amide and polycyclic aromatic hydrocarbon derivatives.

Using the same procedures as described for UV-irradiated cultures, Heflich et al. (16) and Maher et al. (23) showed that the rate of recovery of normally-repairing cells from the cytotoxic effect of a series of reactive aromatic amide derivatives was directly related to the rate of removal of the residues from DNA (Fig. 1). In contrast, in XP12BE cells there was little or no removal of the bound material from cellular DNA and no evidence of recovery from the potentially lethal effects of the

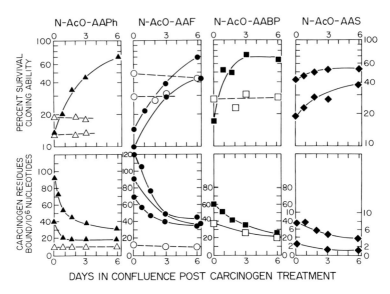

FIG. 1. Comparison of the rates of recovery from the potentially lethal effects of four aromatic amine derivatives with the rate of removal of radioactive labeled residues from the DNA of normal *(closed symbols)* or XP12BE cells *(open symbols)*. Cells were treated at confluence as described and then assayed after the designated period of time in the G_0 state. (Data from ref. 23, with permission.)

compound, even after 6 days in confluence. (Note that the removal of chemical adducts from the DNA took days as opposed to the few hours required for excision of UV-induced lesions.) Yang et al. (44), using this same approach, showed that the potentially cytotoxic and mutagenic lesions induced in confluent cultures of normal human cells by radioactive $7\beta,8\alpha$-dihydroxy-$9\alpha,10\alpha$-epoxy-7,8,9,10-tetrahydrobenzo(a)pyrene (antiBPDE) were removed with approximately the same kinetics as were the total number of DNA adducts (Fig. 2). Again, there was no loss of adducts from the excision-deficient XP12BE cells and no change in survival or mutation frequency. These results strongly suggest that excision repair in human cells can reduce the potentially cytotoxic and potentially mutagenic effects of exposure to these chemical carcinogens, just as in UV irradiated cells.

These results predicted that shortening the time available for excision before DNA synthesis (S-phase) occurred, by synchronizing cells and irradiating them or treating them with chemical carcinogens just prior to the onset of DNA synthesis, should significantly increase the frequency of mutations induced and the cell killing observed in excision-proficient cells, but not in XP12BE cells. We tested these predictions using UV (20) or antiBPDE (45). Cells were synchronized by release from density-inhibition of replication, allowed to attach at lower densities and elongate, treated with carcinogen in early G_1 (about 18 hrs prior to the onset of S) or just prior to S phase, and assayed the frequency of mutations and percent survival. The results are shown in Figures 3 and 4 along with data from cells treated in

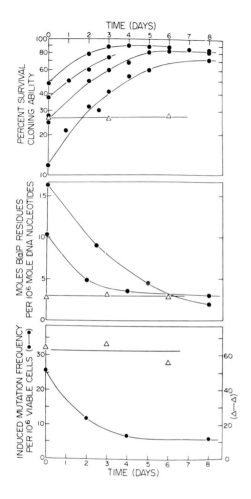

FIG. 2. Kinetics of removal of covalently bound adducts *(center)* and recovery of normal *(circles)* or XP12BE cells *(triangles)* from the potentially cytotoxic *(top)* or mutagenic *(bottom)* effects of anti BPDE. The cells were treated in the G_0 state, released on the designated days, and assayed for survival of colony-forming ability, for the number of residues bound to DNA, and after a suitable expression period, for the frequency of induced mutations to TG resistance. (Data from ref. 44, with permission.)

confluence and then released so as to have at least 24 hrs prior to the onset of S phase. The slope of the dose response for mutations induced in the normal cells treated just prior to S was 8- to 10-fold steeper than that of cells irradiated 18 hrs earlier. As expected, the frequency of mutations induced in the XP cells was the same whether they were treated just before S, 18 hrs prior to S, or 24 hrs before DNA synthesis began (20,45). These results support the idea that mutations are "fixed" by DNA replication, and the frequency is determined by the number of unexcised lesions remaining during DNA replication.

Although the mutagenic effect of these agents in repair-proficient normal human cells was inversely correlated with the amount of time available for excision repair before S-phase, the cell survival results did not show this. There was no significant difference in the slope of the survival curves of the normal cells at various times prior to the onset of S-phase (20,45) (Figs. 3 and 4). The XP12BE cells, of course,

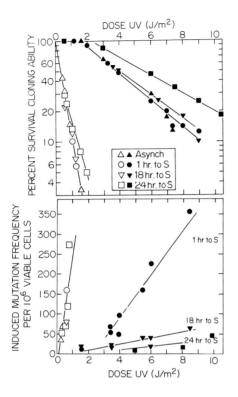

FIG. 3. Cytotoxicity and mutagenicity of UV in normal *(closed symbols)* or XP12BE cells *(open symbols)* irradiated under conditions designed to allow various lengths of time for excision repair to take place prior to the onset of S phase. Cells irradiated in confluence (G_0) and then released and plated at lower densities *(closed, open squares)*; cells released from G_0 and irradiated 6 hrs later *(closed, open triangles)*; cells released and irradiated 24 hrs later *(closed, open circles)*; cell replated from asynchronously growing cultures, and irradiated 16 hrs later *(closed, open triangles)*. (Data from ref. 20, with permission.)

were not expected to exhibit any real difference, but the repair-proficient cells were. We suggested, therefore, that after DNA is damaged by these agents, the time available for repair of potentially lethal lesions is determined by the cell's need for critical cellular proteins and their respective mRNAs (20,45). If the DNA template for transcription of these mRNAs is still blocked by lesions at the time the cell has need of them, reproductive death is the result. This would explain why holding cells in a resting state following exposure to DNA damaging agents before releasing them into the cycling state results in a higher survival than does immediate release. Cells held in confluence have a lower metabolic state than cells in exponential growth, and fewer critical proteins are needed before the cell has time to remove the blocking DNA damage. This explanation for cell death, inability to form a clone, is consistent with the fact that the XP12BE cells, which do not remove such lesions from their DNA, show no dose modifying effect on being held in the resting state.

EVIDENCE THAT NEOPLASTIC TRANSFORMATION OF HUMAN CELLS INVOLVES A MUTAGENIC EVENT

Our Assay for Neoplastic Transformation

The underlying purpose of our research is to determine the number and nature of the steps involved in the transformation of cells in culture in order to understand

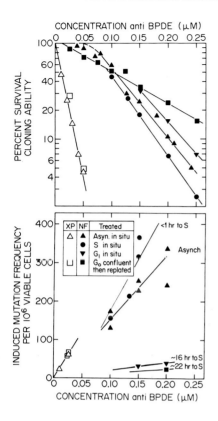

FIG. 4. Cytotoxicity *(upper panel)* and frequency of mutations to thioguanine resistance *(lower panel)* induced by low doses of anti BPDE in normal *(closed symbols)* and XP12BE cells *(open symbols)* treated under conditions designed to allow various lengths of time between treatment and the onset of S phase. The symbols are the same as specified in Figure 3. (Data from ref. 45, with permission.)

the mechanisms of human carcinogenesis. Although results obtained with cells in culture cannot fully represent the *in vivo* process of carcinogenesis, they do provide an opportunity to dissect the steps involved in changing a normal diploid cell into a fully transformed cell capable of giving rise to a malignant tumor in an appropriate host. In our assay, as we are currently using it, diploid fibroblasts derived from neonatal foreskin material or from skin biopsies of older persons, i.e., normal persons, or XP patients, or other persons with a genetic predisposition to cancer are exposed to low doses of carcinogens during exponential growth. [Note that these cells from the cancer-prone persons are not malignant; the skin biopsies from which they are derived are always obtained from normal tissue. Injection of $>2 \times 10^7$ untreated XP cells s.c. into athymic mice never produced a tumor (28).] The dose of radiation (UV or ionizing) or chemicals used are those we have determined will lower the survival, as judged by cloning, to between 80 and 10% of the control population.

The number of target cells is adjusted to insure at least 10^6 survivors. The surviving cells are allowed to undergo 3 to 4 population doublings in the original dishes and are pooled and $\geq 10^6$ subcultured to maintain the progeny in exponential growth for a total of 8 to 10 population doublings to allow full expression of the anchorage-independent phenotype (42). The progeny are then pooled and $\geq 10^6$ are assayed for anchorage independence by plating them as single cells into medium containing 0.33% agar. Within 18 to 22 days, colonies of anchorage independent cells develop to a size which can be counted under low magnification (about 0.1mm).

Cells from these soft agar colonies have repeatedly been tested for tumorigenicity by isolating colonies, propagating them into large populations and injecting 10^7 cells s.c. into immunologically depressed (sub-lethally X-irradiated) athymic mice. Tumors of about 1 cm diameter invariably develop at the site of injection in less than 2 weeks, but then the nodules regress. No tumors have developed in the animals injected with nontransformed control populations ($>2 \times 10^7$/injection) (28,43). Pathology examination identified representative tumors as fibrosarcomas. Cells from several of the tumors have been returned to culture. They have a human karyotype which appears to be diploid.

We suggest that acquisition of anchorage independence is a preliminary or initial step in the transformation of normal human fibroblasts and that cells with this property are partially transformed. We suggest further that acquisition of this particular phenotype occurs as the result of a mutagenic event (see below). Whether a second event is required to allow the progeny of these anchorage independent cells to form tumors (regressing) in immunologically depressed athymic mice is currently under investigation in our laboratory. Preliminary evidence suggests that a second event is not required. However, a second event or step, is required in order for such cells to acquire the ability to cause nonregressing tumors (fully transformed) (34).

DNA Excision Repair Can Decrease the Potentially Transforming Lesions Induced by UV Radiation

Further evidence that loss of anchorage dependence, with its subsequent tumorigenicity, is induced as a genetic event in human diploid cells derives from a recent study in our laboratory comparing the frequency of induction in normal human cells and in cells derived from the two excision repair-deficient xeroderma pigmentosum patients, XP7BE (complementation group D) and XP12BE from group A (28) (Fig. 5). In the majority of these studies, the same population of cells was simultaneously assayed for resistance to thioguanine (middle panel) and for anchorage independence (lower panel). The data indicate that to achieve a particular degree of cell killing, mutagenesis, and transformtion the repair-proficient cells have to be exposed to 8- to 10-fold higher doses of UV radiation than XP cells. As discussed above, this is the result expected if induction of anchorage independence as well as thioguanine resistance results ultimately from DNA damage remaining unexcised in the cell at some critical time after irradiation and if, because of the difference in their respective rates of excision repair, the average number of lesions remaining at this critical time is approximately equal in the three populations.

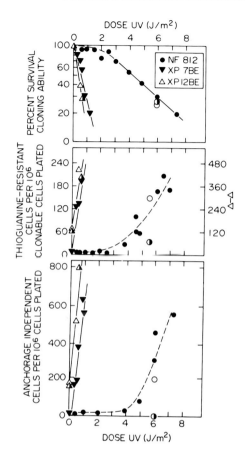

FIG. 5. Cytotoxicity, mutagenicity, and transforming ability of UV radiation in normal *(circles)* and XP cells *(XP12BE, triangles, XP7BE, inverted triangles)*. The frequency of thioguanine resistant cells was assayed after 6 doublings; that of anchorage-independent cells after 9 to 11 doublings. The former were corrected for cloning efficiency on plastic. *Solid symbols,* populations irradiated in exponential growth; *open symbols,* cells synchronized by release after confluence and irradiated shortly before onset of S phase; *half-solid symbols,* cells irradiated 18-20 hrs prior to S. See text for details.

Lengthening the Period Between UV Irradiation and the Onset of DNA Synthesis in Excision Repair Proficient Cells Can Decrease the Frequency of Anchorage Independent Cells

If, like thioguanine resistance, anchorage independence results from an event "fixed" during semiconservative DNA synthesis on a template which still contains unexcised lesions, the frequency of such cells should be much higher in populations of normal human cells UV-irradiated just before the onset of S-phase than in cells irradiated 18 to 20 hrs prior to S-phase. XP12BE cells should not show such a cell-cycle dependence. We tested this prediction and found it to be correct (28). The results are included in Figure 5 as open and half-solid symbols.

The transformation frequencies of the normal cells irradiated with 6 J/m² approximately 3 hrs prior to onset of S phase yielded 200 anchorage-independent cells per 10^6 cells plated; those irradiated 18 hrs prior to S phase showed no colonies out of 10^6 cells plated. The control cells in this experiment also gave no colonies out of 2×10^6. In contrast, the frequency of anchorage independent cells in XP12BE population irradiated in early G_1 did not decrease; in fact it was somewhat higher. In the corresponding mutation experiment, the frequencies of thioguanine resistant XP12BE cells irradiated at the two times were equal. In the mutagenesis experiments with normal cells from which the data in the middle panel were taken, the frequency of mutant cells did not decrease completely to the background level. However, in this mutagenesis experiment, the cells irradiated in G_1 had somewhat less time for excision repair before onset of S than was available in the transformation experiments. The fact that allowing substantial time for excision before DNA synthesis eliminated the potentially mutagenic and transforming effect of UV radiation in normal cells, but not in XP12BE cells, suggests that DNA synthesis on a template still containing unexcised lesions is the cellular event responsible for "fixing" the mutations and transformation.

The similarity of the dose-responses for the two phenotypes is obvious and supports the idea that acquisition of anchorage independence (transformation) in human cells occurs as the result of a single mutational event. The frequencies of mutations and transformation differ by a factor of about 2.5. In our earliest experiments, using propane sultone, the difference was approximately 22-fold (42). However, a ratio of 2.5 is much closer to the ratios we now observe with a number of agents. (See reference 28 for a discussion of possible explanations for this decrease.) If one assumes that anchorage independence results from a mutation, one might be tempted to speculate about the size of the DNA target involved. In computing the data shown in Figure 5, the observed number of thioguanine-resistant colonies (selected on plastic at a density equivalent to 10^4 cells per 60-mm dish) has been multiplied by a factor of 2 to 3 to correct for the cells' intrinsic cloning efficiency (i.e., 30 to 50%). The number of anchorage-independent cells (selected at a density of 10^5 cells per 3 ml of soft agar), on the other hand, was determined directly from the observed number of agar colonies without correction. There is no simple way to determine the "intrinsic cloning efficiency" under these conditions in which 10^5 cells are plated per dish. If the cloning efficiency in agar is less than 100%, these frequencies should be increased accordingly. Nevertheless, the *relationship* between the frequencies observed for thioguanine resistance as well as anchorage independence in the three strains that differ in DNA repair capacity supports the hypothesis that mutations are involved in at least this early step in the transformation process.

CONCLUSIONS

These studies indicate that the transformation of diploid human fibroblasts into tumor-forming cells is a multistepped process and that an initial step, to anchorage independence, occurs as a mutagenic event. The data indicate that excision repair in these fibroblasts is essentially an error-free process and that the ability to excise potentially cytotoxic, mutagenic, or transforming lesions induced in DNA by UV radiation or by several classes of chemical carcinogens determines their ultimate biological consequences. Other classes of carcinogens which form "bulky" lesions in DNA can be expected to give similar results, whereas the results with carcinogens that methylate DNA and with ionizing radiation may be different since the damage produced by these latter agents is repaired by pathways at least partially different from those studied here. Studies with the latter agents are in progress. The data presented here suggest that there is a certain limited amount of time available between the initial exposure and the onset of the cellular events responsible for mutation induction, for cell transformation to anchorage independence, and for cell killing, and that the critical event for the mutation and transformation to anchorage independence is DNA replication on a template containing unexcised lesions (photoproducts, adducts). Cells deficient in excision repair, such as those derived from cancer-prone xeroderma pigmentosum patients, proved abnormally sensitive to the cytotoxic, mutagenic, and transforming effects of carcinogens. The accompanying cytotoxicity studies indicated that, although a population's survival is determined by the extent of excision repair of potentially lethal damage from DNA before some critical cellular event, no single cell cycle-related event, such as DNA synthesis on a damaged template, is responsible for cell death.

ACKNOWLEDGMENTS

We wish to express our indebtedness to our colleagues, A. E. Aust, J. C. Ball, N. R. Drinkwater, R. H. Heflich, J. Howell, B. Konze-Thomas, J. W. Levinson, J. D. Patton, K. C. Silinskas, and L. L. Yang for their invaluable contributions to the research summarized here. The excellent technical assistance of M. R. Antczak, R. C. Corner, D. J. Dorney, R. M. Hazard, S. A. Kateley, T. E. Kinney, L. D. Milam, M. M. Moon, T. G. O'Callaghan, D. L. Richmond, L. A. Rowan, J. E. Tower, and T. Van Noord is gratefully acknowledged. The labeled antiBPDE was provided by the Cancer Research Program of the National Cancer Institute and the labeled aromatic amines by Dr. John Scribner of the Pacific Northwest Research Foundation. The research summarized in this report was supported in part by Contract ES-78-4659 from the Department of Energy and by Grants CA 21247, CA 21253, and CA 21289 and ES 07076 from the Department of Health and Human Services, NIH. Additional financial assistance was provided by the Michigan Osteopathic College Foundation.

REFERENCES

1. Aust, A. E., Falahee, K. J., Maher, V. M., and McCormick, J. J. (1980): Human cell-mediated benzo(a)pyrene cytotoxicity and mutagenicity in human diploid fibroblasts. *Cancer Res.*, 40:4070–4075.
2. Aust, A. E., Zator, R., Yang, L. L., Maher, V. M., and McCormick, J. J.: Comparison of the cytotoxicity and mutagenicity of the 4,5-oxide and the anti 7,8-diol 9,10-epoxide of benzo(a)pyrene in diploid fibroblasts from human skin and Chinese hamster embryos. *Carcinogenesis (submitted 1982)*.
3. Barrett, J. C., Crawford, B. D., and Ts'o, P. O. P. (1980): The role of somatic mutation in a multi-stage model of carcinogenesis. In: *Mammalian Cell Transformation by Chemical Carcinogens*, edited by N. Mishra, V. Dunkel, and M. Mehlman, pp. 467–501. Senate Press Inc., Princeton.

4. Barrett, J. C., and Ts'o, P. O. P. (1978): The relationship between somatic mutation and neoplastic transformation. *Proc. Natl. Acad. Sci. USA*, 75:3297–3301.
5. Barrett, J. C., and Ts'o, P. O. P. (1978): Evidence of the progressive nature of neoplastic transformation in vitro. *Proc. Natl. Acad. Sci. USA*, 75:3761–3765.
6. Bellett, A. J. D., and Younghusband, H. B. (1979): Spontaneous, mutagen-induced and adenovirus-induced anchorage independent tumorigenic variants of mouse cells. *J. Cell Physiol.*, 101:33–48.
7. Berwald, Y., and Sachs, L. (1965): *In Vitro* transformation of normal cells to tumor cells by carcinogenic hydrocarbons. *J. Natl. Cancer Inst.*, 35:641–661.
8. Bouck, N., and diMayorca, G. (1976): Somatic mutation as the basis for malignant transformation of BHK cells by chemical carcinogens. *Nature*, 264:722–727.
9. Bouck, N., and diMajorca, G. (1982): Chemical carcinogens transform BHK cells by inducing a recessive mutation. *Molec. Cell. Biol.*, 2:97–105.
10. Brookes, P., and Lawley, P. D. (1964): Evidence for the binding of polynuclear aromatic hydrocarbons to nucleic acid of mouse skin. Relation between carcinogenic power and their binding to DNA. *Nature*, 202:781–784.
11. Boveri, T. (1929): *The Origin of Malignant Tumors*. Williams and Wilkins Co., Baltimore (First edition Jena, 1914).
12. Cleaver, J. E. (1969): Xeroderma pigmentosum: a human disease in which an initial stage of DNA repair is defective. *Proc. Natl. Acad. Sci. USA*, 63:428–435.
13. Corbett, T. H., Heidelberger, C., and Dove, W. F. (1970): Determination of the mutagenic activity of bacteriophage T_4 of carcinogenic and non-carcinogenic compounds. *Mol. Pharmacol.*, 6:667–679.
14. DiPaolo, J. A., Nelson, R. L., and Donovan, P. J. (1972): *In vitro* transformation of Syrian hamster embryo cells by diverse chemical carcinogens. *Nature*, 235:270–280.
15. Drinkwater, N. R., Corner, R. C., McCormick, J. J., and Maher, V. M.: An *in situ* assay for induced diphtheria toxin resistant mutants of diploid human fibroblasts. *Mutat. Res. (in press)*.
16. Heflich, R. H., Hazard, R. M., Lommel, L., Scribner, J. D., Maher, V. M., and McCormick, J. J. (1980): A comparison of the DNA binding, cytotoxicity and repair synthesis induced in human fibroblasts by reactive derivatives of aromatic amide carcinogens. *Chem. Biol. Interactions*, 29:43–56.
17. Huberman, E., Aspiras, L., Heidelberger, C., Grover, P. L., and Sims, P. (1971): Mutagenicity to mammalian cells of epoxides and other derivatives of polycyclic hydrocarbons. *Proc. Natl. Acad. Sci. USA*, 68:3195–3199.
18. Kukunaga, T. (1977): The transformation of human diploid cells by chemical carcinogens. In: *Origins of Human Cancer, Vol. C*, edited by H. H. Hiatt, J. D. Watson, and J. A. Winsten, pp. 1537–1548. Cold Spring Harbor Laboratory Press, Cold Spring Harbor, New York.
19. Konze-Thomas, B., Levinson, J. W., Maher, V. M., and McCormick, J. J. (1979): Correlation among the rates of dimer excision, DNA repair replication, and recovery of human cells from potentially lethal damage induced by ultraviolet radiation. *Biophys. J.*, 28:315–326.
20. Konze-Thomas, B., Hazard, R. M., Maher, V. M., and McCormick, J. J. (1982): Extent of excision repair before DNA synthesis determines the mutagenic but not the lethal extent of UV radiation. *Mutat. Res.*, 94:421–434.
21. Maher, V. M., Curren, R. D., Ouellette, L. M., and McCormick, J. J. (1976): Role of DNA repair in the cytotoxic and mutagenic action of physical and chemical carcinogens. In: *In Vitro Metabolic Activation in Mutagenesis Testing*, edited by F. J. deSerres, J. R. Fouts, J. R. Bend, and R. M. Philpot, pp. 313–336. Elsevier/North-Holland Biomedical Press, Amsterdam.
22. Maher, V. M., Dorney, D. J., Mendrala, A. L., Konze-Thomas, B., and McCormick, J. J. (1979): DNA excision repair processes in human cells can eliminate the cytotoxic and mutagenic consequences of ultraviolet irradiation. *Mutat. Res.*, 62:311–323.
23. Maher, V. M., Heflich, R. H., and McCormick, J. J. (1981): Repair of DNA damage induced in human fibroblasts by N-substituted aryl compounds. In: *Carcinogenic and Mutagenic N-Substituted Aryl Compounds, Monograph 58*, edited by and S. S. Thorgeirsson, E. K. Weisberger, C. M. King, and J. D. Scribner, pp. 217–222. National Cancer Institute.
24. Maher, V. M., and McCormick, J. J. (1976): Effect of DNA repair on the cytotoxicity and mutagenicity of UV irradiation and of chemical carcinogens in normal and xeroderma pigmentosum cells. In: *Biology of Radiation Carcinogenesis*, edited by J. M. Yuhas, R. W. Tennant, and J. D. Regan, pp. 129–145. Raven Press, New York.

25. Maher, V. M., McCormick, J. J., Grover, P. L., and Sims, P. (1977): Effect of DNA repair on the cytotoxicity and mutagenicity of polycyclic hydrocarbon derivatives in normal and xeroderma pigmentosum human fibroblasts. *Mutat. Res.*, 43:117–138.
26. Maher, V. M., Miller, J. A., Miller, E. C., and Summers, W. C. (1970): Mutations and loss of transforming activity of *Bacillus subtilis* DNA after reaction with esters of carcinogenic *N*-hydroxy aromatic amides. *Cancer Res.*, 30:1473–1480.
27. Maher, V. M., Miller, E. C., Miller, J. A., and Szybalski, W.: Mutations and decreases in density of transforming DNA produced by derivatives of the carcinogens 2-acetylaminofluorene and *N*-methyl-4-aminoazobenzene. *Mol. Pharmacol.*, 4:411–426.
28. Maher, V. M., Rowan, L. A., Silinskas, K. C., Kateley, S. A., and McCormick, J. J. (1982): Frequency of UV-induced neoplastic transformation of diploid human fibroblasts is higher in xeroderma pigmentosum cells than in normal cells. *Proc. Natl. Acad. Sci. USA*, 79:2613–2617.
29. Maher, V. M., Ouelette, L. M., Curren, R. D., and McCormick, J. J. (1976): Frequency of ultraviolet light-induced mutations is higher in xeroderma pigmentosum variant cells than in normal human cells. *Nature*, 261:593–595.
30. McCann, J., Choi, E., Yamasaki, E., and Ames, B. N. (1975): Detection of carcinogens as mutagens in the *Salmonella*/microsome test: Assay of 300 chemicals. *Proc. Natl. Acad. Sci. USA*, 72:5135–5139.
31. McCormick, J. J., and Maher, V. M. (1981): Measurement of colony-forming ability and muta-genesis in diploid human cells. In: *DNA Repair: A Laboratory Manual of Research Procedures, Vol. 1, Part B*, edited by E. C. Friedberg and P. C. Hanawalt, pp. 501–521. Marcel Kekker, Inc., New York.
32. McCormick, J. J., Kateley, S. A., Moon, M. M., and Maher, V. M.: Cells from xeroderma pigmentosum variants are abnormally sensitive to transformation by ultraviolet light. *Mutat. Res. (submitted)*.
33. McCormick, J. J., Silinskas, K. C., Kateley, S. A., Tower, J. E., and Maher, V. M. (1981): The induction of anchorage independent growth and tumor formation of diploid human fibroblasts by carcinogens. *Proc. Amer. Assoc. Cancer Res.*, 21, 122.
34. McCormick, J. J., Silinskas, K. C., and Maher, V. M. (1980): Transformation of diploid human fibroblasts by chemical carcinogens. In: *Carcinogenesis, Fundamental Mechanisms and Environmental Effects*, edited by B. Pullman, P. O. P. Ts'o, and H. Gelboin, pp. 491–498. D Reidel Publ. Co., Dordrecht.
35. Milo, G. E., Jr., and DiPaolo, J. A. (1978): Neoplastic transformation of human diploid cells in vitro after chemical carcinogen treatment. *Nature*, 275:130–132.
36. Patton, J. D., Rowan, L.A., Mendrala, A. L., Maher, V. M., and McCormick, J. J. (1983): Xeroderma pigmentosum fibroblasts including cells from XP variants are abnormally sensitive to the mutagenic and cytotoxic action of broad spectrum simulated sunlight. *Photochem. Photobiol., (in press)*.
37. Perez-Rodrigues, R., Chambard, J. C., Van Obberghen-Schilling, E., Franchi, A., and Pouys-segur, J. (1981): Emergence of hamster fibroblast tumors in nude mice-evidence for in vivo selection leading to loss of growth factor requirement. *J. Cellul. Phys.*, 190:387–396.
38. Perez-Rodrigues, R., Franchi, A., Deys, B. F., and Pouyssegur, J. (1982): Evidence that hamster fibroblast tumors emerge in selections leading to growth factor "relaxation" and to immune resistance. *Int. J. Cancer*, 29:309–314.
39. Petinga, R. A., Andrews, A. D., Tarone, R. E., and Robbins, J. H. (1977): Typical xeroderma pigmentosum complementation group A fibroblasts have detectable ultraviolet light-induced unscheduled DNA synthesis. *Biochim. Biophys. Acta*, 479:400–410.
40. Peto, R. (1977): Epidemiology, multistage models, and short-term mutagenicity tests. In: *The Origins of Human Cancer*, edited by H. H. Hiatt, J. D. Watson, and J. A. Winsten, pp. 1403–1427. Cold Spring Harbor Laboratory Press, Cold Spring Harbor, New York.
41. Robbins, J. H., Kraemer, K. H., Lutzner, M. A., Festoff, B. W., and Coon, H. G. (1974): Xeroderma pigmentosum an inherited disease with sun sensitivity, multiple cutaneous neoplasms, and abnormal DNA repair. *Annals of Internal Medicine*, 80:221–248.
42. Silinskas, K. C., Kateley, S. A., Tower, J. E., Maher, V. M., and McCormick, J. J. (1981): Induction of anchorage independent growth in human fibroblasts by propane sultone. *Cancer Res.*, 41:1620–1627.
43. Simon, L., Hazard, R. M., Maher, V. M., and McCormick, J. J. (1981): Enhanced cell killing

and mutagenesis by ethylnitrosourea in xeroderma pigmentosum cells. *Carcinogenesis*, 6:567–570.

44. Yang, L. L., Maher, V. M., and McCormick, J. J. (1980): Error-free excision of the cytotoxic, mutagenic N^2-deoxyguanosine DNA adduct formed in human fibroblasts by ($\pm$)-7,8-dihydroxy-9,10-epoxy-7,8,9,10-tetrahydrobenzo(a)pyrene. *Proc. Natl. Acad. Sci. USA*, 77:5933–5937.

45. Yang, L. L., Maher, V. M., McCormick, J. J. (1982): Relationship between excision repair and the cytotoxic and mutagenic effect of the "anti" 7,9-diol-9,10-epoxide of benzo(a)pyrene in human cells. *Mutat. Res.*, 94:435–447.

Biochemical Basis of Chemical Carcinogenesis,
edited by H. Greim, R. Jung, M. Kramer,
H. Marquardt, and F. Oesch.
Raven Press, New York © 1984.

Genetic and Developmental Determinants in Neoplastic Transformation

*Sarah A. Bruce, **Khin Khin Gyi, †Shuji Nakano, †Hiroaki Ueo,
††Maria Zajac-Kaye, and *Paul O. P. Ts'o

*Division of Biophysics, School of Hygiene and Public Health, The Johns Hopkins
University, Baltimore, Maryland 21205; **College of Medicine, University of Vermont,
Burlington, Vermont 05401; †School of Medicine, Kyushu University, Fukuoka 812,
Japan; ††Center for Experimental Cell Biology, Mt. Sinai School of Medicine,
New York, New York 10029

The relative contributions of mutational (genetic) and nonmutational (epigenetic or developmental) mechanisms in neoplastic development are unknown. Considerable evidence points to the involvement of mutation, defined as alteration, deletion, or rearrangement of the primary structure of the DNA (40), in the process of carcinogenesis. For example, one characteristic of most tumor cells is that they are aneuploid (22). Indeed it was observations on abnormal development and aneuploidy which led Boveri (12) to postulate the theory of the somatic mutational basis of neoplasia. In some cases, specific chromosomal changes are associated with neoplasia, particularly in the case of the Philadelphia chromosome and chronic myelocytic leukemia (35,38). Although in the latter examples, it is difficult to determine whether the chromosomal alteration is a cause or an effect, there are several other congenital autosomal recessive conditions (Franconi's anemia, ataxia telangiectasia) in which there is both a high frequency of chromosomal abnormality in the normal somatic cells of afflicted individuals and an increased incidence of cancer (25). In addition, dominantly inherited familial cancers such as retinoblastoma and genetic defects affecting DNA damage repair such as xeroderma pigmentosum (25) also provide evidence for a mutational basis of neoplasia. Lastly, the development of the Ames assay to detect mutation in *Salmonella* bacteria has led to the finding that there is a 90% correlation between mutagenicity in bacteria and carcinogenicity in test animals (1).

Another argument for the genetic character of neoplastic development is that cancer represents a stably heritable alteration. In some cases, the stability of a phenotype may have a mutational basis as shown by studies on the development of drug resistance in somatic mammalian cells (40). However, other studies such as those on the development of embryonal carcinoma cells, which can develop alternatively into normal mouse tissue or teratocarcinoma, depending on their environment (31), suggest a nonmutational basis of a stably heritable alteration.

Similarly, during normal development and differentiation, cells acquire stably heritable phenotypes presumably via stable alterations in gene expression rather than in gene structure. Lastly, one clear distinction between mutation and cancer is that, whereas mutation is a single-step phenomenon, carcinogenesis *in vivo* (20,21) and neoplastic transformation *in vitro* (3) are progressive phenomena characterized by multiple, qualitatively different stages. This distinction necessitates the comparative study of mutation versus transitions between different stages in neoplastic progression (as opposed to the entire process of neoplastic transformation), but it also suggests the possibility that neoplastic transformation includes both mutational and nonmutational stages. Superimposed on this, one need also consider the influence of the state of development or differentiation of a cell on its susceptibility to induction of neoplastic transformation.

Recent studies in our laboratory aimed at better understanding neoplastic transformation include additional studies on the relationship between neoplastic transformation and somatic mutation (DNA as the critical target molecule as well as neoplastic transformation induced by nonmutational treatment) and new studies on the interrelationship between neoplastic transformation, cellular differentiation, and senescence and aging.

THE GOLDEN SYRIAN HAMSTER SYSTEM

Our laboratory has previously developed a cell culture system based on the golden Syrian hamster *(Mesocricetus auratus)* for the concomitant study of neoplastic transformation and somatic mutation (4). Current and future studies are focused on the interrelationships among neoplastic transformation, cellular differentiation, and *in vitro* senescence and *in vivo* aging. For these studies, the Syrian hamster (SH) is an excellent animal model and cellular system for the following reasons:

1. Normal diploid cell strains of SH origin exhibit a very low rate of spontaneous establishment into permanent cell lines in contrast to other rodent cell systems, and SH cells can be routinely transformed neoplastically *in vitro* by exposure to chemical carcinogens;

2. Normal cellular differentiation occurs spontaneously and can be manipulated (either enhanced or retarded) in diploid SH cell cultures of 9-day gestation embryonic origin;

3. The pattern of senescence of SH fibroblastic cell strains is qualitatively similar to that in human cell strains in terms of morphologic changes, loss of proliferative capacity, and cellular volume changes; and there is an inverse relationship between the *in vitro* proliferative life span and the *in vivo* age of the donor animal similar to that reported for the senescence of human fibroblastic cell strains (28,39);

4. The entire SH system both at the organismal and cellular level can be manipulated. Variously aged pre-embryonic (morula, blastocyst), embryonic and fetal cells plus all ages of adult tissue are available for use in primary culture; and

5. All types of tissue are available as required and longitudinal aging studies are feasible.

To better relate our studies on Syrian hamster embryonic and fetal cells to their normal development sequence *in utero*, we have begun to define the sequence and timing of developmental stages in the Syrian hamster. The hamster conceptus enters the uterus from oviduct at the morula stage (approximately 16 cells) and implantation occurs between 3.25 to 3.5 days after fertilization (36,37). Embryonic development begins on approximately the sixth day, indicated by the formation of the three embryonic germ layers (37), and is completed by the ninth or tenth day, as indicated externally by the formation of the handplate and microscopically by the presence of all the major organ systems (Fig. 1). Hamster fetal development represents the remaining one-third of the gestation period (15.5 days) and is notable for the rapid increase in the size of the fetus (Fig. 2).

Based on these studies, we designate cell strains isolated from ≤9 days gestation as embryonic and ≥10 days gestation as fetal. This is in agreement with Boyer (11) who concluded that Syrian hamster organogenesis is complete by the ninth day. Since embryonic development is characterized by differentiation and fetal development by growth and maturation, the distinction between embryonic (E) and fetal (F) cell strains may have a direct bearing on our studies on the differentiation, senescence, and spontaneous and induced neoplastic transformation of these cell types.

GENETIC DETERMINANTS: NEOPLASTIC TRANSFORMATION AND SOMATIC MUTATION

DNA as a Critical Target Molecule for Neoplastic Transformation

Evidence for genetic determinants in neoplastic transformation can be derived from determining that DNA is one of the critical target molecules. Our laboratory's approach has been to show that a specific and direct perturbation of DNA is sufficient to induce neoplastic transformation. In early experiments (6), unsynchronized cul-

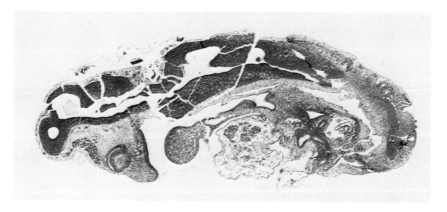

FIG. 1. 9 day SH embryo, whole mount.

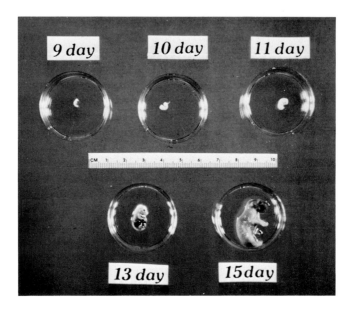

FIG. 2. Development in the SH between 9 and 15 days gestation.

tures of tertiary passage Syrian hamster fibroblastic cells derived from 13 day gestation fetuses (F13 cells) were first exposed to 5-bromo-3'-deoxyuridine (BrdU) to allow incorporation of this analog into cellular DNA; and then the cultures were exposed to near ultraviolet (UV) irradiation resulting in photochemically induced breakage in the BrdU-substituted DNA, primarily DNA single strand breaks as detected by alkaline sucrose gradient analysis. Combined treatment of the cells with BrdU plus irradiation resulted in dose-dependent morphologic transformation and the acquisition of anchorage independence and tumorigenicity after a progression period of 20 to 30 passages (Table 1). In contrast, untreated controls and cultures treated with BrdU or UV alone exhibited no detectable somatic mutation, no morphologic transformation, and, with one exception, senesced by passage 20. Further, similar experiments on synchronized SH fibroblastic cell cultures showed that morphologic and neoplastic transformation could only be induced in cultures treated during early to middle S-phase, while no transformation was observed in late S-phase, G_1 or G_2 (41). This observation was further confirmed by the similar study on the transformation leading to tumorigenic cells (Tsutsui and Ts'o, unpublished results).

   In a second series of experiments, neoplastic transformation resulting from localized damage induced by tritium incorporated into DNA has been investigated (26,27). In these experiments, tertiary passage SH F13 fibroblast cultures were exposed to methyl-^{3}H-thymidine (^{3}H-TdR) for 17 hrs, briefly incubated in medium with deoxycytidine and thymidine, successively passaged at confluence, and assayed

TABLE 1. *Progressive acquisition of neoplasia-associated phenotypes following various perturbations (expressed as posttreatment population doubling level at which phenotype was first detected unless otherwise indicated)*

Phenotype	B(a)P[a]	Transforming agent			
		Spontaneous[b]	BrdU + nrUV[c]	Tritium-thymidine[d]	DNase I[e]
Morphologic transformation	<3	—[f]	~3	3–4	nd[g]
Enhanced fibrinolysis	3	>60	nd	11–16	nd
Cloning in low serum	nd	nd	nd	18–32	41–161
Cloning in soft agar	32–75	≥200	passage 20–30[c]	25–32	39–57
Tumorigenicity	~45–87	>200	passage 20–30[c]	46	≥60

[a]Data from ref. 3.
[b]Data from refs. 2 and 5.
[c]Data expressed as posttreatment passage, from ref. 6.
[d]Data from ref. 27.
[e]Data from ref. 44.
[f]FOL cells used as an example here did not exhibit morphologic transformation.
[g]nd = not determined.

for somatic mutation and the acquisition of neoplasia-associated phenotypes. Treatment with ^{3}H-TdR (about 1.25 pCi/cell incorporation) resulted in cytotoxicity and mutation at the hypoxanthine phosphoribosyl transferase (HPRT) locus but not at the Na^+/K^+ ATPase locus, suggesting that ^{3}H-TdR induces a frameshift or deletion mutation. Tritium incorporation into DNA also resulted in neoplastic transformation with the temporal acquisition of neoplasia-associated phenotypes as shown in Table 1. Untreated control cultures and ^{3}H-uridine treated control cultures did not exhibit somatic mutation or morphologic transformation and did not become tumorigenic.

In recent experiments, we have utilized liposomes to deliver active DNase I into the nucleus of normal cells to provide a third type of direct and specific perturbation to the DNA (43,44). Treatment of SH F13 fibroblastic cells with liposomes containing DNase I results in dose-dependent cytotoxicity and dose dependent induction of somatic mutation at the HPRT locus. Untreated control cultures and control cultures treated with DNase I or liposomes alone exhibited no cytotoxicity and only a background spontaneous frequency of somatic mutation. All eight cultures treated with DNase I encapsulated in liposomes survived crisis and yielded established cell lines which exhibited increased cloning efficiency from low density inocula, increased saturation density, growth in low serum (medium supplemented with 1% fetal bovine serum), growth in 0.3% agar semisolidified medium, and tumorigenicity. In contrast, 32 out of 34 control cultures senesced and the 2 nonsenescent control cultures did not acquire neoplasia-associated growth properties and were not tumorigenic.

These studies provide direct evidence that DNA is one of the critical target molecules for neoplastic transformation by showing that various direct and specific perturbations to DNA alone are sufficient to initiate neoplastic progression. However, the initial treatment alone is insufficient to result in tumorigenicity, the acquisition of which requires >45 posttreatment population doublings regardless of the transforming agent (Table 1).

Neoplastic Transformation by Nonmutational Treatment

Another approach to the question of the interrelationship between neoplastic transformation and somatic mutation is to determine whether nonmutagenic treatment of normal cells can result in neoplastic transformation. For example, L-ethionine, a known rat hepatocarcinogen (19) is not mutagenic in bacterial assays (30); but has been shown to induce cellular differentiation in Friend erythroleukemic (FEL) cells in culture (16). In this system, L-ethionine, along with other known inducers of FEL cell differentiation, has been shown to inhibit DNA methylation (17).

To determine the mutagenicity of L-ethionine in our assay system, secondary passage SH F13 fibroblastic cells were treated with 10^{-2} M L-ethionine for 4 days (85% cytotoxic) or 5×10^{-6} M N-methyl-N'-nitro-N-nitrosoguanidine (MNNG) for 2 hrs (60% cytotoxic). One million cells from each treated and untreated control culture were assayed 4, 7, and 10 days after treatment for mutation at the HPRT and N^+/K^+ ATPase loci by measuring the frequency of 6-thioguanine resistant ($6TG^r$) and ouabain resistant (Oua^r) colonies, respectively. The frequency of mutation at both loci was less than 10^{-6} for the untreated control and L-ethionine treated cells. In contrast, the maximum observed frequency of MNNG-induced mutation was 10.2×10^{-4} (10 day expression time) for $6TG^r$ and 2.9×10^{-4} (7 days expression time) for Oua^r (23). For neoplastic transformation studies, replicate L-ethionine treated cultures (10^{-2}M, 4 days), MNNG treated cultures (5×10^{-6}M, 2 hrs) and untreated control cultures were passaged *in vitro* and analyzed for the acquisition of neoplasia-associated phenotypes. In three separate experiments, treated and control cultures entered crisis 2 to 3 weeks posttreatment. Approximately 60% (13/23) of L-ethionine treated cultures and 80% (15/19) MNNG-treated cultures escaped senescence and became established cell lines, whereas only 9% (2/23) of the control cultures escaped senescence. In addition, upon further passage, the L-ethionine-treated established cell lines acquired the ability to clone in reduced calcium (0.02 mM) medium, low serum (2%) medium and 0.3% agarose semisolidified medium (Gyi, Bignone, Bruce and Ts'o, in preparation). Tumorigenicity assays are in progress on these L-ethionine-induced anchorage independent clones. However, based on our previous observations of a strong correlation between anchorage independence (cloning in semisolid medium) and tumorigenicity (8), these data strongly suggest that L-ethionine is approximately equal to MNNG in terms of its ability to induce neoplastic transformation in this system despite the 100 to 1000 fold lower frequency of mutations induced by L-ethionine compared to MNNG.

Our studies along with similar results with diethylstilbesterol (7) and sodium bisulfite (18) dissociate the phenomena of neoplastic transformation and somatic mutation and suggest that transformation can occur through a nonpoint mutational mechanism.

DEVELOPMENTAL DETERMINANTS: NEOPLASTIC TRANSFORMATION AND CELLULAR DIFFERENTIATION

Cellular Differentiation in Syrian Hamster Embryonic and Fetal Cell Cultures

Contact-Sensitivity

Primary and low passage cultures of SH cells derived from 10 to 13 day gestation fetuses contain a subpopulation of cells which lack contact-sensitivity (CS^- cells). CS^- cells can be detected by their ability to form colonies on irradiated preformed monolayers (cell mats) of contact-sensitive (CS^+) cells. Thus, their frequency can be quantitated as cloning efficiency on cell mat (CEcm) (32). Tumor cells exhibit a similar CS^- phenotype and there is a good rank correlation between cloning efficiency on cell mat and cloning efficiency in soft agar (32) which we have previously shown is highly and quantitatively correlated with tumorigenicity (8). However, the CS^- property of fetal cells is distinct from that of tumor cells. Tumor cells have a permanently heritable CS^- phenotype. In contrast, the CS^- phenotype of fetal cells is transient and its frequency decreases both with gestational age and with passage *in vitro* falling below the level of detection (CEcm <0.001%) after about 5 passages or 6 to 9 population doublings (32).

Further, this decrease in CS^- cells is also observed when the cells are cultured continuously on cell mats which select for CS^- cells. Therefore, negative selection cannot be the explanation for the loss of CS^- cells in the population, leaving two other possibilities: either the loss of proliferative capacity of CS^- cells or the acquisition of sensitivity to postconfluence inhibition of cell division (CS^+) by the CS^- subpopulation during *in vitro* culture and *in vivo* development. To analyze the proliferative capacity of CS^- cells, CS^- clones growing on cell mats were isolated by local trypsinization and about 50 such clones were pooled to yield sufficient cells for analysis. The pooled CS^--enriched clones (>10% CEcm) were serially passaged in parallel under two conditions of substrate surface in culture: cell mats versus plastic dishes. At each passage, under both culture surface conditions, the proportion of CS^- cells and the proliferative capacity of the cells were determined by measuring the cloning efficiency on plastic surface and on cell mat, as well as by measuring the cumulative number of cells attained during serial passage (Fig. 3). CS^- pooled clones grew well under both conditions (Fig. 3, insert); the longer population doubling time of these cells on cell mat is presumably due to CS^+ cells in the population which are not able to grow on cell mat. The proportion of CS^- cells gradually decreased in cultures maintained under both culture surface conditions. However, the rate of decline was more rapid in cultures maintained on plastic

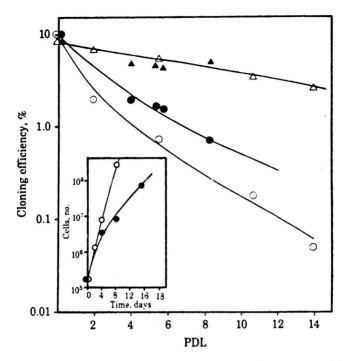

FIG. 3. Cloning efficiency of CS⁻ cell culture grown continuously on cell mats *(closed circle, closed triangle)* and in plastic dishes *(open circle, open triangle)* as assayed on cell mats *(open circle, closed circle)* and on plastic surfaces *(open triangle, closed triangle)*. (Inset) Cumulative number of CS⁻ cells in culture grown in plastic dishes *(open circle)* and on cell mats *(closed circle)*. (Data from ref. 32.)

than in cultures maintained on cell mats. In contrast, the proliferative capacity of CS⁻ pooled clones as measured by cloning efficiency on plastic dishes was not significantly different between the cells maintained under the two culture surface conditions. These results show that CS⁻ cells do not lose their proliferative capacity during *in vitro* passage. The remaining explanation for the loss of CS⁻ cells in culture is that they are converted to CS⁺ cells which results in the dilution of the CS⁻ cells by constantly emerging CS⁺ cells. Further, we have recently shown that the rate of decline of the CS⁻ subpopulation is retarded by promoters [12-0-tetradecanoyl-phorbol-13-acetate (TPA) and phorbol-12,13-didecanoate (PDD)] (42) and enhanced by a noncytotoxic dose of L-ethionine (10^{-3}M) (24). These results, together with the observation that the frequency of the CS⁻ subpopulation also decreases with increased gestational age, suggest that the disappearance of CS⁻ cells is due to the conversion of the CS⁻ cells → CS⁺ cells by a mechanism similar to cellular differentiation.

In Vitro Senescence

Another conversion from one cell type to another which occurs in cultured SH cells is the conversion of small highly proliferative fibroblasts to grossly enlarged nonproliferative senescent fibroblasts (15). Similar patterns of senescence are observed in cultures of SH fibroblastic cells of fetal (F13), 6 month adult (A6) and 20 to 26 month aged adult (A20+) origin. As SH cultures senesce, the previously homogeneous population of actively proliferating cells becomes more heterogeneous, containing increasing proportions of grossly enlarged, frequently multinucleated cells with extensive cytoplastic stress cables (Fig. 4). This increase in size can be quantitated as a decrease in saturation density and an increase in cell volume. F13, A6, and A20+ SH cell cultures all senesce with a very low rate of spontaneous escape from senescence (2 established cell lines (one A6 and one A20+) per 31 analyzed cell strains), and there is an inverse relationship between the *in vivo* age of the donor animal and the *in vitro* proliferative life span of the cells: F13 cells = 20.3 average maximum population doubling level (PDL); A6 cells = 17.0 average maximum PDL; A20+ cells = 10.8 average maximum PDL (14).

Cultures unable to proliferate to confluence within 2 weeks from an inoculum of $0.25 \times 10^6/75$ cm^2 flasks are judged to be senescent. However, these nonproliferative senescent SH cells remain viable for 4 to 8 weeks or longer with biweekly medium changes similar to senescent human fibroblasts. The observation that senescent fibroblasts retain metabolic activity when they are no longer proliferative has led to the hypothesis that *in vitro* senescence may be a form of cellular differentiation (9,10,29).

Adipocyte Differentiation

Recently we have observed a high frequency of spontaneous development of adiopocytes in normal diploid cultures of SH cells derived from 9 day gestation embryos (E9 cells). In contrast, few if any such cells are observed in SH cultures of fetal, neonatal, or adult origin. Adipocytes are detected by phase-contrast and electron microscopic observation as lipid-laden cells or by histochemical staining with the lipid-specific stain, Oil Red O. Developing adipocytes first appear as rounded cells filled with several or many small Oil Red O positive, lipid-containing perinuclear droplets (Fig. 5A). The size of the droplets increases and they coalesce to form fewer, larger droplets. At the terminal stage, a single large droplet is formed which expands to fill the entire cytoplasm pushing the nucleus off to one side to yield the signet ring morphology characteristic of adipocytes *in vivo*.

To quantitate the frequency of cells capable of differentiating into adipocytes during passage *in vitro*, E9 cells at each passage were seeded into replicate cloning plates, incubated for up to 6 weeks, stained with Oil Red O, and counterstained with hematoxylin (Fig. 5B). At passage 1 to 2, up to 20% of the colonies contained Oil Red O positive cells after 5 weeks incubation and the frequency of adipocyte development increased at higher passages, exceeding 50% by passage 4. Another feature of adipocyte development in this system is that it requires a nonproliferative state. Adipocytes are not observed in mass culture until the culture is confluent or senescent; in the clonal assay, adipocytes first develop in the central confluent regions of colonies and are not observed among the peripheral proliferative cells. Further, the differentiation of adipocytes in SH E9 cultures is enhanced by treatment

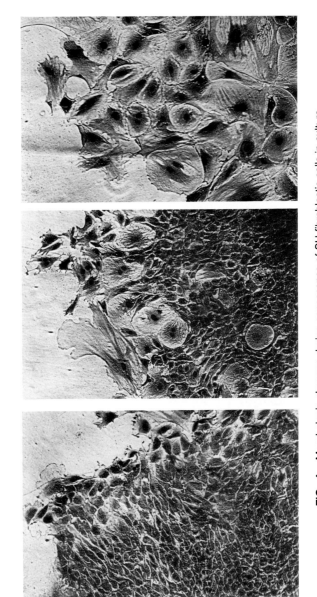

FIG. 4. Morphologic changes during senescence of SH fibroblastic cells in culture.

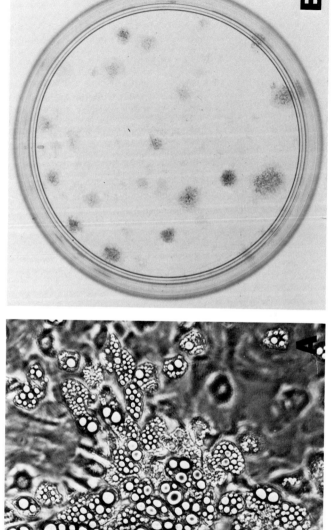

FIG. 5. Adipocyte development in SH E9 cultures: A, unstained, phase contrast; B, Oil Red O stained clones.

with 10^{-3}M L-ethionine (24) and reversibly inhibited by exposure to TPA or PDD at 0.1 μg/ml (42).

The Effect of the Stage of Development and State of Differentiation upon a Cell's Susceptibility to Induction of Neoplastic Transformation

To investigate the influence of differentiation on susceptibility to neoplastic transformation, we have compared the frequency of induced neoplastic transformation and somatic mutation of less differentiated CS$^-$ cells and more differentiated CS$^+$ cells (33,34). Pooled isolated CS$^-$ clones were either used directly (CS$^-$-enriched cultures; %CEcm = >4.0%), cultured on cell mats for 8 days (CS$^-$-enriched cultures; %CEcm = 0.6 to 4.0%), or cultured on plastic for 8 days (CS$^-$-depleted cultures; %CEcm = 0.2 to 0.02%). Cultures thus generated, which varied in their initial percentage of CS$^-$ cells, were exposed to MNNG (1, 5 or 10μM, 2 hrs). The CS$^-$-enriched cultures were less sensitive to the cytotoxic effects of MNNG treatment than the CS$^-$ depleted cultures; 25% versus 12% survival at 10 μM MNNG respectively. The frequency of MNNG-induced somatic mutation at the NA$^+$/K$^+$ ATPase locus is similar at equitoxic doses (about 30% survival) for the CS$^-$-enriched and the CS$^-$-depleted cultures. However, comparing the frequency of MNNG induced morphologic transformation and focus formation at equitoxic doses (30% survival), CS$^-$-enriched cultures are nearly 20-fold more susceptible than CS$^-$-depleted cultures. Further, all MNNG-treated CS$^-$-enriched cultures escaped senescence and acquired anchorage independence; whereas only approximately one-half of the MNNG-treated CS$^-$-depleted cultures escaped senescence and became anchorage independent. These data suggest that the less differentiated CS$^-$ cells are significantly more susceptible to chemically induced neoplastic transformation than more differentiated CS$^+$ cells. In addition, these studies also dissociate the phenomena of neoplastic transformation and somatic mutation, and the results show that neoplastic transformation is strongly influenced by differentiation and can occur via a mechanism other than single locus mutation.

In line with these observations on the influence of the state of differentiation on neoplastic transformation, we are also investigating the influence of the *in vivo* age of cells on their susceptibility to neoplastic transformation. We have previously shown that SH fetal fibroblasts can be neoplastically transformed *in vitro* by exposure to chemical carcinogens and that the acquisition of phenotypes associated with neoplasia occurs progressively over 45 or more posttreatment population doublings (PTPD) (Table 1). To determine whether adult fibroblasts can be neoplastically transformed in a similar manner and to investigate the effects of the *in vivo* cellular age of the cells on transformation, dermal fibroblast cultures derived from young adults (A6) and aged adults (A20+ cells) have been exposed to MNNG (5 μM, 2 hrs) or benzo(*a*)pyrene (10 μg/ml, 24 hrs) passaged *in vitro* and analyzed for neoplasia-related phenotypes (13). Eight weeks (20 to 30 PTPD) after carcinogen treatment, by which time all the controls had senesced, all treated adult cell cultures contained morpoohologically distinct cells which continued to proliferate and exhibited increased saturation density. Anchorage independent growth, analyzed by cloning in semisolid agar, a phenotype which appears late in the neoplastic transformation of fetal cells (Table 1) was detected in adult cells 16 passages posttreatment (about 60 PTPD). However, anchorage independence was detected in only one of three A6 cultures. The other two A6 cultures and the three A20 + cultures did not acquire anchorage independence and eventually exhibited reduced proliferation. This was especially evident in two A20 + cultures which were also still primarily diploid in contrast to the transformed cultures of fetal and young adult origin which showed a heterogeneous karyotype pattern.

In summary, treatment of Syrian hamster fibroblast mass cultures with carcinogens routinely disrupts the senescence pattern of both fetal and adult cells. Escape from senescence is clearly required, and possibly an early event, in neoplastic progression of this system. However, only 1 out of 6 of the treated adult skin fibroblast cultures both escaped senescence and continued to progress to anchorage independence. The adult culture which did transform was derived from a young adult. These results suggest that fetal fibroblasts (75% of cultures neoplastically transform after carcinogen treatment) are more susceptible than adult fibroblasts to chemically induced neoplastic transformation and that young adult cells are more susceptible than old adult cells. Thus, a single carcinogen treatment can result in a perturbation or delay in senescence without necessarily committing adult cells to neoplastic progression.

CONCLUSIONS

In carefully designed and executed experiments, both genetic and developmental determinants in induced neoplastic transformation *in vitro* can be clearly defined and demonstrated. Specific and direct perturbation to DNA alone (such as strand breakage) can cause somatic mutation and initiate the neoplastic transition process, but such direct damage to DNA cannot immediately induce the tumorigenic phenotype; 30 to 40 cell divisions or more are required for the expression of tumorigenicity (or other closely associated phenotypes such as anchorage independent growth). On the other hand, agents such as L-ethionine, which has little or no demonstrable ability to cause single locus mutation, can be nearly as effective in inducing neoplastic transformation as the potent, direct-acting mutagen MNNG. Although MNNG is an effective transforming agent, its effectiveness in transformation can be greatly modified or influenced by the developmental stages of the treated cells. In at least one clear case, while the effect of cellular differentiation on the induced neoplastic transformation is very large (nearly 20-fold), the effect of cellular differentiation on induced somatic mutation is nondetectable, indicating a possible dissociation of these two phenomena induced by the same mutagen. A complex interaction among differentiation (including senescence or aging), neoplastic transformation, and somatic mutation clearly exists, and the Syrian hamster system seems to be an excellent model for this investigation.

The basic understanding of this complex interaction must come from the investigation of the mechanism of heritable changes of mammalian cells *in vivo* and *in vitro*, either changes induced by foreign agents or spontaneous changes governed by the intrinsic genetic determinants in response to the environmental influence. The genetic and epigenetic determinants in neoplastic transformation must be similar if not identical to those in differentiation/development. Current efforts in our laboratory are to redefine these cellular changes (either induced or spontaneous) at the molecular level, particularly in terms of messenger RNA and genomic DNA organization. In other words, the mechanisms of and interaction among neoplastic transformation, somatic mutation, and differentiation will be investigated at the molecular level through studies on the changes and control of the structure, organization, and expression of genes in these defined cellular systems.

ACKNOWLEDGMENTS

The authors acknowledge the excellent technical assistance of Ms. Kathleen McDonald, Mr. Scott Deamond, and Ms. Mary Anne Bury. This research was supported by the National Cancer Institute (CA 16043), the Department of Energy (DE-AC02-76-EV03280), and the National Institute on Aging (AG 01998).

REFERENCES

1. Ames, B. N., Durston, W. E., Yamasaki, E., and Lee, F. D. (1973): Carcinogens are mutagens: A simple test system combining liver homogenates for activation and bacteria for detection. *Proc. Natl. Acad. Sci. USA*, 70:2281–2285.
2. Barrett, J. C. (1980): A preneoplastic stage in the spontaneous neoplastic transformation of Syrian hamster embryo cells in culture. *Cancer Research*, 40:91–94.
3. Barrett, J. C., and Ts'o, P. O. P. (1978): Evidence for the progressive nature of neoplastic transformation in vitro. *Proc. Natl. Acad. Sci. USA*, 75:3761–3765.
4. Barrett, J. C., Bias, N. E., and Ts'o, P. O. P. (1978): A mammalian cellular system for the concomitant study of neoplastic transformation and somatic mutation. *Mutation Research*, 50:121–136.
5. Barrett, J. C., Crawford, B. D., and Ts'o, P. O. P. (1980): The role of somatic mutation in a multistage model of carcinogenesis. In: *Mammalian Cell Transformation by Chemical Carcinogens*, edited by N. Mishra, V. Dunkel, and M. Mehlman, pp. 467–501. Senate Press, Princeton Junction.
6. Barrett, J. C., Tsutsui, T., and Ts'o, P. O. P. (1978): Neoplastic transformation induced by a direct perturbation of DNA. *Nature*, 274:229–232.
7. Barrett, J. C., Wong, A., and McLachlan, J. A. (1981): Diethylstilbestrol induces neoplastic transformation without measurable gene mutation at two loci. *Science*, 212:1402–1404.
8. Barrett, J. C., Crawford, B. D., Mixter, L. O., Schechtman, L. M., Ts'o, P. O. P., and Pollack, R. (1979): Correlation of *in vitro* growth properties and tumorigenicity of Syrian hamster cell lines. *Cancer Research*, 39:1504–1510.
9. Bell, E., Marek, L. F., Levinstone, D. S. Merrill, C., Sher, S., Young, I. T., and Eden, M. (1978): Loss of division potential in vitro: Aging or differentiation? *Science*, 202:1158–1163.
10. Bell, E., Marek, L., Sher, S., Merrill, C., Levinstone, D., and Young, I. (1979): Do diploid fibroblasts in culture age? *International Review of Cytology* [Suppl.]10:1–9.
11. Boyer, C. C. (1968): Embryology. In: *The Golden Hamster*, edited by R. A. Hoffman, P. F. Robinson, and H. Magalhaes, pp. 73–89. Iowa State Univ. Press, Ames.
12. Boveri, T. (1914): *Zur Frage der Entstehung Maligner Tumoren*. Fisher, Jena.
13. Bruce, S. A., and Ts'o, P. O. P. (1981): Neoplastic transformation of Syrian hamster embryo and adult fibroblasts. *J. Supramolec. Struct. and Cell Biochem.* [Supp.], 5:224.
14. Bruce, S. A., Deamond, S. F., and Ts'o, P. O. P. (1981): Relationship between *in vitro* life span and *in vivo* age of Syrian hamster fibroblasts. *In Vitro*, 17:239.

15. Bruce, S. A., Deamond, S. F., Ueo, H., and Ts'o, P. O. P. (1982): Markers of senescence in cultured Syrian hamster cells of fetal and adult origin. *J. Cell Biol.*, 95:58a.

16. Christman, J. K., Price, P., Pedrinan, L., and Acs, G. (1977): Correlation between hypomethylation of DNA and expression of globin genes in Friend erythroleukemia cells. *Eur. J. Biochem.*, 81:53–61.

17. Christman, J. K., Weich, N., Schoenbrun, B., Schneiderman, N., and Acs, G. (1980): Hypomethylation of DNA during differentiation of Friend erythroleukemia cells. *J. Cell Biol.*, 86:366–370.

18. DiPaolo, J. A., DeMarinis, A. J., and Doniger, J. (1981): Transformation of Syrian hamster embryo cells by sodium bisulfite. *Cancer Letters*, 12:203–208.

19. Farber, E. (1963): Ethionine carcinogenesis. *Adv. Cancer Res.*, 7:383–474.

20. Foulds, L. (1969): *Neoplastic Development, Vol. 1.* Academic Press, London.

21. Foulds, L. (1975): *Neoplastic Development, Vol. 2.* Academic Press, London.

22. German, J., editor (1974): *Chromosomes and Cancer.* John Wiley and Sons, New York.

23. Gyi, K. K. (1982): Non-mutational induction of transformation-associated phenotypes in Syrian hamster fibroblasts by L-ethionine. *Proc. Amer. Assoc. for Cancer Res.*, 23:77.

24. Gyi, K. K., Ueo, H., and Ts'o, P. O. P. (1982): Enhancement of cell differentiation in Syrian hamster (SH) cells by L-ethionine. *J. Cell Biol.*, 985:36a.

25. Knudson, A. G., Jr. (1973): Mutation and human cancer. *Adv. Cancer Res.*, 17:317–352.

26. Lin, S. L. (1982): The neoplastic transformation of golden Syrian hamster embryo cells by [methyl-³H] thymidine exposure. Ph.D. Thesis, The Johns Hopkins University.

27. Lin, S. L., Takii, M., and Ts'o, P. O. P. (1982): Somatic mutation and neoplastic transformation induced by [methyl-³H] thymidine. *Radiation Research*, 90:142–154.

28. Martin, G. M., Sprague, C. A., and Epstein, C. J. (1970): Replicative life-span of cultivated human cells. *Laboratory Investigation*, 23:86–92.

29. Martin, G. M., Sprague, C. A., Norwood, T. H., and Pendergrass, W. R. (1974): Clonal selection, attenuation and differentiation in an *in vitro* model of hyperplasia. *Am. J. Path.*, 74:137–154.

30. McCann, J., Choi, E., Yamasaki, E., and Ames, B. N. (1975): Detection of carcinogens as mutagens in the Salmonella/microsome test: Assay of 300 chemicals. *PNAS*, 72:5135–5139.

31. Mintz, B. (1978): Genetic mosaicism and *in vivo* analyses of neoplasia and differentiation. In: *Cell Differentiation and Neoplasia*, edited by G. F. Saunders, pp. 27–53. Raven Press, New York.

32. Nakano, S., and Ts'o, P. (1981): Cellular differentiation and neoplasia: Characterization of subpopulations of cells that have neoplasia-related growth properties in Syrian hamster embryo cell cultures. *PNAS*, 78:4995–4999.

33. Nakano, S., Ueo, H., and Ts'o, P. O. P. (1982): Relationship among neoplastic transformation (NT), differentiation and somatic mutation (SM) in Syrian hamster embryo (SHE) fibroblast. *Proc. Amer. Assoc. Cancer Res.*, 23:77.

34. Nakano, S., Ueo, H., Bruce, S. A., and Ts'o, P. O. P. (1983): A contact-insensitive subpopulation in Syrian hamster cell cultures with a greater susceptibility to chemically induced neoplastic transformation. *(submitted)*.

35. Nowell, P. C., and Hungerford, D. A. (1961): Chromosome studies in human leukemia. II. Chronic granulocytic leukemia. *J. Natl. Cancer Inst.*, 27:1013–1035.

36. Parkening, T. A. (1976): An ultrastructural study of implantation in the golden hamster. I. Loss of the zona pellucida and initial attachment to the uterine epithelium. *J. Anat.*, 121:161–184.

37. Parkening, T. A. (1976): An ultrastructural study of implantation in the golden hamster. II. Trophoblastic invasion and removal of the uterine epithelium. *J. Anat.*, 122:211–230.

38. Rowley, J. D. (1973): A new consistent chromosomal abnormality in chronic myelogenous leukemia identified by quinacrine fluorescence and giemsa staining. *Nature*, 243:290–293.

39. Schneider, E. L., and Mitsui, Y. (1976): The relationship between *in vitro* cellular aging and *in vivo* human age. *Proc. Natl. Acad. Sci. USA*, 73:3584–3588.

40. Siminovitch, L. (1976): On the nature of hereditable variation in cultured somatic cells. *Cell*, 7:1–11.

41. Tsutsui, T., Barrett, J. C., and Ts'o, P. O. P. (1979): Morphological transformation, DNA damage, and chromosomal aberrations induced by a direct DNA perturbation of synchronized Syrian hamster embryo cells. *Cancer Research*, 39:2356–2365.

42. Ueo, H., Bruce, S. A., Gyi, K. K., Nakano, S., and Ts'o, P. O. P. (1982): Effect of phorbol

esters on cellular differentiation of adipocytes and contact-insensitive cells in Syrian hamster (SH) cell culture. *J. Cell Biol.*, 95:58a.

43. Zajac, M., and Ts'o, P. O. P. (1980): *In vitro* neoplastic transformation induced by DNase I encapsulated in liposomes. *Europ. J. Cell Biol.*, 22:533.

44. Zajac-Kaye, M. (1982): The study of the mechanism of neoplastic transformation induced by DNase I encapsulated in liposomes. Ph.D. Thesis, The Johns Hopkins University.

Biochemical Basis of Chemical Carcinogenesis,
edited by H. Greim, R. Jung, M. Kramer,
H. Marquardt, and F. Oesch.
Raven Press, New York © 1984.

Permissive and Protective Factors in Malignant Transformation of Cells in Culture

Carmia Borek

Radiological Research Laboratory, Departments of Radiology and Pathology, Columbia University, College of Physicians & Surgeons, New York, New York 10032

The development of cell culture systems has made it possible to assess at a cellular level the oncogenic potential of a variety of physical, chemical, and viral agents (4,5). These *in vitro* systems free of host-mediated homeostatic influences afford the opportunity to evaluate both qualitative and quantitative aspects of oncogenic transformation. They also allow us to define factors which modulate the effects of the agents either by inhibiting transformation or by serving as permissive and/or potentiating factors in the process of neoplastic development.

The scope of this chapter will be limited to some of our studies involving cellular and extracellular factors which play a role in establishing the competence of cells to be transformed by radiation and some chemicals.

INITIATION AND PHENOTYPIC EXPRESSION OF TRANSFORMATION *IN VITRO*

One of the basic conundrums in cancer research evolves from our inability at the present time to unequivocally distinguish primary events associated with initiation of neoplastic transformation from those which function as secondary events. While we aim to identify the processes in initiation and consequently hope to modulate them we are faced with the fact that at present we determine the occurrence of initiation by its phenotypic expression. Thus, for example, although radiation carcinogenesis was recognized some 85 years ago, we are still relatively ignorant of the mechanisms involved and must judge the events determining neoplastic transformation by a variety of phenomena associated with the neoplastic phenotype. The phenotype appears to be similar irrespective of the initiating oncogenic agent; whether it is a virus or transfected DNA whose contribution is the introduction of new genetic material, a chemical carcinogen which can form adducts with cellular DNA or radiation, whose initiating action on the cell is established and over within a fraction of a second.

We therefore strive at defining various steps within the processes of transformation and try to associate cellular and molecular events with each step.

SEQUENCE OF EVENTS IN TRANSFORMATION *IN VITRO*

One can define the oncogenic process *in vitro*, in a manner similar to that presumed to occur *in vivo* (2), into early and late phases.

Initiation

The early stage is associated with initiation of neoplastic transformation. It is made possible by the interaction of the cell with the oncogenic agent in a manner where the cell is physiologically and genetically competent to be transformed. It must be stated that we remain ignorant of the exact mechanisms; whether the initiation process is induced via direct interaction of radiation and chemicals with cellular DNA with an ensuing alteration in gene expression; or whether some of these events are initiated in part by activation of specific cellular oncogenes (39) as well as by relay from membrane signals due to action of free radicals (4,5,8).

Initiation can be modified by a variety of cocarcinogens which would enhance the frequency by complementing processes or by impinging on the same mechanism.

Fixation

Once cells have been initiated fixation of transformation as a hereditary property of the cells requires cell replication within hours after initiation both in rodent and human cells (3,14,16,17,27,37).

The processes of initiating fixation are cell cycle dependent. Exposure of human cells to radiation or to chemical carcinogens results in a higher transformation rate and a shorter latent period when cells are exposed to the carcinogens at G_1S phase of the cell cycle (3,34) compared to cells exposed in randomly growing cultures (28).

Modification of Fixation

Fixation of the transformed state can be inhibited by preventing cell division after initiation (3,4,5,15). When cells were irradiated under conditions of confluence, in liquid holding, for a period of 5 to 72 hours, before trypsinization and cloning, transformation rate decreased proportionately with the time of incubation. No transformation was observed if cells were inhibited from replication for 72 hrs after exposure to radiation. If cells were maintained at 25°C for the same 72 hr period, where metabolic and repair events are slowed, and then cloned out, transformation was observed.

These results clearly implicate events associated with DNA replication and cellular metabolism in the processes responsible for the oncogenic transformation of the cells.

More direct evidence of DNA metabolism associated with transformation emanates from our recent experiments (7) that 3 amino benzamide, an inhibitor of polyADP ribose, (36) inhibits oncogenic transformation by radiation and methyl methane sulfanate in hamster embryo cells and in the mouse 10T½ cell line (7).

Expression

Later events in the oncogenic process are associated with expression, a period during which promotion can take place by interaction with a variety of enhancing agents similar to the situation *in vivo* (2,4,5) (Fig. 1).

Expression of the transformed state in both rodent and human cells requires several cell replications, depending on the cell type. The results are the growth of a focus or a colony (depending on the assay), which in fibroblasts are some epithelial cells are morphologically distinct from control (4,5) (Fig. 2). It should be added that there is little information on the neoplastic characteristic of exposed fibroblasts which do not differ morphologically from the normal. So far, the assessment of the transformed state in rodent fibroblasts has consistently adhered to the premise that the earliest observable phenotypic change in culture in the process of transformation is morphologic.

However more recent work using human cells in transformation studies indicate that anchorage independence may be a suitable endpoint in evaluating the transformed nature of the cells (1,3,28,32,50) (Fig. 2). In contrast to rodent cells where the acquisition of anchorage independence is observed at late stages in transformation much after altered morphology in culture (10) human cells acquire anchorage independence early after initiation (40,44).

Modification Expression by Cell-Cell Interaction

Expression of oncogenic transformation can be modified by cell-cell interaction with normal cells, the latter being able to inhibit the proliferation of the transformed cells (15). This type of inhibition of expression exerted by direct contact or in part by physiologic interactions among cells can be observed in other studies on transformation:

1. Physiologic competence for transformation can differ within the progeny of a single cell. Thus, irradiation of hamster cells at various stages of clone growth resulted in a fraction of cells within the clone which underwent neoplastic trans-

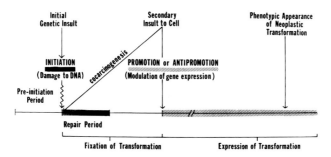

FIG. 1. Diagram of various events which may take place at a cellular level in the course of initiation expression and promotion of neoplastic transformation.

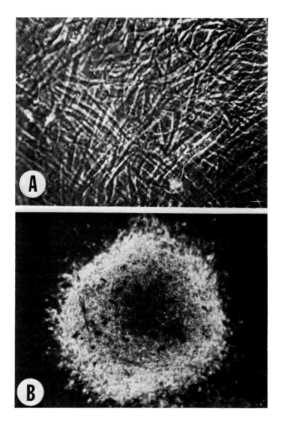

FIG. 2. A, A focus of human skin fibroblasts KD strain transformed by radiographs. **B,** Anchorage independent radiograph transformed KD cells growing in Agar. (Data in part from ref. 3)

formation as indicated by morphologic changes while others maintained the appearance of the normal phenotype (16).

This type of physiologic competence as well as cell-cell relationship may be in fact close to what we observe *in vivo*.

2. Studies *in utero* indicate that exposure of hamster embryo cells *in utero* to 300 rad of radiation and subsequent culture *in vitro* within 24 hrs after exposure resulted in transformation rates which were ten-fold lower than those observed in parallel experiments where cells were exposed *in utero* (13). These results of lower frequency upon irradiation *in utero* are closer to the frequency of oncogenic transformation *in vivo*, and indicate that besides the interaction at cellular level between the oncogenic agent and the single cell other factors are involved in transformation such as host mediation, repair and loss of fixation at high density, inhibition of expression by cell-cell interaction (15), or other influences exerted by the tissue specific organization present *in vivo*, and modifying intercellular communication and other cell-cell relationships (11). When cells are transformed *in vitro* they are

devoid of tissue specific arrangements and are able to replicate under conditions where normally they may remain in a nonreplicating state. Thus, the *in vitro* situation may yield an exaggerated rate of transformation since fixation of transformation can be carried out with ease in log phase cultures.

A number of transformed cell lines were developed from these *in utero* experiments and studied for a variety of phenotypic properties (13). The most striking finding was that injection of the mixed populations of transformed cells into hamsters yielded both carcinomas as well as sarcomas. While these epithelial transformed embryonic cells went undetected in culture, beause of their unaltered morphology they proliferated in the animal to form carcinomas.

GENETIC SYNDROMES PREDISPOSED TO CANCER

Though a defined population of cells is exposed to a variety of carcinogens only a fraction of the surviving cells convert to a negative state. Genetic susceptibility to transformation is clearly essential. This susceptibility is enhanced in certain genetic diseases where DNA metabolism is defective. Two of these syndromes associated with a high rate of cancer are Bloom Syndrome (38) and xeroderma pigmentation (XP) (13). We find that the neoplastic transformation of these human cells by ultraviolet B irradiation, the rays clinically important to man, can be achieved at doses as low as 33 Joules/m^2, while the normal human fibroblasts do not transform at this dose level (1). Similarly, exposure of XP cells to UVC irradiation resulted in a higher transformation in the XP as compared to control (32). Specific defects in DNA metabolism resulting in the inability to adequately repair damage clearly serve as permissive genetic factors in cellular sensitivity to the oncogenic action of agents causing the specific damage which must go unrepaired or misrepaired.

HORMONES AS PERMISSIVE AND POTENTIATING FACTORS *IN VITRO*

Hormones have long been known to exert an important influence in the neoplastic process *in vivo* (24). Yet, underlying mechanisms of their action of neoplastic transformation are hard to define *in vivo* where host homeostatic mechanisms prevail.

Cell cultures afford us the opportunity to study the effect of hormones at a cellular level and to examine sites of action, dose response relationship, and temporal aspects of cell-hormone interaction.

Thyroid Hormones in Transformation

Using two cell systems, short term cultures of diploid hamster embryo cells (14,45) as well as a heteroploid mouse cell line C3H 10T½ (37) we have studied the role of thyroid hormones in radiogenic and chemically induced transformation (8,9,26). Cells were grown and maintained in medium containing serum depleted of thyroid hormones (26), (designated "hypothyroid"), control serum (designated "euthyroid"), and serum depleted of thyroid hormones supplemented with 10^{-7}M triiodothyronine (T_3) (designated "hyperthyroid"). Initial experiments evaluated the role of thyroid hormones in radiograph-induced transformation.

We found that whereas growth kinetics and cell survival following radiation were not influenced by the altered thyroid levels, transformation was greatly modified, indicating that the hormones directly influenced the induction of neoplastic transformation. The results showed that in both cell types transformation was inhibited in the hypothyroid state (Table 1) and that the addition of triiodothyronine (T_3) at physiologic doses (10^{-12} - 10^{-10}M) resulted in transformation which was T_3 dose dependent (Fig. 3).

The effectiveness of making the cells competent for transformation was not mimicked by reverse T_3, an inactive isomer of triiodothyronine indicating the significance of the active hormone. It is of interest to note that there existed a close similarity between the T_3 dependent induction of transformation and that of the membrane associated transport enzyme Na/K ATPase (Fig. 3). T_3 must be present either before or at the time of exposure to radiation (Fig. 4). Addition of T_3 to the medium just 12 hrs before irradiation and removal 12 hrs after irradiation elicits full expression of transformation. Moreover, the addition of T_3 12 or 24 hrs after irradiation yields no transformants even though the cells were maintained in T_3 supplemented media for the entire 6 weeks required for expression of the transformed state. It is important to note that when T_3 is added at the time of irradiation there is a reduction (80%) in transformation frequency. These results indicate that T_3 is required only during initiation of radiograph-induced transformation but not at the late phase of expression. Furthermore, it is evident that the critical period for the

TABLE 1. *The effect of thyroid hormone on radiograph irradiation-induced cell transformation in vitro of C3H/10T½ mouse cells and hamster embryo cells (HE) in culture[a]*

Cells	Treatment[b]	Transformation/ surviving cells	Transformation frequency
C3H/10T½	Eu	0/23313	0
	Eu + 300 rad	29/27737	8.65×10^{-4}
	$-T_3-T_4$[c] + 300 rad	0/33747	0
	$+ T_3$[d] + 300 rad	16/21040	7.60×10^{-4}
HE	Eu	0/2800	0
	Eu + 220 rad	16/4300	3.33×10^{-3}
	$-T_3-T_4$ + 220 rad	0/1500	0
	$+T_3$ + 220 rad	15/3600	4.17×10^{-3}

[a]Data modified from ref. 26.
[b]Eu, euthyroid conditions, medium supplemented with untreated serum.
[c] $-T_3-T_4$, medium containing serum depleted of thyroid hormones (hypothyroid)
[d] $+T_3$, medium containing hypothyroid serum but supplemented with T_3 at 10^{-7} M.

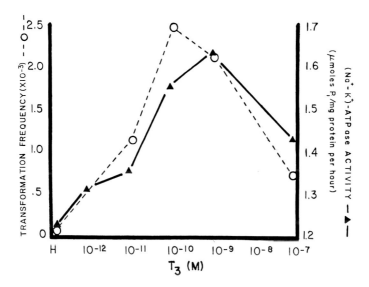

FIG. 3. Effect of various concentrations of T_3 on transformation frequency *(empty circle)* and on Na+/K+ ATPase *(solid triangle)*. (Data from ref. 26, with permission).

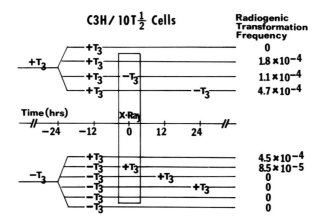

FIG. 4. Time course for thyroid effectiveness in radiation-induced transformation cells were grown incubated in the presence of T_3 or in the absence of T_3 ($-T_3$). T_3 was added or removed at different times in relation to radiograph exposure.

presence of thyroid hormone in the culture medium is the 12-hr period just prior to irradiation.

An important characteristic of thyroid hormone action is the lag time of 8 to 24 hrs between the administration of the hormone and the augmentation of protein synthesis. The time dependent of the action of T_3 on transformation is consistent with a possible induction of a host protein that acts in concert with the events set in motion by irradiation.

The dependence of radiogenic-induced transformation on T_3 concentration falls within the range of hormone levels in the circulation of intact animals under physiologic conditions. Maximal transformation frequency was observed at a T_3 concentration of 0.1 nM with a K½ of 10 pM. It is important to note that thyroid augmentation of Na^+, K^+-ATPase was elicited in the same media (resin-treated fetal calf serum with and without) as was T_3 modulation of neoplastic transformation. Moreover, both responses to T_3 (Na^+, K^+-ATPase and radiograph-induced transformation) appear to have similar latent periods, i.e., 12 to 24 hrs. These analogies raise the possibility that thyroid hormone induces a host protein that mediates irradiation-induced transformation, an inference supported by our finding that T_3 potentiation of radiograph-induced transformation was completely suppressed in the presence of cyclohexamide at 100 µg/ml.

More recent experiments to evaluate further aspects of T_3 involvement in the initiation of radiogenic transformation indicate that whereas the tumor promotors TPA (12-0-tetradecanoyl-phorbol 13 acetate) and teleocidin (23) markedly enhance induced transformation in the C3H10T½ cells, under euthyroid and hyperthyroid conditions no enhancement was seen. Since promotors will enhance initiated cells (4,5) this clearly suggests that no initiation of radiogenic transformation took place when cells were irradiated under hypothyroid conditions.

Thyroid hormones appear to serve as crucial factors also in the initiation of transformation by chemical carcinogens (8,9).

Exposure of hamster embryo cells or C3H10T½ to benzo(a)pyrene (B(a)P) (1 µg/ml) or the N-methyl-N-nitro-N-nitrosoguanidine (MNNG) (0.1 µg/ml) resulted in no observed transformation under hypothyroid conditions (Table 2). The addition of T_3 at physiologic doses of 10^{-12} to 10^{-9} 12 hrs prior to addition of the chemicals resulted in transformation rate which was directly related to the dose of T_3 in a similar manner to the dose response relationship to T_3 dependent radiograph-induced transformation. Peak transformation rate was seen when T_3 was added 12 hours prior to exposure to the chemical carcinogen at a dose of 2×10^{-10}M.

TABLE 2. *The effect of thyroid hormones on MNNG[a] induced neoplastic transformation[b]*

Treatment	C3H/10T½ cells		Hamster embryo cells	
	Transformation/ surviving cells	Transformation frequency	Transformation/ surviving cells	Transformation frequency
Eu[c]	0/15000	0	0/4100	0
Eu + MNNG	37/12300	3.01×10^{-3}	30/2120	1.4×10^{-2}
$-T_3-T_4$[d] + MNNG	0/13100	0	0/5780	0
$+T_3$[e] + MNNG	21/11305	1.86×10^{-3}	34/2614	1.3×10^{-2}

[a]MNNG 0.5 µG/ml
[b]Data in part from ref. 9.
[c]Eu, euthyroid conditions, medium supplemented with untreated serum.
[d]$-T_3-T_4$, medium containing serum depleted of thyroid hormones (hypothyroid).
[e]$+T_3$, medium containing hypothyroid serum but supplemented with T_3 at 10^{-9} M.

A time course study of T_3 effects on B(a)P induced transformation is somewhat more complex than with radiograph-induced transformation. While cellular interaction with radiographs takes place within a fraction of a second, the protocol for chemically induced transformation consisted of a 48 hr incubation time with the carcinogen in media devoid of thyroid hormones or supplemented with T_3. Our result indicates that similar to radiographs, the highest transformation rate is observed when T_3 is added 12 hrs prior to exposure to B(a)P indicating the crucial role of the hormone in early events of initiation. Addition of T_3 to cells grown under hypothyroid conditions concomitantly with B(a)P or 24 hrs after addition resulted in a lower transformation rate.

When T_3 was added to cells exposed to B(a)P, under hypothyroid condition, following the removal of B(a)P no transformation was observed. Similar to the finding and described above in relation to radiogenic transformation we found that reverse T_3 is inactive in substituting for T_3 as a permissive factor for transformation. We also find that cylohexamide at 100 µg/ml greatly inhibits B(a)P induced transformation, indicating the important role of protein synthesis in the action of T_3 in chemically induced transformation.

The observations *in vitro* that thyroid hormones are important permissive factors in neoplastic transformation is supported by *in vivo* data. Hypothyroid animals have been found to develop fewer metastases than hyperthyroid animals (35), and the development of primary tumors is suppressed in a hypothyroid state (47).

Thyroid hormones are also potentiators of ozone toxicity (12). Animals exposed to ozone, a ubiquitous environmental pollutant, are protected from ozone toxicity when they are in a hypothyroid state but suffer severe toxicity under hyperthyroid conditions (21). Though ozone is not a documented oncogenic agent it is a producer of free radicals which may be associated in processes of carcinogenesis (18,46).

Another hormone which appears to serve as a permissive factor at a cellular level in neoplastic transformation is β-estradiol (3,34). The hormone potentiates both radiation and chemically induced transformation in human cells.

PROTECTIVE FACTORS MODIFYING EXPRESSION AND PROMOTION OF TRANSFORMATION

Factors associated with inhibition of late stages in the progress of neoplastic development are essentially an inherent component of the cell. These include retinoids (6,31,42), selenium (4,5,25), and the free radical scavenging enzyme superoxide dismutase (18).

Our findings indicate that Vitamin A analogs β-all-trans-retinoic acid and trimethylmethoxyphenyl analog of *N*-ethyl retinamide inhibit in both hamster embryo cells as well as in the C3H10T½ mouse cells neoplastic transformation induced by x-irradiation, or by the tryptophan pyrolysale 3-amino-1-methyl-5H-pyrido(4,3,b) indol (Trp-P-2) (6). We also found that the retinoids were effective protectors against the enhancement of radiation induced transformation by TPA (4,5,33), while this antagonism was not reflected in modification of sister chromatid exchanges it was reflected at the membrane level in altered levels of the sodium transport enzyme Na/K ATPase. The enzyme level was decreased in the presence of the retinoids; it was enhanced by TPA and when both TPA and the vitamin A analog were present the enzyme level returned to control (Table 3).

The effectiveness of the retinoids in preventing expression and promotion took place within a short time after their addition. Their action in suppressing oncogenesis and promotion was irreversible (6,33).

Similar to the retinoids, selenium (Se) $NaSeO_3$, a ubiquitous element in nature and one used in industry, was an effective inhibitor of transformation induced by radiographs, benzo(a)pyrene and by tryptophan pyrolysate Tr P-P-2 (6) derived from broiled proteins (43,45). Se exerts an inhibitory effect whether added to the cells before exposure to the carcinogen or after exposure. Se is a cofactor in the Se-dependent glutathione peroxidase, an enzyme involved in cellular defense against the toxic action of free radicals on cellular components (22,23). Note that Se is an important cellular protector against ozone toxicity and its toxic effects may be enhanced by interaction with other photochemical pollutants (12).

Recent data seem to suggest more and more that free radicals which cause a variety of cascading events associated with lipid peroxidation (23) play an important role in carcinogenesis especially in promotion, *in vivo* (41) and *in vitro* (4,5,18). We find that superoxide dismutase, a scavenger of free radicals (22), inhibits oncogenic transformation in hamster embryo cells by radiograph and by bleomycin as well as inhibiting the enhancement of transformation by TPA (Table 4).

CONCLUSIONS

When evaluating permissive and protective factors in oncogenic transformation utilizing *in vitro* systems to carry out an assessment we are cognizant of the fact

TABLE 3. *The effect of all-trans retinoic acid (RA)
and TPA on membrane enzyme activities in normal and
radiograph transformed hamster embryo (HE) and
C3H/10T½ cells (C3H)[a]*

	Na^+/K^+-ATPase	Mg^+-ATPase	5'-Nucleotidase
C3H($N=6$)			
Control	1.79 ± 0.32	1.26 ± 0.31	0.56 ± 0.08
RA	1.13 ± 0.20	1.32 ± 0.26	0.68 ± 0.05
TPA	2.18 ± 0.31	1.26 ± 0.26	0.60 ± 0.12
RA + TPA	1.73 ± 0.23	1.23 ± 0.28	0.64 ± 0.10
He ($N=5$)			
Control	1.21 ± 0.21	1.35 ± 0.17	1.73 ± 0.28
RA	0.78 ± 0.19	1.32 ± 0.36	1.75 ± 0.21
TPA	1.53 ± 0.43	1.44 ± 0.45	1.89 ± 0.31
RA + TPA	1.13 ± 0.27	1.19 ± 0.41	1.91 ± 0.32

All values are mean ± standard error in μM P_1/hr/mg protein.

[a]Data in part from ref. 6.

TABLE 4. *The inhibiting effect of superoxide dismutase on hamster embryo cell transformation by radio and bleomycin[a,b]*

Treatment	S.F.	% Transformation
300 rad	0.75	0.70 ± 0.14
300 rad + TPA	0.69	1.82 ± 0.09
300 rad + SOD	0.91	0.17 ± 0.06
300 rad + TPA + SOD	0.89	0.51 ± 0.08
Bleomycin	0.65	1.30 ± 0.09
Bleomycin + SOD	0.75	0.33 ± 0.10

[a]Data in part from ref 18.
[b]SOD was added at 10μg/ml at seeding time. Cells were exposed to radiation or bleomycin treatment (μg/ml) 24 hrs later. SOD was left throughout the experiment (for 14 days). TPA was added 24 hrs after irradiation at 1 μg/ml.

that these systems do not faithfully represent the situation *in vivo*. However, these systems allow us to dissect events under definite conditions.

Clearly, genetic susceptibility to the initiation of cellular transformation by oncogenic agents is a primary factor in carcinogenesis, and it may depend in part on the presence and activation of cellular transforming genes (20). However, transformation of a genetically susceptible cell requires a set of physiologic conditions such as the right hormonal milieu, e.g. adequate thyroid hormone level, as seen in our work. Defective DNA metabolism would enhance the genetic susceptibility as in the UV irradiated XP cells, yet if cells are in nonreplicating state and cannot fix the transformed event, no transformation would take place. Once cells are initiated under favorable conditions of cell cycle and a permissive cellular milieu there are a number of cellular defense systems which modify the progression of the neoplastic event into frank neoplasia and inhibit the effect of promotors. Some of these protectors such as SOD, Se, retinoids play a role in part by modifying the action of free radicals. These radicals which are inherent in living cells may have deleterious effects on a variety of biological molecules resulting in peroxidation of membranes and in a cascade of events of both nuclear and extranuclear nature (23).

The availability of cellular defense systems may vary from one system to another depending on species (18) and probably source of tissue, thus determining along with the other factors the ultimate frequency of malignant transformation.

Some of these agents, such as the retinoids which play a role in differentiation as well as inhibiting neoplasia (31), may exert multiple effects. Their suppressive action on transformation and promotion, which we found to be associated with gene expression, may be in part a result of delicate genetic alterations associated with the expression of the cellular oncogenes (43,48). However, at the present time one cannot exclude the possibility that the action of free radicals in producing DNA strand scission (30) may render them suspect in modifying cellular transforming genes and that retinoids inhibit this action.

ACKNOWLEDGMENTS

This investigation was supported by Contract DE-ACO2-78EVO4733 from the Department of Energy and by Grant No. CA 12536-11 to the Radiological Research Laboratory/Department of Radiology, and by Grant No. CA 13696 to the Cancer Center/Institute of Cancer Research, awarded by the National Cancer Institute, Department of Health and Human Services.

REFERENCES

1. Andrews, A., and Borek, C. (1982): Neoplastic transformation of human xeroderma pigmentosum and Bloom syndrome cells by UVB. *Clinical Res.* 30:574A.
2. Berneblum, I. (1975): Sequential aspects of chemical carcinogenesis: skin. In: *Cancer, a Comprehensive Treatise, Vol. 1*, edited by F. F. Becker, pp. 323–344, Plenum Press, New York.
3. Borek, C. (1980): X-ray induced *in vitro* neoplastic transformation of human diploid cells. *Nature*, 283:776–778.
4. Borek, C. (1982): Radiation oncogenesis in culture. *Adv. in Cancer Res.*, 37:159–232.
5. Borek, C. (1982): Environmental Cancer Hazards; *in vitro* studies on risk, protection and potentiation. In: *Proc. of 13th Internatl. Cancer Congress, Seattle*. Alan Liss, New York.
6. Borek, C. (1982): Vitamin and micronutrients modify carcinogenesis and tumor promotion *in vitro*. In: *Molecular Interactions of Nutrition and Cancer*, edited by M. S. Arnott et al. Raven Press, New York.
7. Borek, C., Morgan, W. F., Ong, A., and Cleaver, E. J.: Inhibition of malignant transformation *in vitro* by inhibitors of Poly (ADP-ribose) synthesis. *Proc. Nat. Acad. Sci. (USA) (in press)*.
8. Borek, C., Guernsey, D. L., and Ong, A. (1981): Thyroid hormones modulates radiation and chemically induced neoplastic transformation *in vitro*. *Proc. Amer. Asso. for Cancer Res.*, 22:139.
9. Borek, C., Guernsey, D. L., Ong, A., and Edelman, I. S. (1982): The crucial role of thyroid hormone in oncogenic transformation induced by chemical carcinogens. Proceedings of the National Academy of Sciences (USA) *(in press)*.
10. Borek, C., Hall, E. J., and Rossi, H. H. (1978): Malignant transformation in cultured hamster embryo ells produced by x-rays, 430-keV mono-energetic neutrons, and heavy ions. *Cancer Res.*, 38:2997–3005.
11. Borek, C., Higashino, S., and Loewenstein, W. R. (1969): Intercellular communication and tissue growth IV. Conductance of membrane functions of normal and cancerous cells in culture. *J. Memb. Biol.*, 1:274–293.
12. Borek, C., and Mehlman, M. A. (1983): Evaluation of Health Effects, Toxicity and Biochemical mechanisms of ozone. In: *The Biomedical Effects of Ozone and Related Photochemical Oxidants*, edited by M. A. Mehlman et al., pp. 325–361. Senate Press, Princeton.
13. Borek, C., Pain, C., and Mason, H. (1977): Neoplastic transformation of hamster embryo cells irradiated *in utero* and assayed *in vitro*. *Nature*, 266:452–454.
14. Borek, C., and Sachs, L., (1966): *In vitro* cell transformation by x-irradiation *Nature*, 210:276–278.
15. Borek, C., and Sachs, L. (1966): The difference in contact inhibition of cell replication between normal cells and cells transformed by different carcinogens. *Proc. Natl. Acad. Sci. USA*, 56:1705–1711.
16. Borek, C., and Sachs, L. (1967): Cell susceptibility to transformation by x-irradiation and fixation of the transformed state. *Proc. Natl. Acad. Sci. USA*, 57:1522–1527 (1967).
17. Borek, C., and Sachs, L. (1968): The number of cell generations required to fix the transformed state in x-ray induced transformation. *Proc. Natl. Acad. Sci. USA*, 59:83–85.
18. Borek, C., and Troll, W.: Modifiers of free radicals inhibit *in vitro* the oncogenic actions of x-rays, bleomycin and the tumor promotor TPA *Proc. Natl. Acad. Sci. USA*, 80:1304–1307.
19. Cleaver, J. E. (1980): DNA damage, repair systems and human hypersensitive disease. *J. Environ. Path. and Toxicol.*, 3:53–68.
20. Cooper, G. M. (1982): Cellular transforming genes. *Science*, 218:801–806.
21. Fairhild, E. J., and Graham, S. L. (1963): Thyroid influence in toxicity of respiratory irritant gases, ozone and nitrogen oxide. *J. Pharmacol. Exp. Therap.*, 139:177–184.

22. Fridovich, I. (1978): The biology of oxygen radicals. The superoxide radical is an agent of oxygen toxicity; superoxide dismutase provide an important defense. *Science*, 201:875–880.

23. Fujiki, H., Mori, M., Nakayasu, M., Terada, M., and Sugimura, T. (1979): A possible naturally ocurring tumor promotor, Teleocidin B from Streptomyces, *Biochem. and Biophys. Res. Comm.*, 90:976–983.

24. Furth, H. (1975): Hormones as etiological agents in neoplasia. In: *Cancer, A Comprehensive Treatise, Vol. 1*, edited by F. F. Becker, pp. 95–112. Plenum Press, New York.

25. Griffin, A. C. (1979): Role of selenium in chemoprevention of cancer. *Adv. Cancer Res.*, 34:419–442.

26. Guernsey, D. L., Ong, A., and Borek, C. (1980): Thyroid hormone modulation of x-ray-induced *in vitro* neoplastic transformation. *Nature*, 288:591–592.

27. Kakunaga, T. (1975): The role of cell division in malignant transformation of mouse cells treated with 3 methy-cholanthrene. *Cancer Res.*, 35:1637–1642.

28. Kakunaga, T. (1978): Neoplastic transformation of human diploid fibroblast cells by chemical carcinogens. *Proc. Natl. Acad. Sci. USA*, 75:1334–1338.

29. Leibovitz, B. E., and Siegel, B. V.(1980): Aspects for free radical reactions in biological systems: Aging. *J. of Gerontology*, 35:45–56.

30. Lesko, S. A., Lorentzen, R. J., and T'so, P. O. P. (1980): The role of superoxide in deoxyribonucleic acid strand scission. *Biochemistry*, 19:3028.

31. Lotan, R. (1980): Effects of vitamin A and its analogs (retinoids) on normal and neoplastic cells. *Biochem. Biophys. Acta*, 605:33–91.

32. Maher, V. M., Rowan, L. A., Silinskas, K. C., Kately, S. A., and McCormick, J. J. (1982): Frequency of UV induces neoplastic transformation of diploid human fibroblasts is higher in xeroderma pigmentosum cells than in normal cells. *Proc. Natl. Acad. Sci. USA*, 8:2613.

33. Miller, R. C., Geard, C. R., Osmak, R. S., Rutledge-Freeman, M., Ong, A., Mason, H., Napholtz, A., Perez, N., Harisiadis, L., and Borek, C. (1981): Modification of sister chromatid exchanges and radiation-induced transformation in rodent cells by the tumor promotor 12-0-tetradecanoylphorbol-13-acetate and two retinoids. *Cancer Res.*, 41:655–659.

34. Milo, G. E. Jr., and DiPaolo, J. A. (1978): Neoplastic transformation of human diploid cells *in vitro* after chemical carcinogen treatment. *Nature*, 275:130–132.

35. Mishkin, S. Y., Pollack, R., Yalovsky, M. A., Morris, H. P., and Mishkin, S. (1981): Inhibition of local and metastatic hepatome growth and prolongation of survival after induction of hypothyroidism. *Cancer Res.*, 41:3040–3045.

36. Morgan, W. F., and Cleaver, J. E. (1982): 3-aminobenzamide synergistically increases sister-chromatic exchanges in cells exposed to methane-sulfanate but not to ultraviolet light. *Mut. Res.*, 104:361–366.

37. Reznikoff, C. A., Bertram, J. S., Brankow, D. W., and Heidelberger, C. (1973): Quantative and qualitative studies of chemical transformation of cloned C3H mouse embryo cells sensitive to postconfluence inhibition of cell division. *Cancer Res.*, 33:3239–3249.

38. Schonberg, S., and Germon, J. (1980): Sister chromatid exchange in cells metabolically coupled to Bloom's syndrome cells. *Nature*, 284:72–74.

39. Shilo, B., and Weinberg, R. A. (1981): Unique transforming gene in carcinogen transformed mouse cells. *Nature*, 289:607–609.

40. Silinskas, K. C., Kately, S. A., Towar, J. E., Maher, V. M., and McCormick, J. J. (1981): Induction of anchorage-independent growth in human fibroblast by propane sultane. *Cancer Res.*, 41:1620–1627.

41. Slaga, T. J., Klein-szanto, A. J. P., Triplatt, L. L., Yotti, L. P., and Trosko, J. E., (1981): Skin tumor-promoting activity of Benzoyl Peroxide, a widely used free radical generating compounds. *Science*, 213:1023–1025.

42. Sporn, M. B., Dunlop, N. M., Newton, D. L. and Smith, J. M. (1976): Prevention of chemical carcinogenesis by vitamin A and its synthetic analogs (retinoids). *Fec. Proc.*, 35:1332–1338.

43. Sugimura, T., Magao, M., Kawachi, T., Honda, M., Yahagi, T., Seino, Y., Sato, S., and Matsukura, N. (1977): Mutagen-carcinogens in food with special reference to highly mutagenic pyrolytic products in broiled foods, In: *Origins of Human Cancer*, edited by H. H. Hiatt, J. D. Watson, and J. Winstein, pp. 1561–1577. Cold Spring Harbor Laboratory, Cold Spring Harbor, New York.

44. Sutherland, B. M., Currino, J. S., Dehilas, N., Shih, A. G., and Oliver, R. P. (1980): Ultraviolet light-induces transformation of human cells to anchorage independent growth. *Cancer Res.*, 40:1934.

45. Takayama, S., Katoh, Y., Tanaka, M., Nagao, M., Wakabayashi, K., and Sugimura, T. (1977): *In vitro* transformation of hamster embryo cells with tryptophan pyrolysis products. Proceedings of the Japan Academy 53:126–129.
46. Troll, W., Witz, G., Goldstein, B., Stone, D., and Sugimura, T. (1982): The role of free oxygen radicals in tumor promotion and carcinogenesis. In: *Carcinogenesis 7*, edited by E. Hecker et al., pp. 593–597. Raven Press, New York.
47. Vonderhaar, B. K., and Greco, A. E. (1982): Effect of thyroid status on development of spontaneous mammary tumors in primiparous C₃H mice. *Cancer Res.*, 42:4553–4561.
48. Westin, E. H., Gallo, R. C., Aria, S. K., Eva, A., Souza, L. M., Belluda, M. A., Aaronson, S. A., and Long-Staal, F. (1982): Differential expression of the amv gene in human hematopoietic cells. *Proc. Natl. Acad. Sci. USA*, 79:2194–2198.
49. Westin, E. H., Long-Staal, F., Gillman, F. P., Dalla Favara, R., Papas, T. S., Lautenberger, J. A., Eva, A., Reddy, E. P., Troniek, G. R., Aaronson, S. A., and Gallo, R. C. (1982): Expression of cellular homologues of retro viral one genes in human hematopoietic cells. *Proc. Natl. Acad. Sci. USA*, 79:2490–2494.
50. Zimmerman, R. J., and Little, J. B. (1981): Factors influencing the induction and expression of oncogenic transformation in human diploid cells. *J. of Supramolecular Struct. and Cell Biochem. (Suppl. 5)*, 603:220.

Biochemical Basis of Chemical Carcinogenesis,
edited by H. Greim, R. Jung, M. Kramer,
H. Marquardt, and F. Oesch.
Raven Press, New York © 1984.

The Mechanisms of Chemically Induced Malignant Transformation: Its Inhibition by Polynucleotides and its Reversion by 5-Bromodeoxyuridine

Hans Marquardt

Department of Toxicology, University of Hamburg Medical School and Fraunhofer Institute of Toxicology and Aerosol Research, D-2000 Hamburg 13, Federal Republic of Germany

The mechanisms of action of chemically induced malignant transformation are unknown (11). Transformation may be the result of a somatic mutation, i.e., a heritable change in nucleotide sequence resulting from an alteration, deletion, or rearrangement in the primary structure of DNA. While this remains the most logical explanation for the permanent and heritable malignant change, a variety of experimental results suggests, however, an alternative explanation, i.e., that malignant transformation may be the result of epigenetic changes in cellular transcription/translation. Such changes are presumed to be also responsible for much of normal development. Thus, it has been shown that thyroid hormone plays a crucial role in radiograph induced neoplastic transformation, presumably by inducing the synthesis of a host protein that is an obligatory participant in transformation (7), and that diethylstilbestrol (1) and 5-azacytidine (8) cause neoplastic transformation of C3H10T1/2 cells without measurable mutation. It is noteworthy that the latter compound inhibits DNA methylation and thereby affects cellular differentiation (17). Moreover, clones of mouse fibroblasts which are resistant to chemical transformation exhibit similar proliferation kinetics and metabolic activity as well as similar susceptibility towards chemically induced cytotoxicity, DNA-repair, and mutagenesis than transformable variant clones (9; *own unpublished results*). These data as well as results obtained with promoting agents (5) and caffeine (4) suggest that, in addition to an initial mutational event, other (epigenetic) cellular processes are a prerequisite of malignant transformation or, alternatively, that malignant transformation and mutagenesis *in vitro* induced by chemicals may not be causally related at all. This view is supported by our observations on inhibition and reversion of chemically induced malignant transformation by polynucleotides and 5-bromodeoxyuridine, respectively.

189

INHIBITION OF TRANSFORMATION BY POLYNUCLEOTIDES

We have previously reported that the synthetic double-stranded RNA, poly-riboinosinic-polyribocytidylic acid [poly(rI:rC)], inhibits the induction of malignant transformation of mouse M2 fibroblasts by chemical carcinogens (10,11). In these experiments, the polymer, to be effective, had to be given for 24 hr at 24 hrs before, at the time of, at 3 days or 8 days after carcinogen treatment; the compound, however, did not affect transformation when used 12 days after carcinogen treatment. These results cannot be explained by poly(rI:rC) providing a selective advantage to nontransformed cells: The concentration of the polymer used was lethal neither to nontransformed nor to transformed cells (10). The inhibitory activity of polynucleotides is not restricted to poly(rI:rC); polyribocytidylic:oligodeoxyriboguanylic acid similarly inhibited malignant transformation induced by the chemical carcinogen, *N*-methyl-*N'*-nitro-*N*-nitro-soguanidine (MNNG) (11).

In contrast, both polymers did not affect the induction of 8-azaguanine-resistant mutants of V79 Chinese hamster cells by chemical carcinogens (11). Likewise, when transformation and mutagenesis were investigated concomitantly in M2 mouse fibroblasts (12), poly(rI:rC) inhibited transformation induced by MNNG without affecting the induction of ouabain-resistant mutants (Table 1) (13).

Since one of the prominent actions of poly(rI:rC) is the induction of interferon, which has been shown to cause reversion of the neoplastic phenotype of transformed cells (2), interferon activity was also investigated: A mouse interferon preparation, which stimulated microsomal metabolism of polycyclic aromatic hydrocarbons and thus effectively penetrated M2 cells, had no significant effect on transformation (10). Moreover, in very preliminary results with mouse M2 fibroblasts we observed that poly(1-methyl-6-thioinosinic acid), a single-stranded polynucleotide (kindly provided by Dr. A. D. Broom, University of Utah), which does not induce interferon but inhibits reverse transcriptase activity (3), also seems to inhibit chemically induced malignant transformation but not mutagenesis (40 μg/ml). In addition, both, cultures of nontransformed and of transformed cells, exhibited neither virus particles nor reverse transcriptase activity.

TABLE 1. *Effect of poly(rI:rC) on mutagenesis and malignant transformation by chemicals in cloned mouse M2 fibroblasts*

Treatment		Mutagenesis	Malignant transformation
poly(rI:rC) (10μg/ml)	MNNG (0,2μg/ml)	(Ou^r/10^6 survival)	(transfer foci/10^6 survival)
–	–	0.7	0
+	–	0.6	0
–	+	94	3600
+	+	92	0

Poly(rI:rC) was added 3 days after MNNG-treatment and was present in cultures for 24 hrs.

The mechanism of action of the inhibitory effect of polynucleotides on chemically induced malignant transformation is unknown. These agents, however, are known to inhibit the activity of reverse transcriptase (3,16). Thus, our results may suggest that reverse transcriptase plays a role not only in transformation by oncogenic RNA viruses but, as visualized by Temin (15), also during normal development and in differentiation as well as in chemical carcinogenesis (11).

REVERSION OF THE NEOPLASTIC PHENOTYPE OF TRANSFORMED CELLS

The view that malignant transformation and differentiation, which is potentially reversible, are causally related is emphasized by the numerous observations that reversion of the neoplastic phenotype of plant, mammalian, and even human transformed cells can occur (11). Particularly noteworthy in this regard are such reversion results obtained by treatment of cells with 5-bromodeoxyuridine (BUdR) since this pyrimidine analog has been shown to affect gene expression and cellular differentiation, too (6). We have observed that by treatment of chemically transformed mouse M2 fibroblasts with nonlethal concentrations of BUdR (thus excluding selection as a possible mechanism of action) a reversion of the transformed phenotype (increased flattening of cells, decreased saturation density, loss of tumorigenicity) can be induced in the entire cell population. This effect of BUdR was not observed when the compound was added to confluent cultures or to cultures in which DNA synthesis had been inhibited by hydroxyurea. When BUdR was removed, the cells did not "back-revert" to the transformed phenotype (11). Together with Dr. A. Ogilvie we have studied the glycoprotein composition of cell membranes during chemically induced transformation and during BUdR- induced suppression of the malignant phenotype of transformed cells (14). Several differences in the concentration of concanavalin A-receptor proteins were observed between transformed and nontransformed cells and between transformed and BUdR-reverted cells. However, these changes in glycosylation are not a general phenomenon associated with reversion of malignancy, since comparative analysis of a mouse erythroleukemic cell line during treatment with DMSO, which triggers differentiation to erythroblasts and also leads to suppression of malignancy, revealed no differences in the glycoprotein pattern.

CONCLUSIONS

The mechanisms of action of chemically induced malignant transformation remain unknown. The limited evidence available suggests that transformation is not caused by conventional mutagenesis; transformation, like differentiation, may represent heritable changes that are phenotypic rather than genotypic in nature. It is also conceivable that the transformation process may consist of two distinct steps, i.e., the fixation of transformation through a mutational mechanism and an obligatory subsequent step which leads to the expression of the transformed phenotype. In this regard, the role in the transformation process of genetic transpositions, i.e.,

DNA rearrangements that result in the increased expression of normal cellular genes, remains to be elucidated.

REFERENCES

1. Barret, J. C., Wong, A., and McLachlan, J. A. (1981): Diethylstilbestrol induces neoplastic transformation without measurable gene mutation at two loci. *Science*, 212:1402–1404.
2. Brouty-Boyé, D., and Gresser, J. (1981): Reversibility of the transformed and neoplastic phenotype. I. Progressive reversion of the phenotype of x-ray-transformed C3H/10T 1/2 cells under prolonged treatment with interferon. *Int. J. Cancer*, 28:165–173.
3. Chan, E. W., Lee, C. K., Dale, P. J., Nortridge, K. R., Horn, S. S., and Seed, T. M. (1981): Antiviral properties of polyinosinic acids containing thiol and methyl substitutions. *J. Gen. Virol*, 52:291–299.
4. Clegg, J. C. S., Glatt, H. R., and Oesch, F. (1981): Coordinate mutation and transformation of mouse fibroblasts: induction by nitroquinoline oxide and modulation by caffeine. *Carcinogenesis*, 2:1255–1259.
5. Fisher, P. B., Miranda, A. F., Mufson, R. A., Weinstein, L. S., Fujiki, H., Sugimura, T., and Weinstein, I. B. (1982): Effects of teleocidin and the phorbol ester tumor promoters on cell transformation, differentiation, and phospholipid metabolism. *Cancer Res.*, 42:2829–2835.
6. Goz, B. (1978): The effect of incorporation of 5-halogenated deoxyuridines into the DNA of eukaryotic cells. *Pharmacol. Rev.*, 29:249–272.
7. Guernsey, D. L., Borek, C., and Edelman, I. S. (1981): Crucial role of thyroid hormone in x-ray induced neoplastic transformation in cell culture. *Proc. Natl. Acad. Sci. USA*, 78:5708–5711.
8. Landolph, J. R., and Jones, P. A. (1982): Mutagenicity of 5-azacytidine and related nucleosides in C3H/10T 1/2 clone 8 and V79 cells. *Cancer Res.*, 42:817–823.
9. Lo, K. Y., and Kakunaga, T. (1982): Similarities in the formation and removal of covalent DNA adducts in benzo(a)pyrene-treated BALB/3T3 variant cells with different induced transformation frequencies. *Cancer Res.*, 42:2644–2650.
10. Marquardt, H. (1973): Polyriboinosinic-polyribocytidylic acid prevents chemically-induced malignant transformation in vitro. *Nature-New-Biology*, 246:228–229.
11. Marquardt, H. (1979): DNA - The critical target in chemical carcinogenesis? In: *Chemical Carcinogens and DNA, Vol. 2*, edited by P. L. Grover, pp. 159–179. CRC Press, Inc., Boca Raton, Florida.
12. Marquardt, H. (1980): Induction of mutation to oubain resistance and of malignant transformation by chemicals in cloned mouse M2 fibroblasts. *Carcinogenesis*, 1:215–218.
13. Marquardt, H. (1981): Inhibition by polyriboinosinic-polyribocytidylic acid of malignant transformation in vitro induced by chemical carcinogens without affecting mutagenesis. *Proc. Amer. Assoc. Cancer Res.*, 22:109.
14. Ogilvie, A., Schrappe, M., Arnold, H.-H., and Marquardt, H. (1982): Alteration in glycoprotein pattern during chemically induced malignant transformation and its reversal by 5-bromo-deoxyuridine. *(in press)*.
15. Temin, H. (1971): The protovirus hypothesis: speculations on the significance of RNA-directed DNA synthesis for normal development and carcinogenesis, *J. Natl. Cancer Inst.*, 46:III–VII.
16. Tuominen, F. W., and Kenney, F. T. (1971): Inhibition of the DNA polymerase of Rauscher leukemia virus by single-stranded polyribonucleotides. *Proc. Natl. Acad. Sci. USA*, 68:2198–2202.
17. Venolia, L., Gartler, S. M., Wassman, E. R., Yen, P., Mohandas, T., and Shapiro, L. J. (1982): Transformation with DNA from 5-azacytidine-reactivated x-chromosomes. *Proc. Natl. Acad. Sci. USA*, 79:2352–2354.

Biochemical Basis of Chemical Carcinogenesis,
edited by H. Greim, R. Jung, M. Kramer,
H. Marquardt, and F. Oesch.
Raven Press, New York © 1984.

Molecular Mechanisms in Multistage Chemical Carcinogenesis

I. Bernard Weinstein, Sebastiano Gattoni-Celli, Paul Kirschmeier,
Michael Lambert, Wendy Hsiao, Joseph Backer, and Alan Jeffrey

*Division of Environmental Sciences and Cancer Center/Institute of Cancer Research,
Columbia University, New York, NY 10032*

In 1882, almost exactly 100 years ago, Robert Koch revealed to the Physiological Society of Berlin his discovery that a bacterium was the cause of human tuberculosis (44). This fundamental insight into causation provided a rational basis for the eventual conquest of a major cause of human suffering and death. It also set a precedent for demonstrating the roles of other microorganisms in the causation of various infectious diseases. At the present time cancer presents a challenge somewhat similar to that presented by tuberculosis at the time of Robert Koch's discovery. However, it seems likely that the most common human cancers are due to complex interactions between environmental (exogenous) and host (endogenous) factors, rather than a single pathogenic microorganism. Despite this complexity, there is reason to be optimistic that current advances in our understanding of fundamental mechanisms of carcinogenesis will provide tools for the eventual conquest of the major human cancers, although the postulates and preventive approaches will be quite different than those employed in the control of tuberculosis and certain other infectious diseases (54).

The task of identifying specific causative factors in the origin of human cancers is complicated by several factors including: (a) the long latent period between exposure to causative agents and the overt appearance of the disease, (b) the multistep nature of the process, and (c) the likelihood that most human cancers result from a complex interaction between multiple environmental and endogenous factors (69,70). Nevertheless, our knowledge of basic biology, and the laboratory tools that are now available, are so much more powerful than those available to Robert Koch that there is considerable reason for optimism in terms of opportunities for primary cancer prevention.

Studies in experimental animals and in humans indicate that most tumors evolve through a multistep process that can occupy a considerable fraction of the lifespan of the species. In some instances the process can be divided into at least three stages, initiation, promotion, and progression, although even these stages are probably divisible into substages (22,31,62). These basic phenomena are also becoming apparent during the transformation of cells in culture, whether the process is induced by chemical carcinogens or certain oncogenic viruses (5,20,49,69,70).

Multistage carcinogenesis and tumor progression are often thought of in terms of a series of successive mutations and selections, eventuating in the clonal outgrowth of a fully malignant tumor. This may, however, be an oversimplification. As discussed in detail elsewhere (69,70), we think that a more suitable model is the multistage process that occurs during normal embryologic development, in which new stem cell populations emerge and develop into specialized cells and tissues. There is considerable evidence that the successive stages in carcinogenesis may involve qualitatively different events, that they can be enhanced or inhibited by quite different types of environmental and host factors, and that at least the early stages are often reversible (62,69,70).

EARLY EVENTS IN THE ACTION OF INITIATING CARCINOGENS

It is now known that several types of chemicals that initiate the carcinogenic process yield highly reactive species or metabolites that bind covalently to cellular DNA (48). Although there is considerable evidence that damage to DNA can play a critical role in carcinogenesis, the subsequent biochemical events that lead to the conversion of a normal cell to a cancer cell are not known. There has been a tendency to think of the initiating event in chemical carcinogenesis as a simple random point mutation resulting from errors in replicating the damaged DNA. Several features of the carcinogenic process, particularly the high efficiency of carcinogen-induced cell transformation, the latent period, and the multistep aspects are not consistent with this mechanism. Alternative mechanisms by which carcinogen-induced DNA damage might induce more complex and frequent genomic changes may include induction of gene rearrangements or gene amplification. Consistent with these possibilities is the increasing evidence that gene amplification and gene rearrangements occur in several normal systems undergoing development and differentiation. Complex biochemical mechanisms must regulate the latter genomic changes. It is possible, therefore, that carcinogen-DNA interactions might disrupt these mechanisms, and thus produce stable aberrations in the control of gene expression (69,70).

We have recently utilized a model system that rather dramatically demonstrates the ability of certain carcinogens to induce a much more complex change in DNA replication than random point mutation (45). The system is one in which DNA damage appears to induce asynchronous replication of an integrated viral genome. In these studies we employed the ts-a H3 cell line, which was derived in the laboratory of C. Basilico by transforming Fischer rat embryo fibroblasts 2408 with a ts-a mutant of polyoma virus (26). Ts-a H3 cells contain 1.3 viral equivalents of polyoma DNA integrated in the cell genome and, because the ts-a mutant produces a temperature sensitive large T antigen, these cells produce free polyoma DNA at 33° (the permissive temperature) but not at 39°. The integrated polyoma DNA has three deletions, and these provide very useful markers for the two major species of free viral DNA that can be induced in this cell line (26,73).

We exposed ts-a H3 cells to 0.25 μg/ml BP for 24, 48, or 72 hrs at either 33° or 30°C. The extrachromosomal DNA was then extracted by the method of Hirt, subjected to electrophoresis in 1% agarose, transferred onto nitrocellulose paper, and then hybridized with a ^{32}P-labeled probe of polyoma DNA prepared by nick-translation. Figure 1 (lanes 1,3,5) indicates that, as expected, simply shifting the temperature from 39 to 33° (in the absence of BP treatment) resulted in increasing production of free polyoma DNA during the subsequent 72 hrs. The addition of benzo[a]pyrene BP at the time of the temperature shift (Fig. 1, lanes 2,4,6) led to a marked enhancement in production of free polyoma DNA. On the other hand, when cells were simply maintained at 39°, either in the absence or presence of BP, and the DNA present in the Hirt extract analyzed at 24, 48, or 72 hrs no free polyoma DNA was detected (Fig. 1, lanes 7 through 10). Thus, both the spontaneous production of free polyoma DNA and the production induced by BP are dependent on the function of the T antigen of polyoma virus, since in cells transformed by the ts-a mutant of polyoma the T antigen functions at 33° but not at 39°C (26,73). Previous studies on the mechanism of production of free polyoma DNA in trans-

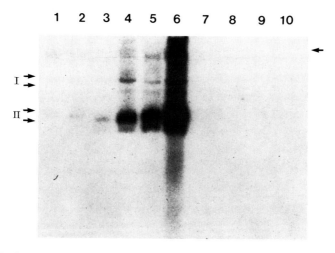

FIG. 1. Blotting patterns obtained with extrachromosomal DNA from ts-a H3 cells and a polyoma DNA probe. Extrachromosomal DNA was extracted by the Hirt procedure, separated by gel electrophoresis, blotted and hybridized to a ^{32}P-labeled polyoma DNA probe, as previously described (26). In lanes 1,3, and 5 the cells were shifted from 39° to 33°C and the DNA extracted at 24, 48, or 72 hrs after the temperature shift, respectively. In lanes 2,4, and 6 the procedure was the same except that BP (0.25 μg/ml) was added to the cultures at the time of the temperature shift. In lane 7 cells were grown continuously at 39°C. In lanes 8, 9, and 10 cells were grown at 39°C in the presence of BP (0.25 μg/ml) for 24, 48, or 72 hrs, respectively. All lanes were loaded with equivalent amounts of Hirt extract DNA. The arrows on the left side of the figure indicate the positions of supercoiled *(Form I, lower arrows)* and relaxed *(Form II, upper arrows)* molecules, of the two major species of free polyoma DNA produced by ts-a H3 cells (26). The arrow on the right indicates the position of the small amount of chromosomal DNA that contaminates the Hirt extract.

formed rat cells (6) are consistent with the onion skin model of viral replication, by which there is *in situ* replication of the integrated viral DNA, followed by excision of these copies and further extrachromosomal replication (10). Presumably, the exposure of cells to BP enhances one or more stages of this process.

Further studies utilizing the highly reactive carcinogenic metabolite of BP, BP-dihydrodiol-9,10-epoxide (BPDE), on a rat cell line transformed by wild type polyoma virus demonstrated that the enhancement of polyoma DNA synthesis persists for at least 5 days after a single exposure to BPDE, despite the rapid decay of this compound. In addition, enhanced synthesis of polyoma DNA could be induced by fusion of normal rat fibroblasts previously exposed to BPDE with polyoma transformed rat fibroblasts not exposed to BPDE. It appears, therefore, that the carcinogen enhancement of polyoma DNA replication is not due to direct damage to the integrated polyoma virus DNA, but may instead involve the induction of a cellular factor(s) that can function in "trans" to enhance asynchronous replication of polyoma DNA (45).

Our results are consistent with other evidence that DNA damaging agents can increase the production of polyoma DNA (37,73) and SV40 DNA (46,57) cells transformed by these viruses. Lavi and Etkin (46) have demonstrated that several types of carcinogens were active in inducing the production of free viral DNA in Chinese hamster embryo cells transformed with SV40 virus. They suggested that this system might be used as a simple screening test for potential carcinogens. Thus, a variety of DNA damaging agents can enhance the asynchronous replication of integrated polyoma or SV40 virus DNA sequences in mammalian cells. On the other hand, our studies suggest that it may be premature to invoke this process as a general mechanism of chemical carcinogenesis, particularly in cells that do not contain an exogenous viral genome, since we found that BP enhancement of polyoma virus DNA production is strictly dependent on the function of the polyoma virus T antigen (45). It is not clear, therefore, whether BP can induce the asynchronous replication of endogenous DNA sequences in normal rat cells. Indeed, in parallel studies we found that under conditions in which BP induced the production of extrachromosomal copies of polyoma DNA it did not induce the production of extrachromosomal DNAs homologous to the endogenous genomes of two rat retroviral sequences, the 30S and rat leukemia virus (45). We have not, of course, excluded the possibility that BP and other carcinogens might induce asynchronous replication and excision of other specific host sequences and this warrants further study. In any case, the ability of BP and other carcinogens to enhance extrachromosomal production, at the population level, of certain viral DNAs is of interest since it demonstrates the complexity of events that may occur when cells are exposed to environmental carcinogens.

Although nuclear events are usually emphasized in the action of chemical carcinogens, there is accumulating evidence that carcinogens can also cause extensive damage to mitochondrial DNA, both in cell culture and in the intact animal (1,3,41,52,72). In addition, we have obtained evidence that the potent tumor promoter 12-0-tetradecanoylphorbol-13-acetate impairs mitochondrial respiration (2,4).

It is possible, therefore, that disturbances in mitochondrial energy metabolism, and/ or related disturbances in intracellular ion homeostatis, may play an important role at specific stages of the carcinogenic process.

Later in this chapter we shall return to the question of the types of nuclear genes that might play a role in chemical carcinogenesis.

MECHANISM OF ACTION OF TUMOR PROMOTERS

Tumor promoters can be defined as compounds which have very weak or no carcinogenic activity when tested alone, but markedly enhance tumor yield when applied repeatedly following a low or suboptimal dose of a carcinogen (initiator)(31). Most of our information on the mechanism of action of this class of agents derives from studies on the potent skin tumor promoter TPA, and related phorbol esters. At the biochemical level, it appears that the major difference between initiators and the phorbol ester tumor promoters is that whereas initiators (or their metabolites) bind covalently to cellular DNA, the primary site of action of the phorbol ester tumor promoters appears to be cell membranes. The phorbol ester tumor promoters can exert highly pleiotropic effects on the growth, function, and differentiation of a variety of cell types. We have found it convenient to classify these effects into three categories: (a) mimicry and enhancement of transformation, (b) modulation of differentiation, and (c) membrane effects (31,69,70).

Utilizing [³H]-phorbol dibutyrate (PDBu), several laboratories have obtained direct evidence for specific high affinity saturable "phorboid receptors" in membrane preparations and intact cells from various avian, rodent, and human tissues (14,17, 31,33,60). We have determined the binding constants and receptor numbers in several types of tissue culture cells (Table 1)(35,36). In general, one or two classes of [³H]-PDBu receptors are found in each cell type. In most cases, a high affinity site, with a K_D in the range of 3 to 17 nmoles is present at 0.1 to 4×10^5 sites per cell. Where a second, lower affinity site is observed the K_D is 300 nmoles or greater, and the number of sites is greater than 1×10^6 per cell. Some variation in receptor number occurs within a cell line depending on the growth state of the cells at the time of assay. When only one binding site is detected the affinity for PDBu appears to be lower (K_D of 12 to 41 nmoles), but the number of sites is, in general, higher. It is of interest that in two rat brain tumor cell lines displaying glial-like properties as many as 2×10^6 high affinity sites per cell are present. This observation is in accord with the results of Nagle et al. (51), showing that brain tissue contains a very large number of phorboid receptors. We have also demonstrated PDBu receptors in normal human keratinocytes and in normal and transformed human melanocytes (29).

In general, the abilities of a series of phorbol esters to compete with [³H]-PDBu for binding to cell surface receptors correlates with their known potencies in cell culture and with their activities as tumor promoters on mouse skin (14,17,33,60). These results provide evidence that the phorboid receptors mediate the biological action of the phorbol esters. We have also found that the antileukemic plant di-

TABLE 1. *Characterization of Phorboid Receptors in various cell types*

		Phorboid receptors			
	Cell type	K_{D1} (nM)	Number/ cell	K_{D2} (nM)	Number/ cell
CREF N	Rat embryo fibroblast	8	1.6×10^5	710	2.8×10^6
CREF A	Rat embryo fibroblast	7	3.8×10^5	1,700	4×10^6
CREF A2	Variant of CREF A	18	1×10^6	—	—
E-11	Adenovirus-transformed rat embryo fibroblast	11	1.5×10^5	1,100	1.4×10^6
K-22	Rat liver epithelial	26	2.5×10^5	1,450	9.4×10^6
TS 19-10	TPA-sensitive friend erythroleukemia cells	8	3×10^4	800	3×10^6
TR 19-4	TPA-resistant friend erythroleukemia cells	8	3×10^4	800	3×10^6
B-35	NEU-transformed rat neuronal cell	25	4.1×10^5	—	—
B-103	NEU-transformed rat neuronal cell	36	4.5×10^5	—	—
B-49	Neu-transformed rat cell with neuronal and glial characteristics	9	1.6×10^5	330	5.4×10^6
B-15	NEU-transformed rat glial cell	40	1.5×10^6	—	—
B-92	Neu-transformed rat glial cell	37	1.4×10^6	—	—
SC-9	RSV-transformed rat cerebellar cells	15	1.8×10^5	700	4.4×10^6
WC-5	RSV-transformed rat cerebellar astrocyte	3	2×10^4	380	1.3×10^6
Ker	Normal human keratinocytes	37	1.3×10^6	4,880	7×10^7
5K-MEL21	Human metastatic melanoma	6	5.6×10^5	900	8×10^6

We thank Dr. G. Giotta of the Salk Institute for cell lines B-35 through WC-5. Lines B-35 through B-92 were isolated by Dr. D. Schubert of the Salk Institute. NEU, N-ethyl nitrosourea; RSV, Rous sarcoma virus.
Data from refs. 20, 29, 32, 33, 36.

terpenes gnidilatin and gnilatimacrin are potent inhibitors of [³H]-PDBu binding (36). As discussed below, it appears that the phorboid receptors also mediate the TPA-like effects of two new classes of tumor promoters, teleocidin (and structurally related indole alkaloids) and aplysiatoxin.

We have partially purified a factor present in normal human and rodent sera that inhibits [³H]-PDBu-receptor binding to both intact cells and isolated cell membranes (33,34). Unlike the phorbol ester tumor promoters, the serum factor does not stimulate the release of choline or arachidonic acid from cellular phospholipids, nor does it inhibit the binding of [¹²⁵I]-labeled epidermal growth factor to cellular receptors. The factor does, however, antagonize the inhibition of epidermal growth factor binding induced by PDBu. It would appear, therefore, that *in vivo* this factor might inhibit certain effects of this class of tumor promoters (34,36).

Until recently, the phorbol esters were the only class of skin tumor promoters that showed marked structure-function specificity and that were active at nanomolar concentrations. Fujiki et al. (23) have found, however, that the indole alkaloids teleocidin (isolated from *Streptomyces*) and dihydroteleocidin and a polyacetate compound aplysiatoxin (isolated from a marine algae) are as potent as TPA in inducing ornithine decarboxylase in mouse skin (23). Dihydroteleocidin and aplysiatoxin have also been demonstrated to be potent tumor promoters on mouse skin (24,25). Teleocidin and aplysiatoxin also induce many of the same effects as TPA in cell culture, including effects on growth, differentiation, and membrane structure and function (21,63). The chemical structures of teleocidin and aplysiatoxin are quite different from those of the phorbol esters. However, the fact that these compounds share similar biological effects suggested to us that they might act by binding to the phorboid receptors. Indeed, in collaborative studies (32,68) we have found that both teleocidin and aplysiatoxin are potent inhibitors of the binding of [³H]-PDBu to membrane receptors. These two compounds are also equipotent with TPA in inhibiting [¹²⁵I]-EGF receptor binding and in stimulating the release of [³H]-arachidonic acid and [³H]-choline from prelabeled cellular phospholipids (32).

These results prompted us to study the stereochemistry of these compounds to see if they might display structural similarities (32). All three types of compounds are amphipathic since they have both hydrophobic and hydrophilic domains. In the case of the phorbol esters there is evidence that all of the biologically active compounds have a highly hydrophobic residue on the 12 position, although the precise chemical structure of this residue is not critical (31,62). Presumably this region of the molecule is required for a relatively nonspecific hydrophilic interaction with a region on the phorboid receptor, or the adjacent lipid microenvironment. The saturated 6 membered ring of teleocidin and the side chain attached to the polyacetate ring of aplysiatoxin might play analogous roles. Extensive structure-activity studies of the phorbol esters on mouse skin and in cell culture indicate that the region of the molecule containing the 3-keto, 4-OH and 6-CH₂OH residues displays marked structural and steric specificity (31,32,62). Our model building studies indicate that the 9-membered lactam region of teleocidin and the macrocyclic polyacetate ring system of aplysiatoxin can assume conformations which are remarkably similar to the corresponding region present in the biologically active phorbol esters. We postulate, therefore, that the respective regions of the phorbol esters, teleocidin, and aplysiatoxin form highly specific chemical bonding and/or steric interactions with the phorboid receptors. These relationships for a phorbol ester and teleocidin are displayed in Fig. 2. Our model is consistent with published data on the stereochemistry of these compounds (32). Precise model building studies with aplysiatoxin cannot be done at the present time because its stereochemistry has not been elucidated. Additional compounds are being examined to obtain further data relevant to this hypothesis. Information of this type could make it possible to rationally design compounds that would either act as agonists or blockers of the phorboid receptor system.

Certain findings lead us to suggest that there may be heterogeneity (or subclasses) of the receptors for phorbol esters and related tumor promoters. Scatchard analyses of [³H]-PDBu-receptor binding to intact cells are consistent with at least two classes of binding sites (33,35,36,65, see also Table 1). Although the compound mezerein is equipotent with TPA with respect to certain biological effects, it competes less well than TPA in inhibiting [³H]-PDBu-receptor binding, and also is much weaker

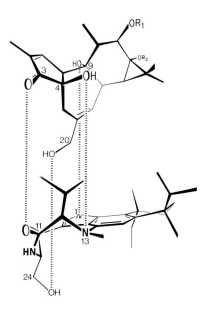

FIG. 2. Perspective drawings of TPA *(top)* and dihydroteleocidin B *(bottom)*. The dotted lines connect heteroatoms whose spatial positions correspond with one another, and represent residues that could form hydrogen bonds with a putative receptor. The hydrophobic R_1 residue on TPA (myristate) and the hydrophobic ring system on the right side of dihydroteleocidin B might interact with a separate hydrophobic domain of the receptor or with its lipid microenvironment. For further details see text and ref. 32.

than TPA as a complete tumor promoter on mouse skin (17,33,61). Therefore, some cell types may have a subset of receptors that discriminate between TPA and mezerein. Differential effects of aplysiatoxin and debromoaplysiatoxin are also consistent with receptor heterogeneity (32). A recent study with C3H10T1/2 cells indicates that the dose response curves for TPA, PDBu, and teleocidin inhibition of the binding of [^{3}H]-PDBu to high affinity receptors were quite different than those obtained when the same compounds were tested for their ability to alter membrane lipid fluidity, as measured with fluorescence polarization probes (65). It is possible that some of the biological effects of these tumor promoters are due to direct interaction with lipid domains in cell membranes. Indeed, specific binding of these compounds to synthetic phospholipid membranes has been demonstrated (15,66). Studies are required to determine the biological significance of these findings. Receptor heterogeneity could contribute to the tissue specificity of these compounds as tumor promoters, and also explain other specific biological effects.

The major limitation in our knowledge of the action of phorbol ester tumor promoters is the mechanism by which, following receptor binding, they induce their highly pleiotropic effects. Elsewhere we have reviewed the known effects of these compounds on ion flux (Na^+, Rb^+, Ca^{++}), nutrient uptake, phospholipid metabolism, and induction of specific enzymes (69,70). In view of the pleiotropic effects of protein kinases, and the evidence that the products of certain oncogenes are protein kinases, an attractive mechanism for mediating the cellular effects of tumor promoters would be through specific protein kinases (69,70). The recent finding of Castagna et al. (12) that low concentrations of TPA (1–5ng/ml) stimulate the *in vitro* activity of protein kinase C, a phospholipid-dependent protein kinase, is of considerable interest.

Since with repeated applications benzo*[a]*pyrene (BP) and certain other polycyclic aromatic hydrocarbon (PAH) carcinogens can act as complete carcinogens on mouse skin, it seemed possible that PAHs might induce certain effects on membranes that are similar to those induced by the phorbol ester tumor promoters. We have indeed found that the exposure of C3H10T1/2 cells to BP and certain other PAHs lead to a loss of EGF-receptor binding (38,39,40). There is evidence that these compounds can also mimic other effects of TPA including increases in membrane phospholipid turnover (40). We have obtained indirect evidence that these responses are mediated via the Ah receptor system (38,39,40). Our results have recently been confirmed and extended by Nebert et al. *(this volume)*. Our findings may also be relevant to recent studies indicating that 2,3,7,8-tetrachlorodibenzo-p-dioxin (TCDD), which binds to the Ah receptor, acts as a potent mouse skin tumor promoter in an appropriate strain of mice (56). It is of interest that the glucorticoid hormones, which are extremely effective inhibitors of tumor promotion on mouse skin, are potent antagonists of some of the membrane-related effects of both TPA and BP (39). Thus reciprocal effects of certain agents on membranes may explain their tumor promoter or tumor inhibitory properties. Additional inhibitors of tumor promotion might be designed based on this rationale.

Before leaving the subject of tumor promoters we should mention that although our group has stressed the membrane and "epigenetic" effects of tumor promoters, other investigators have provided evidence that the phorbol ester tumor promoters may act indirectly to produce chromosomal aberrations and DNA damage, perhaps via activated forms of oxygen (7,18,19,42,50,67). We would stress, however, the importance of determining whether or not these effects are confined to only certain cell types, whether or not they occur at nontoxic concentrations, and whether they can be causally associated with tumor promotion in the intact animal.

CELLULAR GENES INVOLVED IN CHEMICAL CARCINOGENESIS

In contrast to oncogenic viruses, chemical carcinogens, radiation, and tumor promoters cannot introduce new genetic information into cells. During the transformation process they must, therefore, call upon genes already present in the target cells to bring about and maintain the transformed state. Until recently, there did not appear to be a direct method available for the identification of these cellular genes. However, recent findings with retroviruses may provide direct approaches to this problem.

Studies of the RNA acute leukemia and sarcoma viruses have led to the concept that these viruses arose by the recombination of replication proficient retroviruses with specific oncogenes (also called protooncogenes) endogenous to normal vertebrate species (8,71). Infection of cells by these viruses leads to integration (in the proviral DNA form) of the viral oncogenes into the host genome, where they are expressed at high levels and thus lead to the transformed state. The proviral DNAs of retroviruses are flanked by long terminal repeat sequences (LTR) which contain strong promoter signals for controlling transcription and also sequences that might play a role in gene transposition (9,16,30,71).

It is possible that cellular homologs of the viral oncogenes or of the long terminal repeat (LTR) sequences are involved in the transformation of cells by nonviral agents. Perhaps the DNA damage induced by chemical carcinogens or radiation triggers alterations in the state of integration and/or causes a switch-on in the constitutive expression of these DNA sequences, in the absence of a virus vector (Fig. 3)(69,70).

Studies from the laboratories of R. Weinberg, J. Cooper, M. Wigler, and M. Barbacid, utilizing the DNA transfection technique, have provided evidence for a role of specific cellular oncogenes in the causation of human bladder cancer and

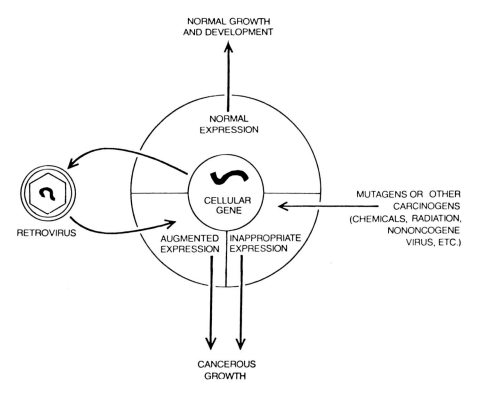

FIG. 3. A unified scheme for genes involved in the transformation of cells by retroviruses, chemical carcinogens, and radiation. In the case of the retroviruses host DNA sequences (oncogenes and/or LTR sequences) were picked up by the viruses during evolution. They become reintegrated into recipient cells during virus infection and are then aberrantly expressed to produce the transformed phenotype. In the case of chemical carcinogens (or radiation) damage to cellular DNA acts on endogenous oncogenes or LTR sequences to produce (via point mutations, gene rearrangement, or altered methylation, etc.) aberrant expression of similar sequences, in the absence of a virus vector. (Figure from ref. 8, with permission.)

certain other human neoplasms (13,47,59,64). However, these findings must be interpreted with caution since the transfection studies were done with a heterologous, aneuploid, and immortal cell line, i.e., NIH 3T3 mouse embryo fibroblasts. In addition, thus far only a limited number of DNA samples from normal human tissues have been studied with this technique, and we do not know the extent of polymorphism of oncogenes in the human population. Furthermore, it is not clear at which stage in a multistage carcinogenic process the changes reported by these investigators may have occurred. We feel that it is essential, therefore, to pursue complementary approaches that employ quite different methods.

Studies on Cellular Oncogenes in Normal and Transformed Murine Cells

We have utilized a cloned DNA fragment representing a portion of the oncogene (v-*mos*) of Moloney murine sarcoma virus (Mo-MSV) as a probe to determine whether or not transformation of rodent cells by chemical carcinogens or radiation is associated with alterations in the state of integration or transcription of the normal cellular sequence (c-*mos*) that is homologous to the v-*mos* gene (28). However, after examining a number of normal rodent cell types and rodent cells transformed by either chemical carcinogens or radiation we found no evidence that transformation by these agents was associated with rearrangement of the c-*mos* sequence within the cell genome. In addition, in all of the normal and transformed cells the c-*mos* sequence was hypermethylated and transcriptionally silent. These results are in contrast to the situation in cells transformed by Mo-MSV in which the exogenous v-mos sequence is integrated at new sites within the host genome, is undermethylated, and is extensively transcribed. In related studies, we have found that another oncogene, c-*ras*, also fails to show any evidence for rearrangement in carcinogen or radiation transformed C3H10T1/2 cells *(unpublished studies)*. Since there is evidence that eukaryotic cells can contain at least 15 oncogenes (8,71), our results do not rule out the possibility that oncogenes other than c-*mos* and c-*ras* may play a role in the transformation of murine cells by chemicals or radiation. Additional studies utilizing probes to other oncogenes are required to evaluate this possibility.

In considering the possible involvement of cellular oncogenes in chemical carcinogenesis it is important to stress that they differ in several respects from their viral homologues. For example, the cellular oncogenes usually contain introns, they are not necessarily flanked by LTR sequences, and they may differ in certain other respects from the oncogenes present in retroviruses (8,71). Therefore, we believe it is likely that they will be expressed at lower levels and under a greater degree of host control in carcinogen-induced tumors than the corresponding oncogenes introduced into cells by the acute transforming viruses. For this reason, cell transformation induced by chemical carcinogens might often depend on changes in the function of multiple cellular oncogenes, as well as other types of host genes, rather than a single dominant gene. The oncogenes present in the acute transforming viruses have had time to evolve, and may have undergone selection, to produce a dominant phenotype. If oncogenes present in normal cellular DNA play a role in chemical carcinogenesis we think that it is unlikely that they do so by undergoing the full evolution in structure that occurred in the origin of viral oncogenes.

Studies Related to LTR Sequences

In a second set of studies we have pursued an alternative approach to identifying retrovirus-related sequences that might be involved in radiation and chemical carcinogenesis. Several types of evidence indicate that the LTR regions of the proviral DNA copies of these viruses play a crucial role in controlling transcription, and that the specific sequences involved are present in the U3 portion of the LTR sequence (16,71). The R region of the LTR defines the site of initiation (at the 5′ end) of viral RNA synthesis, and the U5 region represents the portion of the LTR sequence that is present at the 5′ terminus of the mature viral RNA. The LTR sequence also has structural features similar to transposable elements of bacteria, suggesting that LTR sequences might also be involved in gene transposition (16,71). They could act, therefore, as mobile promoters capable of initiating the transcription of sequences adjacent to sites into which they might become integrated. Consistent with this possibility are recent studies indicating that the insertion of the LTR sequence of an avian leukosis virus at specific sites into the host cell DNA activates transcription of a flanking host oncogene sequence designated c-*myc*, and that this is responsible for the induction of avian lymphomas (30,53). Normal murine cells contain several copies of DNA sequences homologous to the LTR sequence of murine retrovirus proviral DNA (16, also see studies below). These findings suggest that if damage to cellular DNA caused the rearrangement and/or activation of endogenous LTR sequences this could lead to the constitutive expression of host sequences (oncogenes or other genes) whose products might be capable of inducing cell transformation (43). In theory, these events could occur in the absence of a replicating leukemia virus.

To test this hypothesis we have examined whether there are differences between normal C3H10T1/2 cells transformed by radiation or chemical carcinogens in terms of the expression of RNA species containing sequences homologous to a probe prepared to the LTR sequence of Mo-MSV. The polyA$^+$ RNA fraction was purified from these cells, separated by gel electrophoresis, and then hybridized by the "Northern" blotting technique to a [^{32}P]-labeled DNA probe specific for LTR sequences (43).

Figure 4 indicates that with the polyA$^+$ RNA from normal C3H10T1/2 cells there was negligible hybridization to the LTR probe (lane f). On the other hand, the polyA$^+$ RNA from five different transformed C3H10T1/2 cell lines (Fig. 4, lanes a–e) showed appreciable hybridization to this probe. At least five distinct polyA$^+$ RNA species ranging from about 38S to 18S were detected in the transformed lines. We have analyzed a total of eight transformed cell lines that were originally derived from normal C3H10T1/2 cells following exposure to chemical carcinogens, UV, or radiographs, and all of these displayed RNAs homologous to the LTR probe, yielding profiles similar to those shown in Fig. 4. With both an early and late passage clone of normal C3H10T1/2 cells there was always undetectable or only

a   b   c   d   e   f

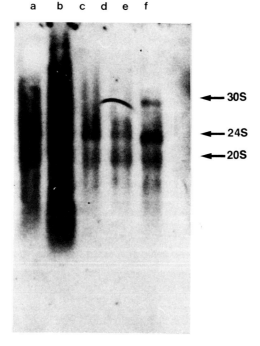

←— 30S

←— 24S

←—20S

FIG. 4. Northern blot analysis showing hybridization of the LTR probe to the polyA+ RNA from normal, transformed, and drug-induced murine cells. The gels contained polyA+ RNAs from the following cell lines: *lane a*, C3H 10T1/2 JL#2 (UV-transformed); *lane b*, C3H 10T1/2 CB#2 (benzo[a]pyrene transformed); *lane c*, C3H 10T1/2 JL#1 (X-ray transformed); *lane d*, C3H 10T1/2 CB#1 (X-ray transformed); *lane 3*, C3H 10T1/2 JL#3 (methylcholanthrene transformed); and *lane f*, normal C3H 10T1/2. Poly A+ RNA was isolated from these cells, denatured with 50% formamide-6% formaldehyde at 65°C and separated on a 0.8% agarose gel containing 6% formaldehyde and 20mM morpholinopropane sulfonic acid at pH 7.0. The RNA was then transferred to nitrocellulose sheets (BA 85, Schleicher and Schuell) and hybridized to a [^{32}P]-labeled LTR probe. (Data from ref. 43.)

slight hybridization to this probe. On the other hand, we have found that the exposure of normal C3H10T1/2 cells to either bromodeoxy-uridine (BrdUrd) or 5-Azacytidine for 24 hrs induced the expression of a series of polyA+ RNAs that were homologous to the LTR probe and were similar in size to those found in the transformed C3H10T1/2 cell lines (43). Thus, it appears that what is unusual in the transformed cells is the constitutive expression of these transcripts rather than the presence of LTR-containing DNA sequences that are unique to the transformed cells.

The polyA+ RNA transcripts detected with the LTR probe in the transformed C3H10T1/2 cell lines could originate from endogenous murine retroviruses genomes and/or from the expression of host genes unrelated to the retroviruses but flanked by LTR sequences. Therefore, we performed a set of experiments to determine whether these transcripts contained, in addition to LTR-like sequences, sequences homologous to the known retrovirus genes *gag, pol, env,* and the *U3* region of the LTR sequence, utilizing the appropriate [^{32}P]-labeled DNA probes. We found that when a probe for the *gag-pol* region of murine retroviruses was hybridized to the polyA$^+$ RNA of carcinogen transformed C3H10T1/2 cell lines there was hybridization to the 30S to 38S RNAs, but there was no detectable hybridization to the lower molecular weight RNAs (24 to 18S) detected with the LTR probe. The probe to the *env* region also hybridized to RNAs of about 30 to 38S, and in addition to an RNA of about 24S, but it did not hybridize to the 20 to 18S RNAs detected with the LTR probe in transformed C3H10T1/2 cells. We also utilized a probe specific to the U3 region of the LTR sequence. This region is usually contained at the 3' end of virally-related messages since it is just proximal to the viral polyadenylation site. We found that the U3 probe hybridized to the 30S–38S and 24S RNAs present in carcinogen-transformed derivatives of C3H10T1/2 cells. However, the 20S and 18S transcripts recognized by the total LTR probe did not hybridize to the probe specific for the U3 region of the LTR. No significant hybridization was detected with either the *gag*, *pol*, *env*, or *U3* probes and the polyA$^+$ RNA from normal C3H10T1/2 cells (43). We suspect that the 20S and 18S transcripts reflect the expression of nonvirally related host sequences that utilize virally-related LTR sequences as promoters. We are currently analyzing the possible role of these mRNAs in initiation or maintenance of the transformed state in rodent systems.

As part of our interest in LTR sequences we have recently developed a transfection and expression vector, in which specific genes can be conveniently inserted between a 5' and 3' LTR sequence present in the vector (55). This construct can then be transfected into rodent cells, and the inserted gene will then be expressed in the recipient cells, utilizing the transcription signals present in the LTR sequences of the vector. This vector also permits the encapsidation of RNA sequences into virus-like particles which then mediate gene transfer with extremely high efficiency. This vector should facilitate the further analysis of genes involved in chemical carcinogenesis.

Studies on Endogenous LTR-Like Sequences in Normal and Transformed Murine Cells

In view of our evidence for the constitutive expression in carcinogen-transformed cells of a series of polyA$^+$ RNAs containing sequences homologous to the LTR sequence of a murine retrovirus (see above) (43), it was of interest to compare the state of integration in cellular DNA of endogenous LTR-like sequences between normal and carcinogen-transformed murine cells (27). We were specifically interested in the possibility that transformation might be associated with rearrangement or amplification of such sequences in the cellular genome.

When DNA from normal C3H10T1/2 cells was cut with the restriction enzyme Bgl II (which does not cut within the Mo-MSV LTR sequence) and the DNA analyzed by the Southern blot procedure, utilizing a [^{32}P]-labeled probe prepared from a cloned Mo-MSV LTR, we obtained a very complex profile consisting of at least 30 distinct bands (Fig. 5)(27). The DNAs from MCA-transformed, BP-transformed, or radiation transformed C3H10T1/2 cells gave similar profiles, and showed no reproducible differences when compared to the profile of normal C3H10T1/2 cells. DNA from normal

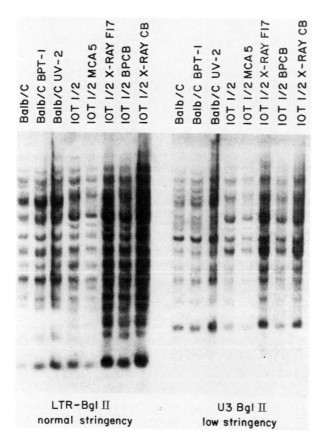

FIG. 5. Southern blots of mouse chromosomal DNA hybridized to [32P]-labeled probes for the Moloney Murine Leukemia Virus LTR and its U3 specific region. Chromosomal DNAs were extracted from mouse cell lines and digested with Bgl II. 15 μg aliquots of each sample were loaded for electrophoresis through 1% agarose gels, followed by transfer to nitrocellulose. The left side of the blot was hybridized with [32P]-labeled LTR probe under conditions of normal hybridization (50% formamide, final concentration) and washed under conditions of normal stringency (0.1X SSC final wash). The right side of the blot was hybridized with a [32P]-labeled U3 specific probe under conditions of low stringency hybridization (40% formamide final concentration) and low stringency washing (2X SSC final wash).

Normal Balb/C 3T3 murine fibroblasts, a BP transformed (BPT-1) and a UV transformed (UV-2) derivative were obtained from Dr. T. Kakunaga. The sources of normal C3H 10T1/2 murine fibroblasts, and the transformed derivatives (MCA5, x-ray F 17, BPCB and x-ray CB) have been previously described (28,43).

Balb/C 3T3 cells also showed a complex LTR profile, and derivatives of this cell line transformed by BP or ultraviolet (UV) light also failed to show any reproducible difference from the normal parental cells (Fig. 5).

When the same cellular DNA samples were hybridized by a similar procedure to a [32P]-labeled probe specific to the U3 region of Mo-MSV LTR (which encompassed about 70% of the total LTR) we obtained no detectable hybridization. This result was surprising since in the carcinogen and radiation transformed C3H10T1/2 cell lines we did detect RNA species homologous to our U3 specific probe (43). We reasoned, therefore, that U3-like sequences must be present in the mouse genome but their sequence differed sufficiently from those present in our probe so that we failed to detect them under the DNA hybridization conditions used. Therefore, we repeated the hybridization studies with the U3 specific probe, utilizing less stringent hybridization conditions (see legend, Fig. 5). Under these conditions we did detect in the DNAs of both the normal and the transformed murine cells approximately 15 bands homologous to the U3 probe (Fig. 5). Each of these bands comigrated with a band detected with the probe to the entire LTR, although only about one-half of the bands detected with the latter probe showed homology with the U3 probe, even under the low stringency condition of hybridization. Comparison of the bands detected with the U3 specific probe in normal and transformed cells failed to show any reproducible differences.

The fact that we detected sequences homologous to the U3 region of the Mo-MSV LTR in the mouse genome only under conditions of low stringency hybridization suggests that these cellular DNA sequences differ considerably from those present in the retrovirus. This finding is consistent with other evidence that the U3 regions of LTR sequences display considerable divergence (11,71). Since the U3 regions contain sequences that promote the transcription of adjoining genes (16,71), variations in the U3 regions of cellular LTR-like sequences may provide important clues to normal mechanisms that control gene transcription. Since we did not find any evidence that carcinogen or radiation induced transformation of murine cells was associated with amplification or rearrangement of endogenous LTR sequences, we suspect that the constitutive expression of these sequences in transformed cells may relate to alterations in DNA methylation, and/or changes in chromatin organization, in regions of cellular LTR-like sequences. We believe that alterations in DNA methylation may play a critical role in this process because of the increasing evidence that activation of transcription is often associated with a decrease in DNA methylation (58). In addition, we have found that the exposure of cells to 5-Azacytidine switches on the transcription of a series of polyA$^+$ RNAs that are similar to those we have detected in carcinogen-transformed cells (43, and Hsiao, W., Gattoni-Celli, S., and Weinstein, I. B., *unpublished studies*). For the reasons mentioned above, changes specifically involving the U3 regions may be particularly critical with respect to aberrations in transcription. Studies are in progress to further explore these possibilities.

ACKNOWLEDGMENTS

This research was supported by DHS, NCI Grants CA 021111 and CA 26056 and a gift from the Dupont Company. The authors wish to acknowledge the valuable collaboration with Drs. T. Sugimura and H. Fujiki of the National Cancer Center Research Institute, Tokyo, K. Umezawa of the Cancer Institute, Tokyo, and R. E. Moore, University of Hawaii in the studies on teleocidin and aplysiatoxin. We thank Patricia Kelly for assistance in preparing this manuscript.

REFERENCES

1. Allen, J. A., and Coombs, M. M. (1980): Covalent binding of polycyclic aromatic compounds to mitochondrial and nuclear DNA. *Nature*, 287:243–245.
2. Backer, J. M., Boersig, M. R., and Weinstein, I. B. (1982): Inhibition of respiration by a phorbol ester tumor promoter in murine cultured cells. *Biochem. Biophys. Res. Commun.*, 105:855–866.
3. Backer, J. M., and Weinstein, I. B. (1982): Interaction of benzo[a]pyrene and its dihydrodiol epoxide with nuclear and mitochondrial DNA in C3H 10T1/2 cell cultures. *Cancer Res.*, 42:2764–2769.
4. Backer, J., and Weinstein, I. B. (1983): A phorbol ester tumor promoter accelerates hydrolysis of ATP by isolated rat liver mitochondria. *Proc. American Assoc. Cancer Res.*, *(Abstract)*.
5. Barrett, J. C., and Ts'o, P. O. P. (1978): Evidence for the progressive nature of neoplastic transformation *in vitro*. *Proc. Natl. Acad. Sci. USA*, 75:3761–3765.
6. Basilico, C., Gattoni-Celli, S., Zouzias, D., and Della Valle, G. (1979): Loss of integrated viral DNA sequences in polyoma transformed cells is associated with an active viral A function. *Cell*, 17:645–459.
7. Birnboim, H. C. (1982): Factors which affect DNA strand breakage in human leukocytes exposed to a tumor promoter, phorbol myristate acetate. *Can. J. Physiol. Pharmacol.*, 60:1359–1366.
8. Bishop, J. M. (1982): Oncogenes. *Scientific American*, 246:81–91.
9. Blair, D. G., Oskarsson, M., Wood, T. G., McClements, W. L., Fischinger, P. J., and Vande Woude, G. F. (1981): Activation of the transforming potential of a normal cell sequence: A molecular model for oncogenesis. *Science*, 212:941–943.
10. Botchan, M., Topp, W., and Sambrook, J. (1978): Studies on SV40 excision from cellular chromosomes. Cold Spring Harbor Symp. *Quant. Biol.*, 43:709–719.
11. Casey, J. W., Roach, A., Mullins, J. I., Burck, K. B., Nicolson, M. O., Gardner, M. B., and Davidson, N. (1981): The U3 portion of feline leukemia virus DNA identifies horizontally acquired proviruses in leukemic cats. *Proc. Natl. Acad. of Sci. USA*, 78:7778–7782.
12. Castagna, M., Takai, U., Kaibuchi, K., Sano, K., Kikkawa, U., and Nishizuka, Y. (1982): Direct activation of calcium-activated, phospholipid-dependent protein kinase by tumor promoting phorbol esters. *J. Biol. Chem.*, 257:7847–7851.
13. Cooper, G. M. (1982): Cellular transforming genes. *Science*, 218:801–806.
14. Delcos, K. B., Nagle, D. S., and Blumberg, P. M. (1980): Specific binding of phorbol ester tumor promoters to mouse skin. *Cell*, 19:1025–1032.
15. Deleers, M., Ruysschaert, J. M., and Malaisse, W. J. (1982): Interaction between phorbol esters and phospholipid in a monolayer model membrane. *Chem. Biol. Interactions*, 42:271–278.
16. Dhar, R., McClements, W. C., Enquist, L. W., and Vande Woude, G. G. (1980): Nucleotide sequences of integrated Moloney sarcoma provirus long terminal repeats and their host and viral junctions. *Proc. Natl. Acad. Sci. USA*, 77:3937–3941.
17. Driedger, P. E., and Blumberg, P. M. (1980): Specific binding of phorbol ester tumor promoters. *Proc. Natl. Acad. Sci. USA*, 77:567–571.
18. Dzarlieva, R. T., and Fusenig, N. E. (1982): Tumor promoter 12-0-tetradecanoyl-phorbol-13-acetate enhances sister chromatid exchanges and numerical and structural chromosome aberrations in primary mouse epidermal cell cultrues. *Cancer Letts.*, 16:7–17.
19. Emerit, I., and Cerutti, P. A. (1982): Tumor promoter phorbol 12-myristate 13-acetate induces a clastogenic factor in human lymphocytes. *Proc. Natl. Acad. Sci. USA*, 79:7509–7513.
20. Fisher, P. B., Bozzone, J. H., and Weinstein, I. B. (1979): Tumor promoters and epidermal growth factor stimulate anchorage-independent growth of adenovirus transformed rat embryo cells. *Cell*, 18:695–705.
21. Fisher, P. B., Mufson, R. A., Miranda, A. F., Fujiki, H., Sugimura, T., and Weinstein, I. B. (1982): Phorbol ester tumor promoters and teleocidin have similar effects on cell transformation, differentiation and phospholipid metabolism. *Cancer Res.*, 42:2829–2835.
22. Foulds, L. (1969,1975): *Neoplastic Development, Vols. 1 and 2*, Academic Press, New York.
23. Fujiki, H., Mori, M., Nakayasu, M., Terada, M., and Sugimura, T. (1979): A possible naturally occurring tumor promoter, teleocidin B from *Streptomyces*. *Biochem. Biophys. Res. Commun.*, 90:976–983.
24. Fujiki, H., Mori, M., Nakayasu, M., Terada, M., Sugimura, T., and Moore, R. E. (1981): Indole alkaloids: Dihydroteleocidin B, teleocidin, and lyngbyatoxin A as members of a new class of tumor promoters. *Proc. Natl. Acad. Sci. USA*, 78:3872–3876.

25. Fujiki, H., Suganama, M., Nakayasu, M., Hoshino, H., Moore, R. E., and Sugimura, T. (1982): The third class of new tumor promoters, polyacetates (debromoaplysiatoxin and aplysiatoxin), can differentiate biological actions relevant to tumor promoters. *GANN*, 73:497–499.
26. Gattoni-Celli, S., Colantuoni, V., and Basilico, C. (1980): Relationship between integrated and non-integrated viral DNA in rat cells transformed by polyoma virus. *J. Virol.*, 34(3):615–626.
27. Gattoni-Celli, S., Kirschmeier, P., Lambert, M. E., and Weinstein, I. B. (1982): Analysis of cellular long terminal repeat (LTR) sequences as potential targets of chemical carcinogens. *(in preparation)*.
28. Gattoni-Celli, S., Kirschmeier, P., Weinstein, I. B., Escobedo, J., and Dina, D. (1982): Cellular moloney murine sarcoma ("c-mos") sequences are hypermethylated and transcriptionally silent in normal and transformed rodent cells. *Mol. Cell Biol.*, 2:42–51.
29. Greenebaum, E. M., Nicolaides, M., Eisinger, M., Vogel, R. H., and Weinstein, I. B. (1983): Binding of phorbol dibutyrate and epidermal growth factor to cultured human epidermal cells. *J. Natl. Cancer Inst.* 70:435–441.
30. Hayward, W. S., Neel, B. G., and Astrin, S. M. (1981): Activation of a cellular *onc* gene by promoter insertion in ALV-induced lymphoid leukosis. *Nature*, 290:475–480.
31. Hecker, E., Fusenig, N. E., Kunz, W., Marks, F., and Thielmann, H. W. (1982): *Carcinogenesis: A Comprehensive Survey, Vol. 7*, Raven Press, New York.
32. Horowitz, A., Fujiki, H., Weinstein, I. B., Jeffrey, A., Okin, E., Moore, R. E., and Sugimura, T. (1983): Comparative effects of aplysiatoxin, debromoaplysiatoxin and teleocidin on receptor binding and phospholipid metabolism. *Cancer Res.* 43:1529–1535.
33. Horowitz, A., Greenebaum, E., and Weinstein, I. B. (1981): Identification of receptors for phorbol ester tumor promoters in intact mammalian cells and of an inhibitor of receptor binding in biologic fluids. *Proc. Natl. Acad. Sci. USA*, 78:2315–2319.
34. Horowitz, A., Greenebaum, E., and Weinstein, I. B. (1982): Inhibition of phorbol ester-receptor binding by a factor from human serum. *Mol. Cell. Biol.*, 2:545–553.
35. Horowitz, A., Nicolaides, M., Greenebaum, E., Woodward, K., Giotta, G., and Weinstein, I. B. (1982): *(in preparation)*.
36. Horowitz, A., and Weinstein, I. B. (1982): Receptor binding and cellular effects of tumor promoters. In: *Prostaglandins and Cancer: First International Conference*, edited by T. J., Powles, R. Bockman, K. Honn, and P. Ramwell, pp. 217–238. Alan R. Liss, Inc., New York.
37. Huberman, E., and Fogel, M. (1975): Activation of carcinogenic polycyclic hydrocarbons in polyoma-virus transformed cells as a prerequisite for polyoma virus induction. *Int. J. Cancer*, 15:91–98.
38. Ivanovic, V., Okin, E., and Weinstein, I. B. (1982): Studies on the mechanism by which benzo[a]pyrene inhibits epidermal growth factor binding to cellular receptors. *Proc. Amer. Assoc. Cancer Res.*, 23(abstract):221.
39. Ivanovic, V., and Weinstein, I. B. (1981): Glucocorticoids and benzo[a]pyrene have opposing effects on EGF receptor binding. *Nature*, 293:404–406.
40. Ivanovic, V., and Weinstein, I. B. (1982): Benzo[a]pyrene and other inducers of cytochrome, P_1-450 inhibit binding of epidermal growth factor to cell surface receptors. *Carcinogenesis*, 3:505–510.
41. Kalf, G. F., Rushmore, T., and Synder, R. (1982): Benzene inhibits RNA synthesis in mitochondria from liver and bone marrow. *Chem. Biol. Interactions*, 42:353–370.
42. Kinsella, A. R., and Radman, M. (1978): Tumor promoter induces sister chromatid exchanges: relevance to mechanisms of carcinogenesis. *Proc. Natl. Acad. Sci. USA*, 75:6149–6153.
43. Kirschmeier, P., Gattoni-Celli, S., Dina, D., and Weinstein, I. B. (1982): Carcinogen and radiation transformed C3H 10T1/2 cells contain RNAs homologous to the LTR sequence of a murine leukemia virus. *Proc. Natl. Acad. Sci. USA*, 79:273–277.
44. Koch, R. (1892): Ueber bakteriologische forschung. In: *Verh. X. International Medical Congress*, Berlin, 1890, p 35.
45. Lambert, M. E., Gattoni-Celli, S., Kirschmeier, P., and Weinstein, I. B. (1983): Benzo[a]pyrene induction of extrachromosomal viral DNA synthesis in rat cells transformed by polyoma virus. *Carcinogenesis*, 4:587–594.
46. Lavi, S., and Etkin, S. (1981): Carcinogen-mediated induction of SV40 DNA synthesis in SV40 transformed hamster embryo cells. *Carcinogenesis*, 2:417–423.
47. Logan, J., and Cairns, J. (1982): The secrets of cancer. *Nature*, 300:104–105.

48. Miller, E. (1978): Some current perspectives on chemical carcinogenesis in humans and experimental animals: Presidential address. *Cancer Res.*, 38:1479–1496.
49. Morris, A. G. (1981): Neoplastic transformation of mouse fibroblasts by murine sarcoma virus: A multi-step process. *J. Gen. Virol.*, 53:39–45.
50. Nagasawa, H., and Little, J. B. (1979): Effect of tumor promoters, protease inhibitors, and repair processes on x-ray-induced sister chromatid exchanges in mouse cells. *Proc. Natl. Acad. Sci. USA*, 76:1943–1947.
51. Nagle, D. S., Jaken, S., Castagna, M., and Blumberg, P. M. (1981): Variation with embryonic development and regional localization of specific [^{3}H]phorbol 12,13-dibutyrate binding to brain. *Cancer Res.*, 41:89–93.
52. Niranjan, B. G., Bhat, N. K., and Avadhami, N. G. (1982): Preferential attack of mitochondrial DNA by aflatoxin B_1 during hepatocarcinogenesis. *Science*, 215:73–75.
53. Payne, G. S., Bishop, J. M., and Varmus, H. E. (1982): Multiple arrangements of viral DNA and an activated host oncogene in bursal lymphomas. *Nature*, 295:209–214.
54. Perera, F. P., and Weinstein, I. B. (1982): Molecular epidemiology and carcinogen-DNA adduct detection: New approaches to studies of human cancer causation. *J. Chron. Dis.*, 35:581–600.
55. Perkins, A., Kirschmeier, P., Gattoni-Celli, S., and Weinstein, I. B. (1983): Development of a new transfection vector containing LTR sequences. *Molecular and Cellular Biology*, 3:1123–1132.
56. Poland, A., Palen, D., and Glover, E. (1982): Tumor promotion of TCDD in skin of HRS/J hairless mice. *Nature*, 300.271–273.
57. Rakusanova, T., Kaplan, J. C., Smales, W. P., and Black, P. H. (1976): Excision of viral DNA from host cell DNA after induction of Simian virus 40 transformed hamster cells. *J. Virol.*, 19:279–285.
58. Razin, A., and Riggs, A. D. (1980): DNA methylation and gene function. *Science*, 210:604–610.
59. Reddy, E. P., Reynolds, R. K., Santos, E., and Barbacid, M. (1982): A point mutation is responsible for the acquisition of transforming properties by the T24 human bladder carcinoma oncogene. *Nature*, 300:149–152.
60. Shoyab, M., and Todaro, G. J. (1980): Specific high affinity cell membrane receptors for biologically active phorbol and ingenol esters. *Nature*, 288:451–455.
61. Slaga, T. J., Fisher, S. M., Nelson, K., and Gleason, G. L. (1980): Studies on the mechanism of skin tumor promotion: Evidence for several stages in promotion. *Proc. Natl. Acad. Sci. USA*, 77:3659–3663.
62. Slaga, T. J., Sivak, A., and Boutwell, R. K. (1978): *Carcinogenesis, Vol. 2: Mechanisms of Tumor Promotion and Cocarcinogenesis*. Raven Press, New York.
63. Sugimura, T. (1982): Potent tumor promoters other than phorbol esters and their significance. *GANN*, 73:499–507.
64. Tabin, C. J., Bradley, S. M., Bargmann, C. I., and Weinberg, R. A. (1982): Mechanism of activation of a human oncogene. *Nature*, 300:143–149.
65. Tran, P. L., Castagna, M., Sala, M., Vassent, G., Horowitz, A. D., Schachter, D., and Weinstein, I. B. (1982): Differential effects of tumor promoters on phorbol ester receptor binding and membrane fluorescence anisotropy in C3H 10T1/2 cells. *European J. of Biochemistry*, 130:155–160.
66. Tran, P. L., Ter-Minassian, L., Madelmont, G., and Castagna, M. (1982): *Biochim. Biophys. Acta (in press)*.
67. Troll, W., Witz, G., Goldstein, B., Stone, D., and Sugimura, T. (1982): The role of free oxygen radicals in tumor promotion and carcinogenesis. In: *Cocarcinogens and Biological Effects*, edited by E. Hecker, N. E. Fusenig, W. Kunz, F. Marks, and H. W. Thielmann, pp. 593–597. Raven Press, New York.
68. Umezawa, K., Weinstein, I. B., Horowitz, A., Fujiki, H., Matsushima, T., and Sugimura, T. (1981): Similarity of teleocidin B and phorbol ester tumor promoters in effects on membrane receptors. *Nature*, 290:411–413.
69. Weinstein, I. B. (1981): Current concepts and controversies in chemical carcinogenesis. *J. of Supramol. Structure and Cellular Biochem.*, 17:99–120.
70. Weinstein, I. B., Horowitz, A. D., Fisher, P. B., Ivanovic, V., Gattoni-Celli, S., and Kirschmeier, P. (1982): Mechanisms of multistage carcinogenesis and their relevance to tumor cell heterogeneity. In: *Tumor Cell Heterogeneity: Origins and Implications*, edited by A. H. Owens, Jr., D. S. Coffey, and S. B. Baylin, pp. 216–238. Academic Press, New York.
71. Weiss, R., Teich, N., Varmus, H., and Coffin, J. (eds) (1982): *Molecular Biology of Tumor*

Viruses, Second Edition, RNA Tumor Viruses, Cold Spring Harbor Laboratory, Cold Spring Harbor, New York.

72. Wunderlich, A., Tetzlaff, A., and Graffi, A. (1971/1972): Studies on nitrosodimethylamine: Preferential methylation of mitochondrial DNA in rats and hamsters. *Chem. Biol. Interactions*, 4:41–49.

73. Zouzias, D., Prasad, I., and Basilico, C. (1977): State of the viral DNA in rat cells transformed by polyoma virus II. Identification of the cells containing non-integrated viral DNA and the effects of viral mutations. *J. Virol.*, 24:142–150.

Biochemical Basis of Chemical Carcinogenesis,
edited by H. Greim, R. Jung, M. Kramer,
H. Marquardt, and F. Oesch.
Raven Press, New York © 1984.

The Role of Retinoids in Differentiation and Carcinogenesis*

Michael B. Sporn and Anita B. Roberts

*Laboratory of Chemoprevention, Division of Cancer Cause and Prevention,
National Cancer Institute, Bethesda, Maryland 20205*

It has been known for more than 50 years that retinoids, the family of molecules comprising both the natural and synthetic analogs of retinol, are potent agents for control of both cellular differentiation and cellular proliferation (63). In their original classic paper describing the cellular effects of vitamin A deficiency in the rat, Wolbach and Howe clearly noted that there were distinct effects on both differentiation and proliferation of epithelial cells. During vitamin A deficiency, it was found that proper differentiation of stem cells into mature epithelial cells failed to occur, and that abnormal cellular differentiation, characterized in particular by excessive accumulation of keratin, was a frequent event. Furthermore, it was noted that there was excessive cellular proliferation in many of the deficient epithelia. Although the conclusion that an adequate level of retinoid was necessary for control of normal cellular differentiation and proliferation was clearly stated in the original paper by Wolbach and Howe, a satisfactory explanation of the molecular mechanisms underlying these effects on both differentiation and proliferation still eludes us more than fifty years later.

It was inevitable that the basic role of retinoids in control of cell differentiation and proliferation would eventually find practical application in the cancer field, and there have been great advances in this area, particularly for prevention of cancer. Many studies have shown that retinoids can suppress the process of carcinogenesis *in vivo* in experimental animals (6,32,48,50,51), and these results are now the basis of current attempts to use retinoids for cancer prevention in man. Furthermore, there is now an extensive literature on the ability of retinoids to suppress the development of the malignant phenotype *in vitro* (5,7,29,30), and these studies corroborate the use of retinoids for cancer prevention. Finally, most recently it has been shown that retinoids can exert effects on certain fully transformed, invasive, neoplastic cells, leading in certain instances to a suppression of proliferation (29), and in other instances to terminal differentiation of these cells, resulting in a more benign, nonneoplastic phenotype (9,10,54,55). Even though there are many types

---

*This article has been published in full in *Cancer Research*, *43*, 3034 (1983).

of tumor cells for which this is not the case (indeed, at present there are only a limited number of instances in which such profound effects of retinoids on differentiation and proliferation of invasive tumor cells have been shown), this finding nevertheless has highly significant implications for the problem of cancer treatment. It emphasizes that in many respects cancer is fundamentally a disease of abnormal cell differentiation (41), and raises the possibility that even invasive disease may eventually be controlled by agents which control cell differentiation, rather than kill cells. Since carcinogenesis is essentially a disorder of cell differentiation, the overall scientific problem of the role of retinoids in either differentiation or carcinogenesis is essentially the same problem, and it will be considered as a single problem in this brief review.

MAJOR PROBLEMS RELATING TO RETINOIDS AND CANCER

In the broadest sense, there are two major domains relating to retinoids and the cancer problem: (a) the practical development and use of retinoids for either cancer prevention or treatment, and (b) the elucidation of the cellular and molecular mechanisms underlying the first domain. The first domain has attracted a great deal of attention in the past 5 years, and requires the coordinated efforts of synthetic organic chemists, cell biologists, investigators in experimental carcinogenesis and chemotherapy, pharmacologists, toxicologists, and clinical investigators in order to synthesize new retinoids, test them both *in vitro* and *in vivo* for useful biological activity, establish their pharmacokinetic and toxicological properties, and then bring the best new retinoids to clinical trial for either prevention or treatment of specific types of malignancy. This is a problem of immense scope, complexity, and expense, which is currently being pursued with vigorous interest throughout the world. We have reviewed some of the key issues in this first domain in previous articles (48,50,51), and will not discuss them further at this point. Instead, we will focus the rest of this short review on the problem of cellular and molecular mechanisms. Studies in this area are not only of great theoretical interest, but should also facilitate the practical development and use of retinoids for prevention and treatment of cancer. Elucidation of the mechanism of action of retinoids may also lead to new applications for their use. It is reasonable to suggest that retinoids may find applications in the prevention or treatment of diseases other than cancer, the pathogenesis of which involves abnormalities of cell differentiation and/or proliferation (49). In terms of the scientific challenge, it is again worth emphasizing that the problem of cellular and molecular mechanism is still unsolved more than 50 years after the initial description of the overall biological activity of the retinoids. The problem of the mechanism of action of retinoids may be studied at three levels, namely in the whole animal, at the cellular level, and finally at the molecular level, which we shall now consider in turn, using effects both on differentiation and carcinogenesis as markers.

MECHANISM OF ACTION OF RETINOIDS IN DIFFERENTIATION AND CARCINOGENESIS STUDIED IN THE WHOLE ANIMAL

Although the earliest studies on retinoid deficiency in the whole animal emphasized their effects on epithelial cell differentiation and proliferation, the possibility that retinoid deficiency caused abnormalities in nonepithelial cells derived from mesenchymal elements was not entirely overlooked by several careful investigators. Indeed, in the 1920s it was reported that there was a reduction in hematopoietic cells in the bone marrow of vitamin A deficient animals (20,63). In the 1930s and 1940s, many studies were performed on the need for retinoids for proper bone formation (33,37), and there was detailed investigation of the control of osteoblasts and osteoclasts (cells derived from mesenchyme) by retinoids (33). However, in the ensuing years, there was a much greater emphasis on studies on the role of retinoids in control of epithelial cell differentiation and proliferation, and the dogma that retinoids were selectively involved in the control of epithelial cells, and were of relatively minor importance with respect to cells of mesenchymal origin, became scientific folklore.

In contrast, in the area of experimental embryology and teratology, there accumulated an impressive body of information which indicated that retinoids had significant, selective teratogenic action on cells of mesenchymal origin in rat, mouse, hamster, and chick embryos; we have reviewed these data elsewhere (52). Particularly striking were the effects of retinol deficiency or retinoic acid excess on the development of the very early vascular system of either the chick or rat embryo. In the one day old chick embryo, retinol deficiency causes failure of mesenchymal cells to proliferate and differentiate to form the early vascular system (59,60, Fig. 1); treatment of rat or chick embryos with excess retinol or retinoic acid has similar effects (38; M. B. Sporn and D. L. Newton, *unpublished results*). Furthermore, in the retinoid deficient chick embryo, normal development of the vascular system can be restored by injection of appropriate amounts of various retinoids, including esters of retinoic acid (59,60). These results indicate a very stringent requirement for retinoids, with either deficiency or excess leading to abnormal development of tissues derived from primitive mesenchyme. The effects of retinoids on the developing vascular system of the early embryo appear to be quite selective, since many other cell types do not appear to be affected to anywhere near the same extent (52,59,60). In the early embryo a common stem cell type has long been believed to be a precursor to both blood cells themselves and those cells which will form the walls of the earliest blood vessels (46). The preceding observations, made with only the simplest of morphologic techniques, suggest that retinoids play a role in controlling the proliferation and differentiation of these mesenchymal precursor cells, or their early progeny; more recent work, using sophisticated cell culture and recombinant DNA techniques, has added important further information, as will be discussed later.

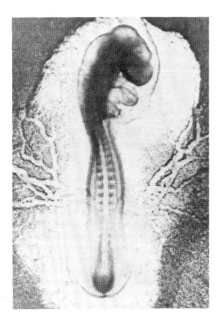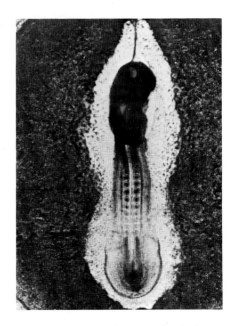

FIG. 1. *(Left)* Normal 3 day avian embryo. Note well developed extraembryonic circulatory system, with large major blood vessels surrounding the embryo. *(Right)* Abnormal 2 day avian embryo, resulting from retinoid deficiency. Although many structures, such as the somites, have formed relatively normally, there is a conspicuous absence of an extraembryonic circulatory system. Treatment of early embryos with retinoic acid methyl ester will restore normal development. (Data from ref. 59, with permission.)

Mechanistic studies in the whole animal on the role of retinoids in prevention of carcinogenesis have dealt largely with the prevention of epithelial carcinogenesis. There are especially convincing data on the efficacy of retinoids in prevention of skin, breast, and bladder cancer in experimental animals (4,6,32,35,36,51,53,58); there are now dozens of experiments in the published literature which document the use of many different retinoids in prevention of cancer at these epithelial sites. Overall, these studies suggest that retinoids exert a hormone-like control of either cell proliferation or cell differentiation. However, in the whole animal, it is extremely difficult to separate these two parameters; they are intimately linked with each other. Some investigators have stressed the role of retinoids as antiproliferative agents (36), while others have emphasized that the role of retinoids in control of differentiation, rather than proliferation, may be more important (3). Whole animal studies do not easily lend themselves to separate analysis of these two parameters. Indeed, the problem of the separation of the effects of retinoids on cell proliferation, as contrasted to effects on cell differentiation, may turn out to be more semantic than real, once a complete genetic analysis, using recombinant DNA methods, is available. The key problem is not to deal with the semantics of whether retinoids preferentially affect cell proliferation or cell differentiation, but to identify the specific genes whose function is ultimately controlled by retinoids, either directly or indirectly. This problem cannot be solved in the whole animal; it requires isolated cellular systems and modern methods of molecular analysis. We will now discuss the application of studies in these areas to understanding the role of retinoids in differentiation and carcinogenesis.

CELLULAR MECHANISM OF ACTION OF RETINOIDS IN DIFFERENTIATION AND CARCINOGENESIS

Significant advances in understanding the mechanism of action of retinoids did not occur until isolated, *in vitro* systems were used as experimental tools. The development of methods for organ culture of tissues, such as the skin and the prostate, in which retinoids are particularly active, was a major advance. In the 1950s the classic studies of Fell and Mellanby showed that the differentiated phenotype of chick epidermis in organ culture could be changed from keratinized to mucus-producing by treatment with retinol or retinyl acetate (19). In cultures treated with retinoids, the keratinizing cells of the epidermis disappeared and were replaced by mucus-producing cells, and in some instances even by ciliated cells, which are not found in normal skin (19). These organ culture experiments were essentially a mirror image to those performed by Wolbach and Howe in the 1920s in the whole animal. In the Wolbach and Howe studies, retinoid *deficiency* caused disappearance of normal mucociliary epithelium, with replacement by keratinizing cells (keratinizing squamous metaplasia); in the Fell and Mellanby experiments, retinoid *excess* caused disappearance of normal keratinizing epithelium, with replacement by mucus and ciliated cells (mucus metaplasia).

The next significant advance in this area also used organ culture methodology. Lasnitzki, working in the same laboratory as Fell and Mellanby, was able to show that the premalignant phenotype of mouse prostate glands that had been treated with the carcinogen, 3-methyl-cholanthrene, could be altered by retinoid treatment (25). The effects of the retinoids were to suppress abnormal cellular differentiation that had been induced by the carcinogen in the epithelium of the prostate gland and to restore a more normal pattern of epithelial differentiation. The atypical epithelial cells that were induced by the carcinogen disappeared upon retinoid treatment of the organ cultures, and they were replaced by cells with more normal morphology (25). In other organ culture studies, Lasnitzki also made the important observation that there were significant morphologic similarities between vitamin A-deficient prostatic epithelium and prostatic epithelium in cultures that had been treated with methyl-cholanthrene (26); these studies provide further evidence for the concept that the mechanisms of action of retinoids in both differentiation and carcinogenesis are closely linked.

In spite of the advances that were made in organ culture studies, these systems have definite liabilities for analysis of mechanism, since they use mixed cell populations, from which it is very difficult, if not impossible, to obtain replicate samples of homogeneous cells. The introduction of cell culture methodology to studies of retinoid mechanism was therefore of great importance, and now is allowing truly molecular investigation of the role of retinoids in differentiation and carcinogenesis. In contrast to the organ culture studies, in which the emphasis was on the role of retinoids in control of epithelial differentiation, cell culture studies have emphasized the role of retinoids in cells of mesenchymal origin, if only because such cells are grown more easily in culture. One may suppose that as better systems are developed for epithelial cell culture, there will be increasing investigation of retinoids in epithelia using these methods; this has already happened with epidermal cell culture (65).

Continuous cell lines of mesenchymal origin have been widely used to study the effects of retinoids on both differentiation and carcinogenesis; the cell lines which have been used are both neoplastic and nonneoplastic. The experiments which opened up this area of investigation were those of Merriman and Bertram (34) and Harisiadis et al. (23), which showed that retinoids can act directly on nonneoplastic cells to suppress the process of malignant transformation induced by either chemicals or radiation. In the case of the experiments done with suppression of chemical carcinogenesis, it was clearly shown that retinoids were effective in suppressing transformation even if they were not applied to cells until a full week after original exposure of the cells to carcinogen. Whatever the genetic damage caused by the carcinogen, it had already occurred, and the role of the retinoids in these experiments was clearly shown to be a suppressor of the expression of the malignant phenotype (34). Furthermore, in these experiments, continuous presence of the retinoids was required to suppress the malignant phenotype; removal of the retinoids from the culture allowed expression of the transformed state.

Retinoids can also change the differentiation of fully neoplastic cells growing in either monolayer or soft-agar culture. The most striking examples of this phenomenon are the induction of terminal differentiation in murine F9 teratocarcinoma cells (54,55) or human promyelocytic leukemia cells (9,10, Fig. 2); in these cases the differentiated phenotype is drastically changed from neoplastic to nonneoplastic, and proliferation of the induced cells is permanently suppressed. In the F9 system, retinoids induce terminal differentiation of teratocarcinoma stem cells to cells which resemble parietal endoderm; a variety of new proteins is induced in the differentiated cells (55,56). In the human promyelocytic leukemia system, retinoids can induce terminal differentiation of malignant leukemia cells, leading to formation of morphologically mature granulocytes, which have functional markers of the mature neutrophil (9,10); these results have been obtained with the established HL-60 cell line (9), as well as with primary cultures of other promyelocytic leukemia cells (10). These studies with neoplastic leukemia cells in turn have had a major influence on studies on possible effects of retinoids on normal myeloid differentiation. Since some of the leukemias may be viewed as diseases in which there is a block or arrest in normal myeloid differentiation and maturation (13,22), and since retinoids can apparently overcome this block in certain leukemia cells, it has been suggested that retinoids may also be involved in normal hematopoiesis (9,17).

The mechanism of all of the effects of retinoids, whether it be to alter the differentiated phenotype in nonneoplastic or preneoplastic epithelial cells in organ

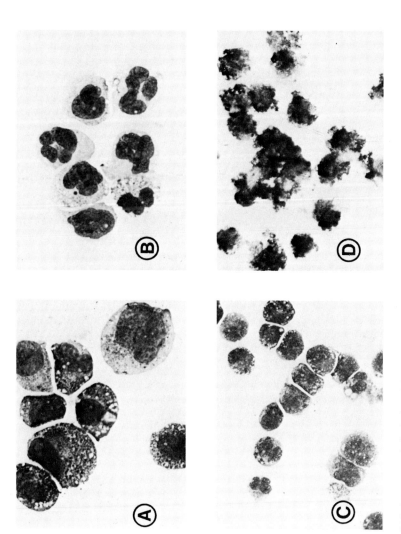

FIG. 2. Retinoic acid induces morphological and functional maturation of leukemic cells obtained from a patient with promyelocytic leukemia. **A,** Cells cultured without retinoic acid consisting of promyelocytes with characteristic cytoplasmic granules (×860). **B,** Cells cultured with retinoic acid showing maturation to banded and segmented neutrophils (×860). **C,** Absence of nitroblue tetrazolium (NBT) reduction by cells cultured without retinoic acid (×315). **D,** NBT reduction by cells incubated with retinoic acid (×315). (Data from ref. 10, with permission.)

culture, to suppress the appearance of the neoplastic phenotype in nonneoplastic mesenchymal cells in monolayer culture, or to induce the terminally differentiated phenotype in fully neoplastic cells in monolayer culture, is not known. It is tempting to believe that there is a common mechanism (or limited number of mechanisms), which underlies all of these phenomena. In cell culture studies, as we noted before in the studies on whole animals, various investigators again have chosen to emphasize the role of retinoids in control of either cell proliferation (29) or cell differentiation (65). It would appear that retinoids control both processes, and that any dispute over which is more important is relatively fruitless at present. Rather it would seem more productive to focus on the specific molecular processes involved, to which we shall now turn.

MOLECULAR MECHANISM OF ACTION OF RETINOIDS IN DIFFERENTIATION AND CARCINOGENESIS

Over the years, numerous hypotheses on the molecular mechanism of action of retinoids in control of differentiation have been proposed, but none have stood up to the experimental data. In particular, any hypothesis relating to molecular mechanism of action must take into account the evidence, now overwhelming, that retinoic acid will support growth in the whole animal fully as effectively as retinol (67), that retinoic acid is more active than retinol or retinal in numerous *in vitro* test systems (9,29,51,55), and that there is no evidence that the mammalian organism can convert retinoic acid to retinol (18). In many test systems retinoic acid is at least 100 to a 1,000 times more active than retinol (9,51,55), and biological activity can be measured at levels as low as 10^{-11} Molar (51). Thus, the hypothesis, proposed in the 1960s, that retinol directly modifies membrane structure (15) to exert its biological effects is now of only historical interest.

More recently it has been suggested that a primary biological role of the retinoids is to participate in sugar transfer reactions by means of the intermediate retinyl phosphate mannose, which is a metabolite of retinol (1,14,64). This hypothesis cannot be rationalized with the experimental data that retinoic acid is more active than retinol in many test systems and that no evidence for conversion of retinoic acid to retinol exists. Neither is there any convincing evidence at present for a metabolite of retinoic acid which is involved in sugar transfer reactions. The recent synthesis of a new series of retinoids (28), which may be viewed as retinoidal benzoic acid derivatives (Fig. 3), and which are even more potent than retinoic acid in many test systems, both *in vivo* and *in vitro*, provides even further exper-

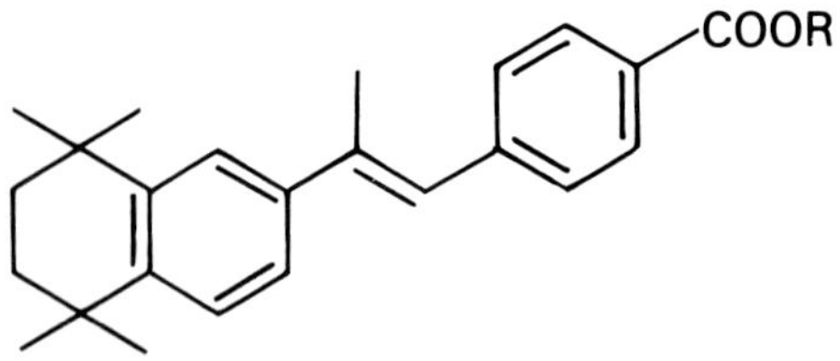

FIG. 3. Structure of a new retinoidal benzoic acid derivative, which is 1,000 times more active than retinol or retinyl acetate in several test systems, both *in vitro* and *in vivo*, when R = H.

imental evidence against any significant role for retinyl phosphate mannose in control of differentiation of carcinogenesis. The new analog shown in Fig. 3 (or its derivatives) will support growth in the whole animal fed a vitamin A-deficient diet (28), is at least 1,000 times more active than retinol in suppressing skin carcinogenesis in the mouse (28), is more than 100 times as active as retinol in the hamster tracheal organ culture system (51), and more than 1,000 times as active as retinol or retinyl acetate in the F9 teratocarcinoma or HL-60 promyelocytic leukemia test systems (Strickland, Breitman, Frickel, Nürrenbach, and Sporn, *unpublished results*). With data such as these at hand, it is unreasonable to believe that retinyl phosphate mannose plays any universally critical role in control of differentiation or carcinogenesis. Although one cannot exclude the possibility that there may be some situations in which retinyl phosphate mannose may play some role, the data at hand at best would relegate this metabolite to a minor role in control of differentiation and carcinogenesis.

If one wishes to develop a molecular hypothesis of retinoid mechanism that is compatible with the broadest range of experimental data, then the simplest one that can be proposed at present is to suggest that retinoids modify gene expression. This, of course, is not a new idea. If one takes this as a general proposition, then two important questions follow: (a) *which genes* are controlled by retinoids? and (b) *how* are these genes controlled by retinoids? (is the mechanism one of direct or indirect control?) We will provide only an outline of what is known regarding these two questions.

With respect to which genes are known to be controlled by retinoids, one is impressed by the number of recent reports which indicate that retinoids control the expression of many proteins which are either direct constituents of the cytoskeleton and extracellular matrix, or participate in the formation of cytoskeleton and matrix. These proteins include keratins (21), collagen (55,56), collagenase (11), transglutaminase (47,66), and laminin (56). Determination of the specific types of cytoskeletal or matrix proteins which are produced in cells is now being used as a specific marker for cell differentiation, and it would appear that retinoids are intimately involved in this process. Other proteins whose expression is known to be controlled by retinoids include plasminogen activator (55,56), alkaline phosphatase (45,56), and the receptor for epidermal growth factor (24,44). Furthermore, the important observation has recently been made in the HL-60 system that retinoic acid controls the expression of the *myc*-oncogene. Using a specific molecular probe for the *myc*-gene, it has been shown that physiological levels of all-*trans*-retinoic acid suppress *myc*-gene expression in HL-60 cells (61, Fig. 4). Although the specific molecular function for the *myc*-gene product has not yet been elucidated, it is presumed that in some way the excessive expression of this gene and its product is correlated with the excessive proliferation (and perhaps with the arrested differentiation) of the HL-60 cell.

Thus, at the gene level, it appears that retinoids affect the expression of genes or gene products involved with both differentiation and proliferation. The remaining, and most difficult, question is: how do they do it? The overall problem of the

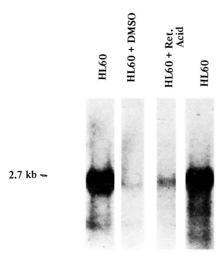

2.7 kb →

FIG. 4. Hybridization of *myc* probe to RNA from HL-60 cells induced to differentiate. Degree of differentiation was judged by the percentage of cells able to reduce NBT, as well as morphologic criteria (see Fig. 2). Lanes are as follows, from left to right: RNA from uninduced HL-60 (less than 2% of cells NBT positive), RNA from HL-60 induced to differentiate with dimethyl sulfoxide (87% of cells NBT positive), RNA from HL-60 induced to differentiate with retinoic acid (40% of cells NBT positive), and a second isolate of RNA from uninduced HL-60 (less than 2% of cells NBT positive). On a molar basis, retinoic acid is approximately a million times more active than dimethyl sulfoxide in inducing differentiation in HL-60 (9). (Data from ref. 61, with permission.)

control of gene expression is beyond the scope of this chapter: one may conceive of both direct and indirect mechanisms that involve either regulation of gene transcription itself, regulation of processing of primary gene transcripts, or regulation of translation of processed message. Little is known about retinoids in any of these areas. By analogy with the steroids, it has been suggested that the effects of retinoids in controlling gene expression are mediated by specific intracellular binding proteins (12). However, retinoids have significant effects in control of both differentiation and carcinogenesis in two important cell systems, namely HL-60 and 10T1/2 fibroblasts, in which no retinoid binding protein (analogous to steroid binding proteins) can be detected (16;27; T. R. Breitman, *personal communication*).

The alternative to a steroid-like mechanism for retinoids is to suggest that they control gene expression via interactions with protein kinases, both cyclic AMP-dependent and cyclic AMP-independent. Retinoids have been shown to increase cyclic AMP-dependent protein kinase activity in B16 melanoma cells (31), which are highly sensitive to their antiproliferative effects (29), as well as in F9 teratocarcinoma cells which are induced to differentiate by retinoic acid (42). Furthermore, dibutyryl cyclic AMP markedly potentiates the differentiating effects of retinoic acid in both F9 teratocarcinoma cells (56) and HL-60 leukemia cells (40). Very recent work has also suggested that a secondary effect of retinoic acid may be the induction in the F9 system of a calcium and phospholipid-dependent, cyclic AMP-independent, protein kinase activity (2,39,57), and that some of the interactions between retinoids and phorbol esters may be mediated through this system (2). These latest studies on a calcium-dependent protein kinase system provide an important link between retinoids and calcium, which is now assuming an increasing importance in control of cell proliferation and differentiation (43,62). Thus, although studies on the interactions between retinoids and the various protein kinase systems of the cells have only recently begun, they have already yielded significant new data which will need to be integrated into an overall hypothesis of mechanism of action.

Ultimately it would appear that the problem of the molecular mechanism of action of retinoids in control of differentiation and carcinogenesis is converging on one of the central problems in all of biology, namely the control of gene expression. There may be new mechanisms, yet to be discovered, that may be critically involved in this process. For example, yet another question that awaits further experimentation is the functional relationship between retinoids and polypeptide growth factors that control cell proliferation and differentiation (52). The role of peptide growth factors in controlling these processes is of fundamental importance (8). Clearly, any future hypothesis dealing with mechanism of action of retinoids will need to integrate the role of retinoids, peptide growth factors, and specific genes controlling differentiation and proliferation. The breadth, potency, and specificity of retinoids in control of cell function all suggest that retinoids will be valuable tools for the experimental scientist to unravel molecular mechanisms, in addition to their practical usefulness in controlling differentiation and carcinogenesis.

ACKNOWLEDGMENT

We thank Ruth Morsillo for expert assistance with the preparation of the manuscript.

REFERENCES

1. Adamo, S., De Luca, L. M., Silverman-Jones, C. S., and Yuspa, S. H. (1979): Mode of action of retinol—Involvement in glycosylation reactions of cultured mouse epidermal cells. *J. Biol. Chem.*, 254:3279–3287.
2. Anderson, W. B., and Kraft, A. S. (1983): Effect of retinoic acid and phorbol ester treatment of embryonal carcinoma cells on calcium, phospholipid-dependent protein kinase activity. *Cold Spring Harbor Conferences on Cell Proliferation*, 10: (in press).
3. Astrup, E. G., and Paulsen, J. E. (1982): Effect of retinoic acid pretreatment on 12-0-tetradeca-noylphorbol-13-acetate-induced cell population kinetics and polyamine biosynthesis in hairless mouse epidermis. *Carcinogenesis*, 3:313–320.
4. Becci, P. J., Thompson, H. J., Grubbs, C. J., Squire, R. A., Brown, C. C., Sporn, M. B., and Moon, R. C. (1978): Inhibitory effect of 13-*cis*-retinoic acid on urinary bladder carcinogenesis induced in C57BL/6 mice by N-butyl-N-(4-hydroxybutyl)-nitrosamine. *Cancer Res.*, 38:4463–4466.
5. Bertram, J. S., Mordan, L. J., Domanska-Janik, K., and Bernacki, R. J. (1982): Inhibition of in vitro neoplastic transformation by retinoids. In: *Molecular Interrelations of Nutrition and Cancer*, edited by M. S. Arnott, J. van Eys, and Y. M. Wang, pp. 315–335. Raven Press, New York.
6. Bollag, W. (1979): Retinoids and cancer. *Cancer Chemother. Pharmacol.*, 3:207–215.
7. Borek, C. (1982): Vitamins and micronutrients modify carcinogenesis and tumor promotion in vitro. In: *Molecular Interrelations of Nutrition and Cancer*, edited by M. S. Arnott, J. van Eys, and Y. M. Wang, pp. 337–350. Raven Press, New York.
8. Bradshaw, R. A., and Sporn, M. B., editors (1983): Polypeptide growth factors and the regulation of cell growth and differentiation. *Fed. Proc.*, 42:2590–2634.
9. Breitman, T. R., Selonik, S. E., and Collins, S. J. (1980): Induction of differentiation of the human promyelocytic leukemia cell line (HL-60) by retinoic acid. *Proc. Natl. Acad. Sci. USA*, 77:2936–2940.
10. Breitman, T. R., Collins, S. J., and Keene, B. R. (1981): Terminal differentiation of human promyelocytic leukemic cells in primary culture in response to retinoic acid. *Blood*, 57:1000–1004.

11. Brinckerhoff, C. E., and Harris, E. D. Jr. (1981): Modulation by retinoic acid and corticosteroids of collagenase production by rabbit synovial fibroblasts treated with phorbol myristate acetate or poly(ethylene glyol). *Biochim. Biophys. Acta*, 677:424–432.
12. Chytil, F., and Ong, D. E. (1979): Cellular retinol- and retinoic acid-binding proteins in vitamin A action. *Fed. Proc.*, 38:2510–2514.
13. Clarkson, B. D. (1972): Acute myelocytic leukemia in adults. *Cancer*, 30:1572–1582.
14. De Luca, L. M., Bhat, P. V., Sasak, W., and Adamo, S. (1979): Biosynthesis of phosphoryl and glycosyl phosphoryl derivatives of vitamin A in biological membranes. *Fed. Proc.*, 38:2535–2539.
15. Dingle, J. T., and Lucy, J. A. (1965): Vitamin A, carotenoids, and cell function. *Biol. Rev.*, 40:422–461.
16. Douer, D., and Koeffler, H. P. (1982): Retinoic acid—Inhibition of the clonal growth of human myeloid leukemia cells. *J. Clin. Invest.*, 69:277–283.
17. Douer, D., and Koeffler, H. P. (1982): Retinoic acid enhances growth of human early erythroid progenitor cells in vitro. *J. Clin. Invest.*, 69:1039–1041.
18. Dowling, J. E., and Wald, G. (1960): The biological function of vitamin A acid. *Proc. Natl. Acad. Sci. USA*, 46:587–608.
19. Fell, H. B., and Mellanby, E. (1953): Metaplasia produced in cultures of chick ectoderm by high vitamin A. *J. Physiol.*, 119:470–488.
20. Findlay, G. M., and McKenzie, R. D. (1922): The bone marrow in deficiency diseases. *J. Path. Bact.*, 25:402–403.
21. Fuchs, E., and Green, H. (1981): Regulation of terminal differentiation of cultured human keratinocytes by vitamin A. *Cell*, 25:617–625.
22. Gallo, R. C. (1974): On the origin of human acute myeloblastic leukemia: Virus-"hot spot" hypothesis. In: *Modern Trends in Human Leukemia*, edited by R. Neth, R. C. Gallo, S. Spiegelman, and F. Stohlman, pp. 227–236. J. F. Lehmanns Verlag, Munich.
23. Harisiadis, L., Miller, R. C., Hall, E. J., and Borek, C. (1978): A vitamin A analogue inhibits radiation-induced oncogenic transformation. *Nature*, 274:486–487.
24. Jetten, A. M. (1980): Retinoids specifically enhance the number of epidermal growth factor receptors. *Nature*, 284:626–629.
25. Lasnitzki, I. (1955): The influence of A hypervitaminosis on the effect of 20-methylcholanthrene on mouse prostate glands grown in vitro. *Br. J. Cancer*, 9:434–441.
26. Lasnitzki, I. (1962): Hypovitaminosis-A in the mouse prostate gland cultured in chemically defined medium. *Exp. Cell Res.*, 28:40–51.
27. Libby, P. R., and Bertram, J. S. (1982): Lack of intracellular retinoid-binding proteins in a retinol-sensitive cell line. *Carcinogenesis*, 3:481–484.
28. Loeliger, P., Bollag, W., and Mayer, H. (1980): Arotinoids, a new class of highly active retinoids. *Eur. J. Med. Chem.*, 15:9–15.
29. Lotan, R. (1980): Effects of vitamin A and its analogs (retinoids) on normal and neoplastic cells. *Biochim. Biophys. Acta.*, 605:33–91.
30. Lotan, R., Thein, R., and Lotan, D. (1983): Suppression of the transformed cell phenotype expression by retinoids. In: *The Modulation and Mediation of Cancer by Retinoids*, edited by F. L. Meyskens and K. Prasad, S. Karger, Basel, *(in press)*.
31. Ludwig, K. W., Lowey, B., and Niles, R. M. (1980): Retinoic acid increases cyclic AMP-dependent protein kinase activity in murine melanoma cells. *J. Biol. Chem.*, 255:5999–6002.
32. Mayer, H., Bollag, W., Hanni, R., and Ruegg, R. (1978): Retinoids, a new class of compounds with prophylatic and therapeutic activities in oncology and dermatology. *Experientia*, 34:1105–1119.
33. Mellanby, E. (1947): Vitamin A and bone growth: the reversibility of vitamin A deficiency changes. *J. Physiol.*, 105:382–399.
34. Merriman, R. L., and Bertram, J. S. (1979): Reversible inhibition by retinoids of 3-methylcholanthrene-induced neoplastic transformation in C3H/10T 1/2 CL8 cells *Cancer Res.*, 39:1661–1666.
35. Moon, R. C., Grubbs, C. J., Sporn, M. B., and Goodman, D. G. (1977): Retinyl acetate inhibits mammary carcinogenesis induced by N-methyl-N-nitrosourea. *Nature*, 267:620–621.
36. Moon, R. C., Thompson, H. J., Becci, P. J., Grubbs, C. J., Gander, R. J., Newton, D. L., Smith, J. M., Phillips, S. L., Henderson, W. R., Mullen, L. T., Brown, C. C., and Sporn, M. B. (1979):

N-(4-Hydroxyphenyl)retinamide, a new retinoid for prevention of breast cancer in the rat. *Cancer Res.*, 39:1339–1346.

37. Moore, L. A. (1939): Relationship between carotene, blindness due to constriction of the optic nerve, papillary edema, and nyctalopia in calves. *J. Nutr.*, 17:443–459.

38. Morriss, G. M., and Steele, C. E. (1977): Comparison of the effects of retinol and retinoic acid on postimplantation rat embryos in vitro. *Teratology*, 15:109–119.

39. Nishizuka, Y., and Takai, Y. (1981): Calcium and phospholipid turnover in a new receptor function for protein phosphorylation. *Cold Spring Harbor Conferences on Cell Proliferation*, 8:237–249.

40. Olsson, I. L., Breitman, T. R., and Gallo, R. C. (1982): Priming of human myeloid leukemic cell lines HL-60 and U-937 with retinoic acid for differentiation effects of cyclic adenosine 3′:5′-monophosphate-inducing agents and a T-lymphocyte-derived differentiation factor. *Cancer Res.*, 42:3928–3933.

41. Pierce, G. B., Shikes, R., and Fink, L. M. (1978): *Cancer—A Problem of Developmental Biology*, Prentice Hall, Englewood Cliffs, N.J.

42. Plet, A., Evain, D., and Anderson, W. B. (1982): Effect of retinoic acid treatment of F9 embryonal carcinoma cells on the activity and distribution of cyclic AMP-dependent protein kinase. *J. Biol. Chem.*, 257:889–893.

43. Rasmussen, H. (1981): *Calcium and cAMP as Synarchic Messengers*, John Wiley, New York.

44. Rees, A. R., Adamson, E. D., and Graham, C. F. (1979): Epidermal growth factor receptors increase during the differentiation of embryonal carcinoma cells. *Nature*, 281:309–311.

45. Reese, D. H., Fiorentino, G. J., Claflin, A. J., Malinin, T. I., and Politano, V. A. (1981): Rapid induction of alkaline phosphatase activity by retinoic acid. *Biochem. Biophys. Res. Comm.*, 102:315–321.

46. Romanoff, A. L. (1960): *The Avian Embryo*, Macmillan, New York.

47. Scott, K. F. F., Meyskens, F. L., and Russell, D. H. (1982): Retinoids increase transglutaminase activity and inhibit ornithine decarboxylase activity in Chinese hamster ovary cells and in melanoma cells stimulated to differentiate. *Proc. Natl. Acad. Sci. USA*, 79:4093–4097.

48. Sporn, M. B., Dunlop, N. M., Newton, D. L., and Smith, J. M. (1976): Prevention of chemical carcinogenesis by vitamin A and its synthetic analogs (retinoids), *Fed. Proc.*, 35:1332–1338.

49. Sporn, M. B., and Harris, E. D. Jr. (1981): Proliferative diseases. *Amer. J. Med.*, 70:1231–1236.

50. Sporn, M. B., and Newton, D. L. (1979): Chemoprevention of cancer with retinoids. *Fed. Proc.*, 38:2528–2534.

51. Sporn, M. B., and Newton, D. L. (1981): Retinoids and chemoprevention of cancer. In: *Inhibition of Tumor Induction and Development*, edited by M. S. Zedeck, and M. Lipkin, pp. 71–99, Plenum Publishing, New York.

52. Sporn, M. B., Newton, D. L., Roberts, A. B., De Larco, J. E., and Todaro, G. J. (1981): Retinoids and suppression of the effects of polypeptide transforming factors—a new molecular approach to chemoprevention of cancer. In: *Molecular Actions and Targets for Cancer Chemotherapeutic Agents*, edited by A. C. Sartorelli, J. S. Lazo, and J. R. Bertino, pp. 541–554, Academic Press, New York.

53. Sporn, M. B., Squire, R. A., Brown, C. C., Smith, J. M., Wenk, M. L., Springer, S. (1977): 13-*cis*-retinoic acid: inhibition of bladder carcinogenesis in the rat. *Science*, 195:487–489.

54. Strickland, S. (1981): Mouse teratocarcinoma cells: prospects for the study of embryogenesis and neoplasia. *Cell*, 24:277–278.

55. Strickland, S., and Mahdavi, V. (1978): The induction of differentiation in teratocarcinoma stem cells by retinoic acid. *Cell*, 15:393–403.

56. Strickland, S., Smith, K. K., and Marotti, K. R. (1980): Hormonal induction of differentiation in teratocarcinoma stem cells: generation of parietal endoderm by retinoic acid and dibutyryl cAMP. *Cell*, 21:347–355.

57. Takai, Y., Kishimoto, A., Kawahara, Y., Minakuchi, R., Sano, K., Kikkawa, U., Mori, T., Yu, B., Kaibuchi, K., and Nishizuka, Y. (1981): Calcium and phosphatidylinositol turnover as signalling for trans-membrane control of protein phosphorylation. *Adv. Cyclic Nucleotide Res.*, 14:301–308.

58. Thompson, H. J., Becci, P. J., Brown, C. C., and Moon, R. C. (1979): Effect of the duration of retinyl acetate feeding on inhibition of 1-methyl-1-nitrosourea-induced mammary carcinogenesis in the rat. *Cancer Res.*, 39:3977–3980.

59. Thompson, J. N. (1969): The role of vitamin A in reproduction. In: *The Fat-Soluble Vitamins*,

edited by H. F. DeLuca, and J. W. Suttie, pp. 267–281. The University of Wisconsin Press, Madison.

60. Thompson, J. N., Howell, J. M., Pitt, G. A. J., and McLaughlin, C. I. (1969): The biological activity of retinoic acid in the domestic fowl and the effects of vitamin A deficiency on the chick embryo. *Brit. J. Nutr.*, 23:471–490.

61. Westin, E. H., Wong-Staal, F., Gelmann, E. P., Dalla Favera, R., Papas, T. S., Lautenberger, J. A., Eva, A., Reddy, E. P., Tronick, S. R., Aaronson, S. A., and Gallo, R. C. (1982): Expression of cellular homologues of retroviral *onc* genes in human hematopoietic cells. *Proc. Natl. Acad. Sci. USA*, 79:2490–2494.

62. Whitfield, J. F., Boynton, A. L., MacManus, J. P., Rixon, R. H., Sikorska, M., Tsang, B., and Walker, P. R. (1980): The roles of calcium and cyclic AMP in cell proliferation. *Annals N.Y. Acad. Sci.*, 339:216–240.

63. Wolbach, S. B., and Howe, P. R. (1925): Tissue changes following deprivation of fat soluble A vitamin. *J. Exp. Med.*, 42:753–777.

64. Wolf, G., Kiorpes, T. C., Masushige, S., Shreiber, J. B., Smith, M. J., and Anderson, R. S. (1979): Recent evidence for the participation of vitamin A in glycoprotein synthesis. *Fed. Proc.*, 38:2540–2543.

65. Yuspa, S. H. (1983): Retinoids and tumor promotion. In: *Diet and Cancer: From Basic Research to Policy Implications*, edited by D. A. Roe, Alan R. Liss, New York, *(in press)*.

66. Yuspa, S. H., Ben, T., and Steinert, P. (1982): Retinoic acid induces transglutaminase activity but inhibits cornification of cultured epidermal cells. *J. Biol. Chem.*, 257:9906–9908.

67. Zile, M., and DeLuca, H. F. (1968): Retinoic acid: some aspects of growth-promoting activity in the albino rat. *J. Nutr.*, 94:302–308.

Biochemical Basis of Chemical Carcinogenesis,
edited by H. Greim, R. Jung, M. Kramer,
H. Marquardt, and F. Oesch.
Raven Press, New York © 1984.

The Role of Genetic Transposition in Carcinogenesis

Jack Spira

Department of Tumor Biology, Box 60400, 104 01 Stockholm

Exposure of an experimental animal to a single dose of a tumor inducing agent, whether a chemical, physical or viral, requires a major period of the animal's life span until the overt tumor develops. The inducing agent is usually not present or active in the body during the whole latent period, and the exposed subject is healthy after the initial assault. It is therefore conceivable that the initiating event alone is not enough for tumor development. Further events, some probably at the genetic level, are required for tumorigenesis. The exact nature of these events, however, are unknown. But results from experimentally induced tumors and also human tumors suggest that genetic transposition, visualized either at the chromosome level (chromosome banding) or at the molecular level, plays a significant role in the genesis of certain lymphoid tumors (2,14).

CHROMOSOME CHANGES (TRISOMY 15) IN MURINE LYMPHOMAS

A high frequency of mouse T-cell lymphomas have as sole abnormality a trisomy of chromosome 15, irrespective whether the inducing agent is x-ray (3), chemical (32), or viral (7,30). By chromosome banding studies of leukemias induced in a translocation stock of mice, CBAT6T6 (31) and in the SJL strain (25) it was determined that the genes that need to duplicate during leukemogenesis are located in the distal third of chromosome 15, below band C1. The crucial role of trisomy 15 is visualized in Robertsonian translocation mice that carry the 15 chromosome centromerically attached to chromosome number 1,5, or 6 resp. In the lymphomas, the whole translocation element became trisomic (11,24). In other Robertsonian stocks, where the 15 chromosome is "free" and two other autosomes are fused, only the free, nonattached 15 chromosome is duplicated in the lymphomas (27). These results strongly emphasize that it is the genetic content of the 15 chromosome that is important for leukemia development. Trisomy 15 is also the most regular change in murine B-cell lymphomas (9,34). Usually these cells also had other abnormalities as well.

Recent experiments performed in our laboratory indicate that the 15 chromosome from a tumor are qualitatively different from those of a normal cell. Cell hybrids were made by fusing chromosome 15 trisomic T-cell line (TIKAUT) with normal lymphocytes or fibroblasts of CBAT6T6 origin. In the hybrids it is possible to distinguish cytogenetically between tumor derived chromosome 15 and the normal derived homologue T(14:15). High and low tumorigenic hybrids were compared by banding. There was a remarkable difference in the number of 15 chromosomes present. High tumorigenic hybrids had five-six copies of the tumor derived 15 and one-two copies of the normal derived T(14;15). Low tumorigenic hybrids had an opposite pattern with two-three tumor derived 15 chromosomes and two T(14;15). The few *in vivo* tumors of the low tumorigenic hybrids increased their number of tumor derived chromosome 15 and decreased the number of normal T(14;15). These results show that the genetic content of tumor and normal derived chromosome 15 homologue is not the same since the tumor derived chromosome was preferentially duplicated in the high tumorigenic hybrids. It also indicates that the normal 15 homologue carries a gene that can counteract the tumorigenic behavior (26).

We have hypothesized that the qualitative change in the tumor derived chromosome 15 can be due to either mutation or proviral promotor insertion in the vicinity of a cellular oncogene. Duplication of the altered 15 oncogene may be a simple way of overcoming the transacting regulation of the normal 15 (26).

TRANSLOCATION IN MURINE PLASMACYTOMAS

The most commonly seen aberration in both IgA kappa and lambda producing murine plasmacytomas (PC) is a translocation of the distal chromosome 15 (below band D2/3) to chromosome 12 (22,33). In a minority of the kappa producers a reciprocal translocation between the same chromosome 15 segment and chromosome 6 was seen (22). Not all but the majority of plasmacytomas have one of these translocations, (Ohno, *personal communication*). The translocated segment is within the same portion of the 15 chromosome that is duplicated in the lymphomas.

The immunoglobulin heavy chain genes of the mouse have been mapped to distal chromosome 12 (5,21) and kappa light chain genes to chromosome 6 (29) and lambda genes to 16 (6). The distal 15 was thus transposed to chromosomes carrying immunoglobulin chain genes and in the T(12;15) case, cytogenetically close to the chromosomal location of the heavy chain genes (21,22). The PC might be generated by activation of an oncogene localized on chromosome 15. After its translocation to the highly active immunoglobulin promotor the oncogene would be highly transcribed and transform the cell.

HUMAN BURKITT LYMPHOMAS AND
CHROMOSOME TRANSLOCATIONS

A remarkably analogous situation to the mouse plasmacytomas is seen in human Burkitt Lymphomas (BL), also a B-cell derived tumor. Ninety percent of BL tumor cells regardless of immunoglobulin chain type expressed and presence of Epstein-Barr virus, carry a specific translocation between distal chromosome 8 and chromosome 14:8q24,14q32 (35). The translocation is specific always involving the same brakepoints. The human heavy chain locus is mapped to chromosome 14 (4), band q32 (19). Approximately 5% of BL tumor cells, however only tumors expressing kappa chains, have the same distal piece of chromosome 8 translocated to chromosome 2. In the remaining 5%, tumors expressing only kappa light chains, the same distal segment from chromosome 8 was translocated to chromosome 22 (17). Chromosome 2 carries the kappa chain locus (20), close to the tumor related brakepoint (18) and on chromosome 22 the lambda chain genes are located (8,20). The location on the chromosome is not yet known. The 8:14 and 8:2 translocation are comparable to the mouse PC T(12;15). In all cases the distal segment of a chromosome is translocated in the close neighborhood of an immunoglobulin gene. In the human BL, a chromosome 8 located oncogene could become activated after its translocation to an active immunoglobulin related promotor on the recipient chromosome (15), just as was visualized in the mouse case. Although probably more experiments are needed to support this hypothesis.

PROMOTOR INSERTION EVENTS

Another line of evidence favoring genetic transposition in tumor development comes from findings with certain RNA tumor viruses (1). RNA tumor viruses induce tumors with either a short latency, 3 to 4 weeks, or a long latency, 4 to 12 months. The acute transforming viruses are replicative defective (except Rous Sarcoma virus) and contain within them a cellular derived transforming gene called oncogene. The slow acting viruses are replication competent and do not contain the transforming oncogene.

Recently it was shown that in some lymphomas induced by one of the slow acting viruses, Avian Leukosis Virus (ALV), the ALV provirus has integrated adjacent to one of the cellular oncogenes called c-*myc*. C-*myc* is the transforming gene of avian myelomatoses virus (MC 29) that is associated with chicken B-cell lymphomas. The tumor cells also had an increased level of c-*myc* transcription (10).

Since the number of cellular oncogenes are rather few, about 20, the promotor insertion event at the right site must be a rather rare event and hence the long latency. The basis for that activation of an oncogene as a mechanism for tumor development is supported by further findings in this and other RNA tumor virus experimental systems (1).

CHROMOSOME DELETION IN HUMAN RETINOBLASTOMA

Retinoblastoma is regarded as existing in two different forms. One is inherited autosomal dominant, is usually bilateral with multiple foci in the both eyes. The other one is spontaneous, unilateral, and usually single foci of transformation. Knudsson (16) has suggested that two sequential mutational events are necessary for the malignant transformation. Could one of them be a chromosomal aberration? Recently a family was described that indicates that one of these events may be a chromosome deletion. The family had a high incidence of unilateral retinoblastoma. Chromosome analysis revealed that development of tumors was associated with a constitutional deletion of chromosome 13(q13.1;q14.5) and that unaffected individuals transmitting the risk had an insertional deletion that was balanced, i.e., the chromosome 13 deleted segment was translocated to chromosome 3 (28). Only individuals with loss of the chromosome 13 derived specific segment were predisposed to retinoblastoma development.

The 13q deletion does not have to be the transforming step. It could just as well be a predisposing step for a secondary genetic change (by mutation or recombination) at the homologue chromosome (13).

However deletion of the 13q14 segment has also been found in the tumor cells of both unilateral and bilateral retinoblastomas, here presenting itself as a tumor related chromosome aberration (12,23) and not constitutionally present. 13q deletions may thus be a final event in the two step model of Knudsson. One could speculate that with the deletion of a regulatory gene at the homologue chromosome is lost and the activated retinoblastoma related gene is fully expressed and has transformed the cell.

CONCLUSIONS

It is conceivable that genetic transposition, detectable either at the chromosomal level or at the molecular level plays an important role during carcinogenesis of certain tumors. The transposition would lead to activation of cellular oncogenes by installing them close to and under the influence of strong cellular promotors. Although probably further experimental evidence is needed to support this model.

ACKNOWLEDGEMENT

This investigation was supported by grant 83:151 from the Swedish Society against Cancer and PHS grant number 5 RO1-CA14054-09 awarded by the National Cancer Institute, DHHS.

REFERENCES

1. Bishop, J. M. (1981): Retroviruses and cancer genes. *Advances in Cancer Research (in press)*.
2. Cairns, J. (1981): The origin of human cancers. *Nature*, 289:353–357.
3. Chang, T. D., Biedler, J. L., Stockert, E., and Old, L. J. (1977): Trisomy of chromosome 15 in X-ray induced mouse leukemia. *Proc. of the American Assoc. for Cancer Res.*, 18:225.
4. Croce, C. M., Shander, M., Martinis, L., Cicurel, L., D'Ancona, G. G., Dolby, T. W., and Koprowski, H. (1979): Chromosomal location of the genes for human immunoglobulin heavy chains. *Proc. Natl. Acad. Sci. USA*, 76:3416–3419.
5. D'Eustachio, P., Pravtcheva, D., Marcu, K., and Ruddle, F. H. (1980): Chromosomal location of the structural gene cluster encoding murine immunoglobulin heavy chains. *J. Exp. Med.*, 151:1545–1550.
6. D'Eustachio, P., Bothwell, A. L. M., Takaro, A. R., Baltimore, D., and Ruddle, F. H. (1981): Chromosomal location of structural genes encoding murine immunoglobulin lambda light chains. *J. Exp. Med.*, 153:793–800.
7. Dofoku, R., Biedler, J. L., Spengler, B. A., and Old, L. J. (1975): Trisomy of chromosome 15 in spontaneous leukemia of AKR mice. *Proc. Natl. Acad. Sci. USA*, 72:1515–1517.
8. Eriksson, J., Martinis, J., and Croce, C. M. (1981): Assignment of the human genes for lambda immunoglobulin chains to chromosome 22. *Nature*, 294:173–175.
9. Fialkow, P. J., Reddy, A. L., and Bryant, J. I. (1980): Clonal origin and trisomy of chromosome 15 in murine B-cell malignancies. *Int. J. Cancer*, 26:603–608.

10. Hayward, W. S., Neel, B. G., and Astrin, S. M. (1981): Activation of a cellular oncogene by promotor insertion in ALV-induced lymphoid leukosis. *Nature*, 290:475–479.

11. Herbst, E. W., Gropp, A., and Tvetzen, C. (1981): Chromosome rearrangements involved in the origin of trisomy 15 in spontaneous T-cell leukemia of AKR mice. *Int. J. Cancer*, 28:805–810.

12. Johnson, M. P., Ramsey, N., Cervenka, J., and Wang, N. (1982): Retinoblastoma and its association with a deletion in chromosome 13: A survey using high-resolution chromosome techniques. *Cancer Genetics and Cytogenetics*, 6:29–37.

13. Kinsella, A. R., and Radman, M. (1978): Tumor promotor induces sister chromatid changes: Relevance to mechanisms of carcinogenesis. *Proc. Natl. Acad. Sci. USA*, 75:6419–6513.

14. Klein, G. (1981): The role of gene dosage and genetic transposition in carcinogenesis. *Nature*, 294:313–318.

15. Klein, G., and Lenoir, G. (1982): Translocation of specific chromosome fragments to Ig-locus carrying chromosomes in B-cell derived neoplasia:alternative model for permanent oncogene activation in tumorigenesis? *Adv. Cancer Res.*, 37:381–387.

16. Knudsson, J. A. G. (1971): Mutation and cancer: Statistical study of retinoblastoma. *Proc. Natl. Acad. Sci. USA*, 68:820–823.

17. Lenoir, G. M., Preudhomme, J. L., Bernheim, A., and Berger, R. (1982): Correlation between immunoglobulin light chains expression and variant translocation in Burkitts Lymphoma. *Nature*, 1998:474–476.

18. Malcom, S., Barton, P., Bentley, D. L., Ferguson-Smith, M. A., Murphy, C. S., and Rabbits, T. H. (1982): Localization of human immunoglobulin kappa chain variable region genes to the short arm of chromosome 2 by *in situ* hybridization. *Proc. Nat. Acad. Sci. (USA)*, 79:4957–4961.

19. McBride, O. W., Swan, D., Leder, P., Hieter, P., and Hollis, G. (1981): *Human Gene Mapping*, edited by V. I. Karger and S. Basel, New York *(in press)*.

20. McBride, O. W., Heiter, P. A., Hollis, G. F., Swan, D., Ohy, M. C., and Leder, P. (1982): Chromosomal location of human kappa and lambda immunoglobulin light chain constant region genes. *J. Exp. Med.*, 155:1480–1490.

21. Meo, T., Johnson, J., Beechey, C. V., Andrews, S. J., Peters, J., and Searle, A. G. (1980): Linkage analyses of murine immunoglobulin heavy chain and serum prealbumin genes establish their location on chromosome 12 proximal to the T(5;12) breakpoint in band 12F1. *Proc. Natl. Acad. Sci. USA*, 77:550–553.

22. Ohno, S., Babonits, M., Wiener, F., Spira, J., Klein, G., and Potter, M. (1979): Nonrandom chromosome changes involving the Ig gene carrying chromosomes 12 and 6 in pristane-induced mouse plasma-cytomas. *Cell*, 18:1001–1007.

23. Sandberg, A. A. (1980): *The Chromosomes in Human Cancer and Leukemias*. Elsevier North Holland, New York.

24. Spira, J., Wiener, F., Ohno, S., and Klein, G. (1979): Is trisomy cause or consequence of murine T cell leukemia development? Studies on Robertsonian translocation mice. *Proc. Natl. Acad. Sci. USA*, 76:6619–6621.

25. Spira, J., Babonits, M., Wiener, F., Ohno, S., Wirschubski, Z., Haran-Ghera, N., and Klein, G. (1980): Non-random chromosome changes in Thy-1 positive and Thy-1 negative lymphomas induced by 7,12-dimethyl-benzanthracene in SJL mice. *Cancer Res.*, 40:2609–2616.

26. Spira, J., Wiener, F., Babonits, M., Gamble, J., Miller, J., and Klein, G. (1981): The role of chromosome 15 in murine leukemogenesis. I. Contrasting behaviour of the tumor vs. the normal parent derived chromosomes no. 15 in somatic hybrids of varying tumorigenicity. *Int. J. Cancer*, 28:785–798.

27. Spira, J., Wiener, F., and Klein, G. (1983): Robertsonian translocation studies on the significance of chromosome 15 trisomy in murine T-cell leukemia. *Cancer Genetics and Cytogenetics*, 9:45–50.

28. Strong, L. C., Riccardi, V. M., Ferrel, R. E., and Sparkes, R. S. (1981): Familial retinoblastoma and chromosome 13 deletion transmitted via an insertional translocation. *Science*, 213:1501–1503.

29. Swan, D., DÈustachio, P., Leinwand, L., Seidman, J., Keithley, D., and Ruddle, F. H. (1979): Chromosomal assignment of the mouse kappa light chain genes. *Proc. Natl. Acad. Sci. USA*, 76:2735–2739.

30. Wiener, F., Ohno, S., Spira, J., Haran-Ghera, N., and Klein, G. (1978): Chromosome changes (trisomies 15 and 17) associated with tumor progression in leukemias induced by radiation leukemia virus. *J. Natl. Cancer Inst.*, 61:227–238.

31. Wiener, F., Ohno, S., Spira, J., Haran-Ghera, N., and Klein, G. (1978): Cytogenetic mapping of the trisomic segment of chromosome 15S in murine T-cell leukemia. *Nature*, 275:658–660.
32. Wiener, F., Spira, J., Ohno, S., Haran-Ghera, N., and Klein, G. (1978): Chromosome changes (trisomy 15) in murine T-cell leukemia induced by 7,12-dimethylbenz(a)antracene (DMBA). *Int. J. Cancer*, 22:447–453.
33. Wiener, F., Babonits, M., Spira, J., Klein, G., and Potter, M. (1980): Cytogenetic studies on IgA lambda producing murine plasmacytomas: regular occurrence of a T(12;15) translocation. *Somatic Cell Genetics*, 6:731–738.
34. Wiener, F., Babonits, M., Spira, J., Bregula, U., Klein, G., Merwin, R. M., Asofsky, R., Lynes, M., and Haghton, G. (1981): Chromosome 15 trisomy in spontaneous and carcinogen-induced lymphomas of B-cell origin. *Int. J. Cancer*, 27:51–58.
35. Zech, L., Haglund, U., Nilsson, K., and Klein, G. (1976): Characteristic chromosomal abnormalities in biopsies and lymphoid cellines from patients with Burkitt and Non-Burkitt lymphoma. *Int. J. Cancer*, 17:47–56.

Since submission of this chapter, a number of investigators have in detail described the transposition of C-myc in murine and human neoplasias of B-cell lineage. A mini-review of these has been published by Klein, G. (1983): In *Cell*, 32:311–315.

Biochemical Basis of Chemical Carcinogenesis,
edited by H. Greim, R. Jung, M. Kramer,
H. Marquardt, and F. Oesch.
Raven Press, New York © 1984.

Enzymology of DNA Repair: A Survey*

Heinz Walter Thielmann

German Cancer Research Centre, Institute of Biochemistry, D-6900 Heidelberg, Federal Republic of Germany

The rapid advances in the field of carcinogen-induced DNA repair have been influenced by two key discoveries:

1. the covalent binding of chemical carcinogens to DNA (7) together with the apparent relation between carcinogenic power and extent of carcinogen/DNA binding, and
2. the fundamental repair reactions following radiation damage to DNA in bacteria (4,49,64,104,122,130), which are proved to pertain to chemical DNA damage as well (57,120).

During the last two decades studies on the nature of carcinogen/DNA adducts have been greatly expanded; it was established that exposure of cells to carcinogens resulted in a variety of DNA modifications (80,95), some of which may be relatively harmless, e.g., phosphotriesters, others which drastically interfere with replicative DNA synthesis and the precision in the copying of DNA (75). Concomitant investigations of the DNA repair pathways revealed that several mechanisms exist, the purpose of which is the maintenance of the accurate genetic information. With the refinement of methods for analyzing DNA a steadily increasing number of chemically distinct DNA adducts were discovered. Thus a great discrepancy became apparent between the multitude of possible DNA modifications and the limited number of repair mechanisms which cope with these modifications. Indeed, with every new DNA adduct discovered the question could be asked: Is there an enzyme which would specifically recognize this type of damage? In many cases this question must be answered negatively, despite the considerable number of known enzymes recognizing structural DNA alterations.

Today there is little doubt that DNA damage accounts for most mutagenesis and, with exception, carcinogenesis. Mutagenesis and carcinogenesis may occur in cells in which DNA repair mechanisms are well functioning. Repair-deficient cells are more prone to neoplastic transformation than repair-proficient ones (77). It thus appears that mutagenesis and carcinogenesis have to be seen through a screen of

---

*Gratefully dedicated to Professor Dr. Otto Westphal on the occasion of his seventieth birthday.

avoidance reactions. Thus, it follows that repair enzymes and repair mechanisms are of primary importance for experimental and clinical cancer research.

Excellent reviews are available on photoreactivation (110,111), DNA repair in bacteria and mammalian cells (36,38), DNA repair enzymes in mammalian cells (28,29,30) and on DNA repair enzymes (66,67).

The purpose of this survey is to summarize carcinogen-induced DNA repair in mammalian cells, with special emphasis on the enzymes involved. However, it will be unavoidable to refer incidentally to *E. coli*, because our knowledge of repair mechanisms and enzymes in mammalian cells is limited. Insofar as the term DNA repair is indiscriminately used to describe a variety of cellular responses to DNA damage, such as excision repair, postreplication repair, adaptive repair, and SOS repair, it is misleading. In the case of SOS repair the DNA damage remains; cell lethality is decreased but mutations are increased (129). Postreplication repair is a bypass mechanism which facilitates tolerance of persisting DNA damage (37). Therefore, this survey will be restricted to the type of DNA repair which can be defined as removal of potentially mutagenic or lethal DNA damage. DNA is not a stable molecule. Potentially mutagenic alterations arise by spontaneous hydrolysis in nonreplicating DNA under physiological conditions. Lindahl and Nyberg (63) have estimated that the genome of a mammalian cell loses about 12,000 purine bases within a generation time, that is 20 hrs. These bases have to be substituted, otherwise the decreased information in the template would affect fidelity in replication. About 200 residues of both cytosine and adenine spontaneously deaminate per genome per day forming uracil and hypoxanthine. Again deamination, if unrepaired, is a mutagenic event. Within the life time of a nonreplicating human cell, e.g., a nerve cell, 300 million bases are spontaneously released from DNA, and that is about 2% of a total bases present. Given the thermodynamic instability of DNA, it is no wonder that compensating mechanisms have evolved which have the function of preserving the accurate genetic information.

DNA REPAIR MECHANISMS

Photoreactivation

Photoreactivation is a special case of repair, whereby a single enzyme, called photolyase, monomerizes ultraviolet-induced pyrimidine dimers in DNA *in situ* without any associated excision (99). Visible light is required for this process. The nature of the light-absorbing cofactor is still unknown. The enzyme was first detected in bacteria and lower eukaryotes, and more recently in mammalian cells (109). It was also shown that photoreactivation contributes to the removal of pyrimidine dimers in human skin and thus mediates biological recovery (110). However, despite extensive debate the actual contribution of this repair mechanism still remains unclear.

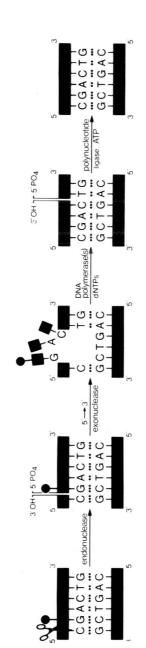

FIG. 1. Schematic representation of DNA excision repair. A chemically modified site on one of the DNA strands is recognized by an endonuclease; the enzyme incises on the 5′ side of the modified site. Starting from the nick, a 5′——3′ exonuclease liberates the modified base either as a mononucleotide (together with a limited number of unaltered nucleotides) or as a part of an oligonucleotide. In a coordinated fashion, the DNA strand being degraded is resynthesized by DNA polymerase. This enzyme uses the intact opposite strand as a template. Finally a ligase links the newly synthesized DNA strand to the old one.

DNA Excision Repair

The very important repair mechanisms have in common that they recognize chemically modified bases in DNA as being nonphysiologic, and replace them with normal ones. The basic principle of the excision repair mechanism is very simple (Fig. 1). The scheme as shown in Fig. 1 has almost become commonplace. Nevertheless, the enzymology behind it is not at all trivial. Within the excision repair cascade, one can discriminate between incision, excision, polymerization and ligation.

Incision

Incision can be achieved by classical endonucleases which cleave a sugar-phosphate bond close to the damaged base. The base is removed as a nucleotide and thus the mechanism is called *nucleotide excision repair*. Incision can also be catalyzed by DNA glycosylases which liberate incorrect or damaged bases as free bases, just by hydrolyzing the *N*-glycosyl bond. This step initiates what is called *base excision repair*. It leaves behind an apurinic site (AP site) which in turn is converted into a single-strand break by an apurinic endonuclease (AP endonuclease). One of the exciting recent developments in the field of DNA repair is the purification of a rapidly increasing number of DNA glycosylases. So far, at least seven (probably 9) distinct types of enzymes have been described and others may be discovered in the near future. All DNA glycosylases share the following properties: they are small proteins; they do not seem to have subunit structure; they do not require cofactors such as divalent cations, and they apparently act by simple hydrolytic cleavage of the *N*-glycosyl bond. Figure 2 shows a cabinet of molecular horrors in DNA, all of which can be recognized by respective DNA glycosylases.

DNA glycosylases were first purified from *E. coli*, but more recent investigations have shown that all but one of these enzymes have mammalian equivalents. Table 1 shows a juxtaposition of enzymes from prokaryotic and eukaryotic origin. Pyrimidine dimer-DNA glycosylase is the exception. It has been purified from *Micrococcus luteus* and phage T4-infected *E. coli* and as yet no counterpart in mammalian cells has been found (54). It acts by hydrolyzing the 5'-glycosyl bond of the dimer, thereby creating an apyrimidinic site which is then attacked by a concomitant apurinic (AP) endonuclease. AP endonuclease will be presented below in detail.

Each DNA glycosylase has a very strict substrate specificity, e.g., two different glycosylases are required to eliminate deaminated cytosine, and deaminated adenine and cannot replace each other. Furthermore, two distinct enzymes serve to remove

FIG. 2. Schematic representation of chemically modified DNA. The base residues are as follows (from top right downwards, shifting to the antiparallel strand and going upwards again): hypoxanthine; 3-methyladenine; cyclobutylcytosine dimer; 3,7-dimethylguanine (because of space limitations the diadduct is depicted which does not occur normally. It is meant to represent both 3-methylguanine and 7-methylguanine); a former 7-methylguanine, the imidazole ring of which opened spontaneously, resulting in a formamido-pyrimidine residue; ring-saturated glycol which is a common base lesion in DNA exposed to ionizing radiation; urea, the product of pyrimidine ring opening and fragmentation due to ionizing radiation.

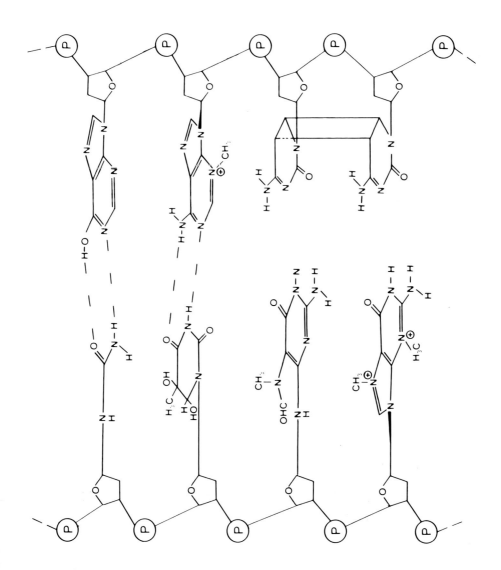

TABLE 1. *DNA glycosylases from prokaryotic and eukaryotic sources*

DNA glycosylase	Source	Molecular weight (dalton)	Reference no.
1. Uracil-DNA glycosylase	*E. coli*	25,000	65
	B. subtilis	24,000	18,19
	M. luteus	16,000	119
	HeLa cells	17–18,000	52
	KB cells	n.d.	1
	WI-38 human fibroblasts	n.d.	35
	Human lymphoblasts	30,000	13
2. Hypoxanthine-DNA glycosylase	*E. coli*	30,000	45
	Calf thymus	31,000	46
3. 3-Methyladenine-DNA glycosylase I	*E.coli*	20,000	96
	M. luteus	20,000	55,105
3-Methyladenine-DNA glycosylase II	*E. coli*	27,000	118
	Human lymphoblasts	34,000	6,44
4. 7-Methylguanine-DNA glycosylase	*E. coli, M. luteus*	n.d.	56
	Human lymphoblasts	n.d.	106
	Rodent liver	n.d.	78
5. Formamido-pyrimidine-DNA glycosylase	*E. coli*	30,000	15,16
	Rodent liver	n.d.	78
6. Urea-DNA glycosylase	*E. coli*	20–25,000	5
	Mammalian cells	n.d.	cited according to 67
7. Thymine glycol-DNA glycosylase	*E. coli* (endonuclease III)	27,000	21
	Mouse plasmocytoma cells ?	28,000	40,85,86
8. Pyrimidine dimer-DNA glycosylase	Bacteriophage T4	16,800	3,39,93
	M. luteus	18,000	21,32,33a

M. luteus, Micrococcus luteus; B. subtilis, Bacillus subtilis; n.d., not determined.

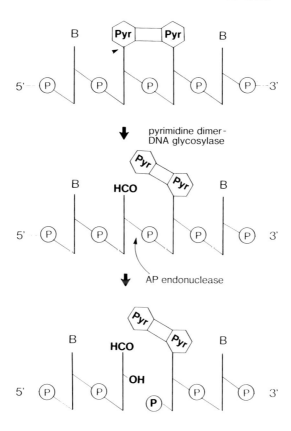

FIG. 3. Two-step incision of a DNA strand containing a pyrimidine dimer. (Data redrawn from ref. 39.)

7-methylguanine on the one hand and its derivative with an opened imidazole ring on the other.

Assuming that a DNA glycosylase has removed the chemically altered base and has left behind an AP site, how does the cell further proceed with this structural problem? The correction of AP sites is initiated by AP endonucleases that cleave the phosphodiester backbone next to them. These AP endonucleases were first discovered in *E. coli* and, originally it was assumed that their main substrates were AP sites resulting from spontaneous hydrolysis of DNA bases. However, with the detection of the various DNA glycosylases which generate the vast majority of AP sites, the increasing importance of the AP endonucleases was recognized (Fig. 3).

Table 2 summarizes the properties of 3 principle AP endonucleases from *E. coli* as well as those from *Hemophilus influenzae* and *Saccharomyces cerevisiae*. Some selected AP endonucleases from mammalian sources are shown in Table 3. In extensive studies Linn and collaborators showed that two classes of enzymes exist, e.g., in human fibroblasts, a type I AP endonuclease that cleaves at the 3′ side of

TABLE 2. *AP endonucleases from prokaryotes and lower eukaryotes*

Designation and source	M_r (kdal)	Cofactor	Substrate	Incision with regard to AP site	Class	Reaction products (termini)	Exonuclease activity	Reference no.
Endonuclease III *E.coli*	22–27	no cation	AP sites in ds, ds with thymine glycol residues	3'	I	3'OH deoxyribose 5'P nucleotide	no	94,31,126
Endonuclease IV *E. coli*	33	no cation; stimulated by 0.2–0.3 M NaCl	AP sites in ds (no ss, no ds)	5'	II	3'OH nucleotide 5'P deoxyribose	no	74
Endonuclease VI or exonuclease III *E. coli*	32	Mg^{2+} (20mM)	AP sites in ds (no ds, no ss, no alkylated sites)	5'	II	3'OH nucleotide 5'P deoxyribose	yes, exonuclease III (3'—5'), 3'-phosphatase	121,33,97
Hemophilus influenzae	30	Mg^{2+}, Mn^{2+} (5 mM)	AP sites in ds (no ds, probably no alkylated sites)	5'	II	3'OH nucleotide 5'P deoxyribose	yes, (3'—5'), 3'-phosphatase	17
Saccharomyces cerevisiae	31	stimulated by Mg^{2+} (3–6 mM)	AP sites in ds (no ds, no methylated sites)	n.d.	–	n.d.	no	116

ss, single-stranded DNA; ds, double-stranded DNA; n.d., not determined.

TABLE 3. *AP endonucleases from mammalian sources*

Source	M_r (kdal)	Cofactor	Substrate	Incision with regard to AP site	Class	Reaction products (termini)	Exonuclease activity	Reference no.
Calf thymus	32	stimulated by Mg^{2+} (3 mM), Mn^{2+} (0.3 mM)	AP sites in ds (no ss, no ds, no m⁷Gua residues)	3'	I	3'OH (deoxyribose ?) 5'P nucleotide	no	71,72,73
Human placenta	27–31 (multiple forms)	Mg^{2+} (3 mM)	AP sites in ds (no ss, no ds, no methylated sites)	5'	II	3'OH nucleotide 5'P deoxyribose	no	70
	37	Mg^{2+} (3mM) stimulated by Mn^{2+} (1 mM)	AP sites in ds	3' and 5'	I, II	3'OH deoxyribose 5' nucleotide 3'CH nucleotide 5'P deoxyribose	no	33b,105a
Mouse epidermal cells	31	stimulated by Mg^{2+} (3–10 mM)	AP sites in ds (no ss, no ds, no methylated sites)	n.d.	n.d.	n.d.	no	76
Human fibroblasts	(3.3 S)	stimulated by Mg^{2+} (10mM)	AP sites in ds	3'	II	3'OH deoxyribose 5'P nucleotide	no	53,69,84
Human fibroblasts	(2.8 S)	stimulated by Mg^{2+} (10mM)	AP sites in ds	5'	II	3'OH nucleotide 5'P deoxyribose	no	53,69,84
HeLa cells	32–41	Mg^{2+} (10 mM)	AP sites in ds and ss (no ss, no ds, no methylated sites)	5'	II	3'OH nucleotide 5'P deoxyribose	no	44a

ss, single-stranded DNA; ds, double-stranded DNA; n.d., not determined.

the AP site producing a 3′ deoxyribose and a 5′ phosphomonoester terminus, and a type II enzyme that cleaves at the 5′ side of the AP site to produce a nucleotide terminus with a free 3′ hydroxyl group and a 5′ phosphomonoester terminus (Fig. 4). Using DNA polymerase I from *E. coli* for defining the terminal structures at the cleavage site, it was demonstrated that termini produced by the type II enzymes were good primers for DNA synthesis. Termini produced by type I enzymes were ineffective (84) due to the fact that DNA polymerase I removes the 3′ terminal deoxyribose slowly. However, the type II AP endonuclease can activate the type I incision products: it removes the 3′ terminal deoxyribose residue as deoxyribose 5′ phosphate and thus paves the way for DNA polymerase (84). At present the question remains open whether or not there is a strict discrimination between type I and type II enzymes, as AP endonucleases capable of incising at either side of the AP site exist (33b,105).

AP endonuclease, type I, seems to be involved in the human genodermatosis Xeroderma pigmentosum (XP). Kuhnlein et al. (53) made the interesting observation that this enzyme is missing in fibroblasts from XP patients belonging to complementation group D. In general, XP patients show only dermatological manifestations of the disease. Group D patients (but also some patients of group A) exhibit in addition, neurologic abnormalities, e.g., low intelligence, hearing loss, ataxia. It

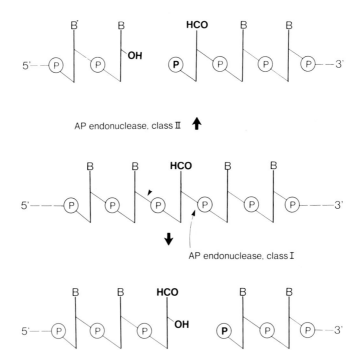

FIG. 4.   Incision by type I or type II AP endonuclease of a DNA strand containing an AP site. (Data redrawn from ref. 84.)

is easily understandable that there might be a causal link between these neurologic symptoms and the lack of AP endonuclease, type I. Considering the 300 million DNA bases which are spontaneously lost during the lifetime of a nerve cell, it appears that a deficiency in the repair of AP sites would lead to premature death of nerve cells and that in fact would explain the symptoms. However, through a comparison of 8 fibroblast lines from normal donors with 6 fibroblast lines from our XP group D patients [Mannheim Collection (25)], we have not been able to demonstrate decreased colony-forming ability or decreased unscheduled DNA synthesis in XP group D strains following treatment with methyl methanesulfonate, although great care was taken to accurately quantitate the biological end points (117).

Strand Incision at Pyrimidine Dimers

Very little is known about this topic with regard to mammalian cells. Waldstein et al. (123) partially purified a UV endonuclease from calf thymus. However, the specific activity achieved as a result of purification was low because the enzyme was very labile. The enzyme required Mg^{++} as cofactor, had a M_r (molecular weight) greater than 200,000 and incised DNA near pyrimidine dimers. These features essentially comprise our knowledge of UV endonucleases in mammalian cells. For further information we have to turn to E. coli. The E. coli UV endonuclease is a multiprotein complex consisting of 3 components, the products of the uvr genes A, B, and C (102). These subunits do not show independent activity. They can only catalyze cleavage as a complex including Mg^{++} and ATP (103). The complex has a broad substrate specificity, as it recognizes a variety of DNA lesions (in addition to pyrimidine dimers) caused by bulky carcinogens such as N-acetoxy-2-acetyl aminofluorene, 7-bromomethylbenz(a)anthracene (114), K-region epoxides of polycyclic aromatic hydrocarbons (115) etc., so it might be sensitive towards helix distortions. The uvrA gene product has been purified to homogeneity; its M_r is 114,000, it possesses DNA-dependent ATPase activity and binds to double-stranded DNA only in the presence of Mg^{++} (102,103). The uvrB and C genes have been cloned and the protein products analyzed: They have molecular weights of 84,000 and 68,000, respectively (100,131). Figure 5 illustrates how DNA incision near pyrimidine dimers could occur: The uvrA subunit could recognize the lesion first and bind; the uvrB and C proteins could then interact with the uvrA subunit to form the incision complex. After cleavage the uvrC subunit would prevent the nick from being sealed before the dimer is excised. The equivalents of these subunits have not been isolated in a eukaryote, and moreover, the enzymology of incision near pyrimidine dimers in mammalian cells is probably by far more complicated than in E. coli. In this context it is important to recall that XP has at least 7 subforms, called complementation groups. Probably all of them are defective at the level of incision. Recently an eighth complementation group, which is also incapable of incising dimer-containing DNA, has been discovered (25). If the complementation groups represent defective genes like uvrA, B, or C, one could postulate that

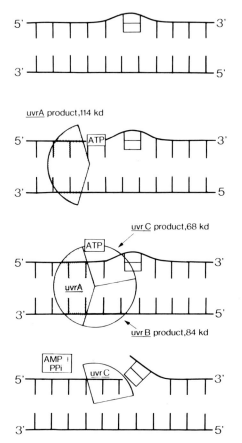

FIG. 5. Sequence of steps possibly involved in the incision at a pyrimidine dimer by *E. coli* UV endonuclease (*uvrABC* endonuclease). The size of the subunits reflects their M$_r$.

the functional incising complex in mammalian cells is composed of 7 or even 8 subunits. This postulate, however, does not imply that the incision defect in XP is restricted to a UV endonuclease, as the defect could be due to steps which precede phosphodiester bond cleavage.

Excision

Unlike the *E. coli* DNA polymerases, the mammalian DNA polymerases α and β lack associated exonuclease activities (see Table 5). An exception is polymerase δ, but this enzyme has only 3'—5' proof-reading activity (59). Therefore, excision must be performed by independent exonucleases. However, it would be difficult to understand that excision and repolymerization would be entirely uncoordinated processes. Mammalian cells contain exonucleases capable of excision whether the damage is on the 5' terminus or the 3' terminus of the nick (Fig. 6, see also Table 4). Damage on the 5' terminus is excisable by the 5'—3' directed exonucleases such as DNase IV, DNase VIII and correxonuclease (the latter enzyme being bidirectional). Damage on the 3' terminus of the nick can be excised by 3'—5' directed exonucleases, mainly DNase VII and correxonuclease (Fig. 6). A compilation of exonucleases which might contribute to excision of DNA damage is given in Table 4. In addition, a few characteristic examples from Table 4 will further be discussed: DNase IV is a representative of the group of exonucleases that degrade duplex DNA in the 5'—3' direction. The enzyme was first isolated by Lindahl (60). It has a M_r of 42,000, requires Mg^{++} and liberates pyrimidine dimers from double-stranded UV-irradiated DNA as oligonucleotides, 5 to 8 residues in length. This enzyme has a striking resemblence to the 5'—3' exonucleolytic activity of DNA polymerase I from *E. coli*. DNase VII is a representative of the group of enzymes which degrades single-stranded and duplex DNA in the 3'—5' direction. It is able to liberate monoadduct-type DNA damage (41). However, diadduct damage, such as pyrimidine dimers, is not excised. Human correxonuclease also has DNA repair capabilities, as it hydrolyzes UV-irradiated nicked duplex DNA in both directions (3'—5' as well as 5'—3'), liberating pyrimidine dimers as a part of oligonucleotides. Intact duplex DNA is not degraded.

DNA Polymerization

The DNA polymerase closely associated with DNA repair is polymerase β (see Table 5 and ref. cited therein). However, polymerase α was also shown to contribute to repair synthesis elicited by UV irradiation and alkylating agents (81). This

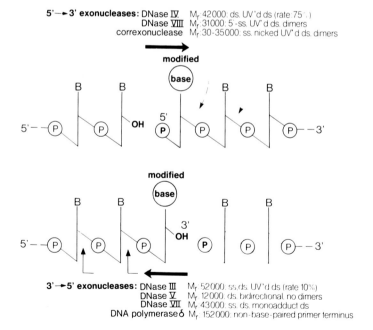

FIG. 6. Degradation of carcinogen-modified DNA strand by 5'——3' or 3'——5' directed exonucleases. For further details, see Table 4.

TABLE 4. *Mammalian exonucleases*

Exonuclease	Source	M_r (kdal)	Cofactor	Substrate	Direction of hydrolysis	Reaction products	Reference no.
DNase III	rabbit bone marrow, liver, spleen (cell nuclei)	52	Mg²⁺ (4mM) or Mn²⁺ (2 mM)	ss: 3'OH 3'P (rate 50%) ds: (rate 25%) UV'd ds (rate 4%)	3'——5'	5'-dNMPs and 5'-dinucleotides dimers as parts of oligornucleotides 3-4 residues long	60 62
DNase IV	rabbit lung (cell nuclei)	42	Mg²⁺ (3 mM)	ds: nicked ds UV'd ds (rate 75%)	5'——3'	5'-dNMPs dimers as part of oligonucleotides 5-8 residues long	61, 62
DNase V (copurifies with DNA polymerase β)	Novikoff hepatoma	12	Mg²⁺ (5-10 mM) or Mn²⁺ or Co²⁺	ds: OH or P terminus UV'd ds nicked UV'd ds	3'——5' 5'——3' bidirectional	5'-dNMPs no dimers n.d.	83
DNase VI	human cell line	50	Mg²⁺ (0.5-2 mM)	ss superhelical ds (partially unmatched areas) no ds no nicked ds no UV'd ds	n.d.	5'P-oligonucleotides nicked circular ds	89

Enzyme	Source		Metal (conc.)	Substrate	Direction	Products	Ref.
DNase VII	human placenta	43	Mg²⁺ (1 mM)	ss: 3'OH 3'P nicked ds (3'OH,5'P) monoadduct ds UV'd ds	$3' \longrightarrow 5'$	5'dNMPs monoadduct 5'-dNMPs no dimers	41
DNase VIII		31		ss: 5'P ds: 5'P UV'd ds	$5' \longrightarrow 3'$	dimers as part of 5'-oligonucleotides (gaps 10 dNMPs long)	cited according to 34
Correxonuclease (similar to exonuclease VII of E.coli)	human placenta		Mg²⁺ (1 mM)	ss: 3' or 5' P OH or P no ds no UV'd unnicked ds nicked ds (DNase I)	$3' \longrightarrow 5'$ $5' \longrightarrow 3'$ bidirectional	5'-P oligonucleotides, 4 residues long gaps 30—40 nucleotides long, dimers	23
DNA polymeraseδ	rabbit bone marrow calf thymus	152	Mn²⁺ (0.2 mM)	nicked UV'd ds ds with mismatched primer terminus	$3' \longrightarrow 5'$	5'-dNMPs	58,59

ss, single-stranded DNA; ds, double-stranded DNA; UV'd ds, UV-irradiated double-stranded DNA; n.d., not determined.

TABLE 5. *Mammalian DNA polymerases*

DNA polymerase	α	β	γ	δ
Subcellular location	nucleus	nucleus	mitochondria, nucleus	n.d.
M_r (kdal)	140	43	150	152
Subunits	75;65	none	n.d.	49;60
Function	replication	repair	replication of mtDNA	replication
Preferred primer template	duplex DNA with gaps 40–60 nucleotides long (gaps are not filled completely)	duplex DNA with base-paired 3′OH terminus and gaps 10 nucleotides long (gaps are filled completely)	mtDNA, ribohomopolymers	poly (dA-dT), non-base paired primer terminus, ssDNA
		nicked duplex DNA (15 dNMPs at each nick under strand displacement)		
Exonuclease	none	none	none	3′——5′ (proof-reading activity)
Cofactor	Mg^{2+}	Mg^{2+} Mn^{2+} (rate 20%)	Mg^{2+}	Mn^{2+}
pI	acidic	basic	acidic	acidic
Inhibitors:				
N-ethylmaleimide	+++	+	++	++++
aphidicolin	+++	–	–	++
arabinosyl NTPs	+++	+	+	+++
2′–3′-dideoxy NTPs	+	+++	+++	+
Source	calf thymus, human, murine, hamster cells	calf thymus, KB cells	HeLa cells, human tissue, calf thymus	rabbit bone marrow, calf thymus
Reference no.	2, 26, 27, 42, 51, 88, 128, 132; see also 14	127, 11, 12, 125, 51	50,132	8, 58, 59

ss DNA, single-stranded DNA; n.d. not determined; pI, isoelectric point.

observation suggests that it might be the nature of the DNA damage that determines the involvement of a particular DNA polymerase in the repair process. Polymerase β is a remarkably small enzyme with a M_r of around 43,000 dalton (51). The preferred template-primer is DNA with gaps about 10 nucleotides long with a base-paired 3'-hydroxyl primer-terminus. The enzyme can also use nicked duplex DNA to perform a limited DNA synthesis, producing DNA stretches of 15 nucleotides at each nick, under strand displacement (51). These features make polymerase β the appropriate enzyme for repair polymerization.

Ligation

Mammalian cells contain at least two antigenically distinct ligases. Ligase I is the dominant form in proliferating cells. Ligase II is the principal activity in resting cells (43, 113 and ref. cited there). Ligase II, $M_r = 85,000$, is most probably the enzyme related to DNA repair. Activation of the 5'-phosphate terminus occurs by adenylyl transfer just as in prokaryotic ligases. By way of a three-step mechanism the 5'-phosphoryl terminus is covalently linked to a 3'-hydroxyl terminus and thus with this ligation, damaged DNA is once again restored to its original state.

Adaptive Response

The adaptive response, an inducible repair of alkylated DNA, should be mentioned. The mechanism, first discovered in *E. coli*, is quite unusual and it seems to occur in mammalian cells as well.

In 1977 Samson and Cairns (98) observed that continuous exposure of *E. coli* to low doses of *N*-methyl-*N*'-nitro-*N*-nitrosoguanidine caused resistance to the mutagenic and killing effects of alkylating agents. This adaptation was found to be largely due to an induced repair function which removed O^6-methylguanine from DNA. The activity has been purified and identified as a methyltransferase with a M_r of 18,000 (22,68,87): the enzyme transfers the methyl group [or ethyl group (101)] from O^6 of alkylguanine to a cysteine residue of its own. It reacts only once and inactivates itself upon methylation. A DNA glycosylase ($M_r = 27,000$) with a strikingly broad substrate specificity is induced simultaneously with the transferase. It recognizes 3-methyladenine, 3-methylguanine, and 7-methylguanine (48). The induced adaptive mechanism as a whole is very effective because it lowers the mutation rate of adapted bacteria by a factor of 6000 as compared to that of unadapted bacteria (9,10).

At present the evidence for adaptive repair in mammalian cells analogous to that in *E. coli* is subject to some controversy. Certainly O^6-alkylguanine can be actively removed from DNA of mammalian cells (90,92). Moreover, this DNA lesion is removed at a faster rate from rat liver cells after chronic treatment with dimethylnitrosamine than after a single treatment with a challenging dose (82). However, it has also been reported that noncarcinogenic substances such as thioacetamide, or noncarcinogenic treatment, e.g., partial hepatectomy, enhance the removal of O^6-methylguanine from rat liver DNA (91). From this and other evidence (112) it was concluded that the enhancement of alkyl transferase activity was due to cell proliferation rather than to the presence of specific DNA lesions.

Karran et al. (47) were not able to associate biological end points (such as cell survival, decrease in mutation induction) with any increase in DNA repair (as quantitated by O^6-methylguanine transferase or 3-methyladenine-DNA glycosylase) in human fibroblasts. Their data led them to infer that adaptation does not occur in human fibroblasts.

Mehta et al. (79) characterized a chromatin factor from rat liver which catalyzes the transfer of the ethyl group of O^6-ethylguanine from DNA to a cysteine residue of an acceptor protein. A similar transferase has been isolated from the human lymphoid cell line, Raji, and its M_r was found to be 20,000 (68).

XP fibroblast lines may be either proficient (mex$^+$) or deficient (mex$^-$) in removing O^6-methylguanine from their DNA (107). The same holds true for human tumor cell lines and for SV40-transformed strains (20). At present it has to remain open whether the mex phenotype is due to a genetic or epigenetic mechanism. However, Waldstein et al. (124) showed that mex proficiency or deficiency does not arise from differences in the constitutive levels of O^6-methyltransferase activity but from the ability to replenish acceptor protein (i.e. transferase) once it is used up by suicide inactivation. It thus appears that mex$^-$ strains are sensitive to the killing effect of alkylating agents because they cannot perform adaptive resynthesis of alkyltransferase. The sensitivity of mex$^-$ tumor cell lines to alkylating antineoplastic drugs (provided they bind to O^6 of guanine) might be therapeutically exploitable, as mex$^-$ tumors could be successfully attacked with appropriate drugs (24). Hence there is evidence that repair studies and cancer therapy may be more closely related than one could anticipate.

ACKNOWLEDGMENT

I wish to express my thanks to Ms. J. Faberman for reading the manuscript and making helpful suggestions.

REFERENCES

1. Anderson, C. T. M., and Friedberg, E. C. (1980): The presence of nuclear and mitochondrial uracil-DNA glycosylase in extracts of human KB cells. *Nucleic Acids Res.*, 8:875–889.
2. Bollum, F. J. (1975): Mammalian DNA polymerases. *Prog. Nucleic Acid Res. Mol. Biol.*, 15:109–144.
3. Bonura, T., Radany, E. H., McMillan, S., Love, J. D., Schultz, R. A., Edenberg, H. J., and Friedberg, E. C. (1982): Pyrimidine dimer-DNA glycosylases: studies on bacteriophage T4-infected and on uninfected *Escherichia coli*. *Biochimie*, 64:643–654.
4. Boyce, R. P., Howard-Flanders, P. (1964): Release of ultraviolet light-induced thymine dimers from DNA in E. coli K-12. *Proc. Natl. Acad. Sci. USA*, 51:293–300.
5. Breimer, L., and Lindahl, T. (1980): A DNA glycosylase from *Escherichia coli* that releases free urea from a polydeoxyribonucleotide containing fragments of base residues. *Nucleic Acids Res.*, 8:6199–6211.
6. Brent, T. P. (1979): Partial purification and characterization of a human 3-methyladenine-DNA glycosylase. *Biochemistry*, 18:911–916.
7. Brookes, P., and Lawley, P. D. (1964): Evidence for the binding of polynuclear aromatic hydro-

carbons to the nucleic acids of mouse skin: relation between carcinogenic power of hydrocarbons and their binding to deoxyribonucleic acid. *Nature*, 202:781–784.

8. Byrnes, J. J., Downey, K. M., Black, V. L., and So, A. G. (1976): A new mammalian DNA polymerase with 3' to 5' exonuclease activity: DNA polymerase δ. *Biochemistry*, 15:2817–2823.

9. Cairns, J. (1980): Efficiency of the adaptive response of *Escherichia coli* to alkylating agents. *Nature*, 286:176–178.

10. Cairns, J., Robins, P., Sedgwick, B., and Talmud, P. (1981): The inducible repair of alkylated DNA. *Prog. Nucleic Acid Res. Mol. Biol.*, 26:237–244.

11. Chang, L. M. S., and Bollum, F. J. (1971): Low molecular weight deoxyribonucleic acid polymerase in mammalian cells. *J. Biol. Chem.*, 246:5835–5837.

12. Chang, L. M. S. (1973): Low molecular weight deoxyribonucleic acid polymerase from calf thymus chromatin. *J. Biol. Chem.*, 248:3789–3795.

13. Caradonna, S. J., and Cheng, Y.-C. (1980): Uracil DNA-glycosylase. *J. Biol. Chem.*, 255:2293–2300.

14. Chen, Y.-C., Bohn, E. W., Planck, S. R., and Wilson, S. H. (1979): Mouse DNA polymerase α. *J. Biol. Chem.*, 254:11678–11687.

15. Chetsanga, C. J., and Lindahl, T. (1979): Release of 7-methylguanine residues whose imidazole rings have been opened from damaged DNA by a DNA glycosylase from *Escherichia coli*. *Nucleic Acids Res.*, 6:3673–3683.

16. Chetsanga, C. J., Lozon, M., Makaroff, C., and Savage, L. (1981): Purification and characterization of *Escherichia coli* formamidopyrimidine-DNA glycosylase that excises damaged 7-methylguanine from deoxyribonucleic acid. *Biochemistry*, 20:5201–5207.

17. Clements, J. E., Rogers, S. G., and Weiss, B. (1978): A DNase for apurinic/apyrimidinic sites associated with exonuclease III of *hemophilus influenzae*. *J. Biol. Chem.*, 253:2990–2999.

18. Cone, R., Duncan, J., Hamilton, L., and Friedberg, E. C. (1977): Partial purification and characterization of a uracil DNA N-glycosidase from *Bacillus subtilis*. *Biochemistry*, 16:3194–3201.

19. Cone, R., Bonura, T., and Friedberg, E. C. (1980): Inhibitor of uracil-DNA glycosylase induced by bacteriophage PBS2. *J. Biol. Chem.*, 255:10354–10358.

20. Day III, R. S., Ziolkowski, C. H. J., Scudiero, D. A., Meyer, S. A., Lubiniecki, A. S., Girardi, A. J., Galloway, S. M., and Bynum, G. D. (1980): Defective repair of alkylated DNA by human tumour and SV40-transformed human cell strains. *Nature*, 288:724–727.

21. Demple, B., and Linn, S. (1980): DNA N-glycosylases and UV repair. *Nature*, 287:203–208.

22. Demple, B., Jacobsson, A., Olsson, M., Robins, P., and Lindahl, T. (1982): Repair of alkylated DNA in *Escherichia coli*. *J. Biol. Chem.*, 257:13776–13780.

23. Doniger, J., and Grossman, L. (1976): Human correxonuclease. *J. Biol. Chem.*, 251:4579–4587.

24. Erickson, L. C., Laurent, G., Sharkey, N. A., and Kohn, K. W. (1980): DNA cross-linking and monoadduct repair in nitrosourea-treated human tumour cells. *Nature*, 288:727–729.

25. Fischer, E., Thielmann, H. W., Neundörfer, B., Rentsch, F. J., Edler, L., and Jung, E. G. (1982): Xeroderma pigmentosum patients from Germany: clinical symptoms and DNA repair characteristics. *Arch. Dermatol. Res.*, 274:229–247.

26. Fisher, P. A., and Korn, D. (1979): Enzymological characterization of KB cell DNA polymerase-α. *J. Biol. Chem.*, 254:11040–11046.

27. Fisher, P. A., and Korn, D. (1979): Enzymological characterization of DNA polymerase-α: basic catalytic properties, processivity and gap utilization of the homogeneous enzyme from human KB cells. *J. Biol. Chem.*, 54:6136–6137.

28. Friedberg, E. C., Cook, K. H., Duncan, J., and Mortelmans, K. (1977): DNA repair enzymes in mammalian cells. In: *Photochemical and Photobiological Reviews, Vol. 2*, edited by K. L. Smith, pp. 263–322. Plenum Press, New York, London.

29. Friedberg, E. C., Anderson, C. T. M., Bonura, T., Cone, R., Radany, E. H., and Reynolds, R. J. (1981): Recent developments in the enzymology of excision repair of DNA. *Prog. Nucleic Acid Res. Mol. Biol.*, 26:197–215.

30. Friedberg, E. C., Bonura, T., Love, J. D., McMillan, S., Radany, E. H., and Schultz, R. A. (1981): The repair of DNA damage: recent developments and new insights. *J. Supramol. Struct. Cell Biol.*, 16:91–103.

31. Gates III, F. T., and Linn, S. (1977): Endonuclease from *Escherichia coli* that acts specifically upon duplex DNA damaged by ultraviolet light, osmium tetroxide, acid, or X-rays. *J. Biol. Chem.*, 252:2802–2807.

32. Gordon, L. K., and Hasetine, W. A. (1980): Comparison of the cleavage of pyrimidine dimers

by the bacteriophage T4 and *Micrococcus luteus* UV-specific endonuclease. *J. Biol. Chem.*, 255:12047–12050.

33. Gossard, F., and Verly, W. G. (1978): Properties of the main endonuclease specific for apurinic sites of *Escherichia coli* (endonuclease VI). *Eur. J. Biochem.*, 82:321–332.

33a. Grafstrom, R. H., Park, L., and Grossman, L. (1982): Enzymatic repair of pyrimidine dimer-containing DNA. *J. Biol. Chem.*, 257:13465–13474.

33b. Grafstrom, R. H., Shaper, N. L., and Grossman, L. (1982): Human placental apurinic/apyrimidinic endonuclease. *J. Biol. Chem.*, 257:13459–13464.

34. Grossman, L. (1981): Enzymes involved in the repair of damaged DNA. *Arch. Biochem. Biophys.*, 211:511–522.

35. Gupta, P. K., and Sirover, M. A. (1981): Stimulation of the nuclear uracil DNA glycoslyase in proliferating human fibroblasts. *Cancer Res.*, 41:3133–3136.

36. Hanawalt, P. C., Cooper, P. K., Ganesan, A. K., and Smith, C. A. (1979): DNA repair in bacteria and mammalian cells. *Ann. Rev. Biochem.*, 48:783–836.

37. Hanawalt, P. C., Cooper, P. K., and Smith, C. A. (1981): Repair replication schemes in bacteria and human cells. *Prog. Nucleic Acid Res. Mol. Biol.*, 26:181–196.

38. Hanawalt, P. C., Cooper, P. K., Ganesan, A. K., Lloyd, R. S., Smith, C. A., and Zolan, M. E. (1982): Repair responses to DNA damage: Enzymatic pathways in *E. coli* and human cells. *J. Cell. Biochem.*, 18:271–283.

39. Haseltine, W. A., Gordon, L. K., and Lindan, C. P. (1980): Cleavage of pyrimidine dimers in specific DNA sequences by a pyrimidine dimer DNA-glycosylase of *M. luteus*. *Nature*, 285:634–640.

40. Helland, D., Nes, I. F., and Kleppe, K. (1982): Mammalian DNA-repair endonuclease acts only on supercoiled DNA. *FEBS Letters*, 142:121–124.

41. Hollis, G. F., and Grossman, L. (1981): Purification and characterization of DNase VII, a 3′→5′-directed exonuclease from human placenta. *J. Biol. Chem.*, 256:8074–8079.

42. Holmes, A. M., Hesslewood, I. P., and Johnston, I. R. (1974): The occurrence of multiple activities in the high-molecular-weight DNA polymerase fraction of mammalian tissues. *Eur. J. Biochem.*, 43:487–499.

43. Inoue, N., and Kato, T. (1980): Nuclear DNA ligase and its action on chromatin DNA in neuronal, glial, and liver nuclei isolated from adult guinea pig. *J. Neurochem.*, 34:1574–1583.

44. Ishiwata, K., and Oikawa, A. (1979): Actions of human DNA glycosylases on uracil-containing DNA, methylated DNA and their reconstituted chromatins. *Biochim. Biophys. Acta*, 563:375–384.

44a. Kane, C. M., and Linn, S. (1981): Purification and characterization of an apurinic/apyrimidinic endonuclease from HeLa cells. *J. Biol. Chem.*, 256:3405–3414.

45. Karran, P., and Lindahl, T. (1978): Enzymatic excision of free hypoxanthin from polydeoxynucleotides and DNA containing deoxyinosine monophosphate residues. *J. Biol. Chem.*, 253:5877–5879.

46. Karran, P., and Lindahl, T. (1980): Hypoxanthine in deoxyribonucleic acid: generation by heat-induced hydrolysis of adenine residues and release in free form by a deoxyribonucleic acid glycosylase from calf thymus. *Biochemistry*, 19:6005–6011.

47. Karran, P., Arlett, C. F., and Broughton, B. C. (1982): An adaptive response to the cytotoxic effects of *N*-methyl-*N*-nitrosourea is apparently absent in normal human fibroblasts. *Biochimie*, 64:717–721.

48. Karran, P., Hjelmgren, T., and Lindahl, T. (1982): Induction of a DNA glycosylase for N-methylated purines is part of the adaptive response to alkylating agents. *Nature*, 296:770–772.

49. Kelner, A. (1949): Effect of visible light on the recovery of *streptomyces griseus conidia* from ultraviolet irradiation injury. *Proc. Natl. Acad. Sci. USA*, 35:73–79.

50. Knopf, K.-W., Yamada, M., and Weissbach, A. (1976): HeLa cell DNA polymerase γ: further purification and properties of the enzyme. *Biochemistry*, 15:4540–4548.

51. Korn, D., Fisher, P. A., and Wang, T. S.-F. (1981): Mechanisms of catalysis of human DNA polymerase α and β. *Prog. Nucleic Acid Res. Mol. Biol.*, 26:63–81.

52. Krokan, H., and Wittwer, C. U. (1981): Uracil DNA-glycosylase from HeLa cells: general properties, substrate specificity and effect of uracil analogs. *Nucleic Acids Res.*, 9:2599–2613.

53. Kuhnlein, U., Lee, B., Penhoet, E. E., and Linn, S. (1978): Xeroderma pigmentosum fibroblasts of the D group lack an apurinic DNA endonuclease species with a low apparent K_m. *Nucleic Acids Res.*, 5:951–960.

54. La Belle, M., and Linn, S. (1982): In vivo excision of pyrimidine dimers is mediated by a DNA N-glycosylase in *Micrococcus luteus* but not in human fibroblasts. *Photochem. Photobiol.*, 36:319–324.
55. Laval, J. (1977): Two enzymes are required for strand incision in repair of alkylated DNA. *Nature*, 269:829–832.
56. Laval, J., Pierre, J., and Laval, F. (1981): Release of 7-methylguanine residues from alkylated DNA by extracts of *Micrococcus luteus* and *Escherichia coli*. *Proc. Natl. Acad Sci. USA*, 78:852–855.
57. Lawley, P. D., Orr, D. J., and Shah, S. A. (1971): Reaction of alkylating mutagens and carcinogens with nucleic acids: N-3 of guanine as a site of alkylation by *N*-methyl-*N*-nitrosourea and dimethyl sulphate. *Chem.-Biol. Interactions*, 4:431–434.
58. Lee, M. Y. W. T., Tan, C.-K., So, A. G., and Downey, K. M. (1980): Purification of deoxyribonucleic acid polymerase α from calf thymus: partial characterization of physical properties. *Biochemistry*, 19:2096–2101.
59. Lee, M. Y. W. T., Tan, C.-K., Downey, K. M., and So, A. C. (1981): Structural and functional properties of calf thymus DNA polymerase δ. *Prog. Nucleic Acid Res. Mol. Biol.*, 26:83–97.
60. Lindahl, T., Gally, J. A., Edelman, G. M. (1969): Properties of deoxyribonuclease III from mammalian tissues. *J. Biol. Chem.*, 244:5014–5019.
61. Lindahl, T. (1971): The action pattern of mammalian deoxyribonuclease IV. *Eur. J. Biochem.*, 18:415–421.
62. Lindahl, T. (1971a): Excision of pyrimidine dimers from ultraviolet-irradiated DNA by exonucleases from mammalian cells. *Eur. J. Biochem.*, 18:407–414.
63. Lindahl, T., and Nyberg, B. (1972): Rate of depurination of native deoxyribonucleic acid. *Biochemistry*, 11:3610–3618.
64. Lindahl, T. (1976): New class of enzymes acting on damaged DNA. *Nature*, 259:64–66.
65. Lindahl, T., Ljungquist, S., Siegert, W., Nyberg, B., and Sperens, B. (1977): DNA *N*-glycosidases. *J. Biol. Chem.*, 252:3286–3294.
66. Lindahl, T. (1979): DNA glycosylases, endonucleases for apurinic/apyrimidinic sites, and base excision repair. *Prog. Nucleic Acid Res. Mol. Biol.*, 22:135–193.
67. Lindahl, T. (1982): DNA repair enzymes. *Ann. Rev. Biochem.*, 51:61–87.
68. Lindahl, T., Karran, P., Demple, B., Sedgwick, B., and Harris, A. (1982): Inducible DNA repair enzymes involved in the adaptive response to alkylating agents. *Biochimie*, 64:581–583.
69. Linn, S., Demple, B., Mosbaugh, D. W., Warner, H. R., Deutsch, W. A. (1981): Enzymatic studies of base excision repair in cultured human fibroblasts and in *Escherichia coli*. In: *Chromosome Damage and Repair*, edited by E. Seeberg and K. Kleppe, pp. 97–112. Plenum Press, New York, London.
70. Linsley, W. S., Penhoet, E. E., Linn, S. (1977): Human endonuclease specific for apurinicic/apyrimidinic sites in DNA. *J. Biol. Chem.*, 252:1235–1242.
71. Ljungquist, S., and Lindahl, T. (1974): A mammalian endonuclease specific for apurinic sites in double-stranded deoxyribonucleic acid. *J. Biol. Chem.*, 249:1530–1535.
72. Ljungquist, S., Andersson, A., and Lindahl, T. (1974): A mammalian endonuclease specific for apurinic sites in double-stranded deoxyribonucleic acid. *J. Biol. Chem.*, 249:1536–1540.
73. Ljungquist, S., Nyberg, B., and Lindahl, T. (1975): Mammalian DNA endonuclease acting at apurinic sites: absence of associated exonuclease activity. *FEBS Letters*, 57:169–171.
74. Ljungquist, S. (1977): A new endonuclease from *Escherichia coli* acting at apurinic sites in DNA. *J. Biol. Chem.*, 252:2808–2814.
75. Loeb, L. A., and Kunkel, T. A. (1982): Fidelity of DNA synthesis. *Ann. Rev. Biochem.*, 51:429–457.
76. Ludwig, G., and Thielmann, H. W. (1979): Apurinic acid endonuclease activity from mouse epidermal cells. *Nucleic Acids Res.*, 6:2901–2917.
77. Maher, V. M., Rowan, L. A., Silinskas, C., Kateley, S. A., and McCormick, J. J. (1982): Frequency of UV-induced neoplastic transformation of diploid human fibroblasts is higher in xeroderma pigmentosum cells than in normal cells. *Proc. Natl. Acad. Sci. USA*, 79:2613–2617.
78. Margison, G. P., and Pegg, A. E. (1981): Enzymatic release of 7-methylguanine from methylated DNA by rodent liver extracts. *Proc. Natl. Acad. Sci. USA*, 78:861–865.
79. Mehta, J. R., Ludlum, D. B., Renard, A., and Verly, W. G. (1981): Repair of O⁶-ethylguanine in DNA by a chromatin fraction from rat liver: transfer of the ethyl group to an acceptor protein. *Proc. Natl. Acad. Sci. USA*, 78:6766–6770.

80. Miller, E. C. (1978): Some current perspectives on chemical carcinogenesis in humans and experimental animals: presidential address. *Cancer Res.*, 38:1479–1496.
81. Miller, M. R., and Chinault, D. N. (1982): The roles of DNA polymerase α, β, and γ in DNA repair synthesis induced in hamster and human cells by different DNA damaging agents. *J. Biol. Chem.*, 257:10204–10209.
82. Montesano, R., Brésil, H., Planche-Martel, G., Margison, G. P., and Pegg, A. E. (1980): Effect of chronic treatment of rats with dimethylnitrosamine on the removal of O⁶-methylguanine from DNA. *Cancer Res.*, 40:452–458.
83. Mosbaugh, D. W., and Meyer, R. R. (1980): Interaction of mammalian deoxyribonuclease V, a double strand 3'→5' and 5'→3' exonuclease with deoxyribonucleic acid polymerase-β from the Novikoff Hepatoma. *J. Biol. Chem.*, 255:10239–10247.
84. Mosbaugh, D. W., and Linn, S. (1982): Characterization of the action of *Escherichia coli* DNA polymerase I at incisions produced by repair endodeoxyribonucleases. *J. Biol. Chem.*, 257:575–583.
85. Nes, I. F. (1980): Purification and properties of a mouse-cell DNA-repair endonuclease, which recognizes lesions in DNA induced by ultraviolet light, depuriniation, γ-rays and OsO₄ treatment. *Eur. J. Biochem.*, 112:161–168.
86. Nes, I. F. (1980): Purification and characterization of an endonuclease specific for apurinic sites in DNA from a permanently established mouse plasmocytoma cell line. *Nucleic Acids Res.*, 8:1575–1589.
87. Olsson, M., and Lindahl, T. (1980): Repair of alkylated DNA in *Escherichia coli. J. Biol. Chem.*, 255:10569–10571.
88. Pedrali-Noy, G., and Spadari, S. (1980): Aphidicolin allows a rapid and simple evaluation of DNA-repair synthesis in damaged human cells. *Mutat. Res.*, 70β389–394.
89. Pedrini, A. M., Ranzani, G., Pedrali-Noy, G., Spadari, S., and Falaschi, A. (1976): A novel endonuclease of human cells specific for single-stranded DNA. *Eur. J. Biochem.*, 70:275–283.
90. Pegg, A. E. (1978): Enzymatic removal of O⁶-methylguanine from DNA by mammalian cell extracts. *Biochem. Biophys. Res. Comm.*, 84:166–173.
91. Pegg, A. E., and Perry, W. (1981): Stimulation of transfer of methyl groups from O⁶-methylguanine in DNA to protein by rat liver extracts in response to hepatotoxins. *Carcinogenesis*, 2:1195–1200.
92. Pegg, A. E., Roberfroid, M., Bahr von, C., Foote, R. S., Mitra, S., Bresil, H., Likhachev, A., and Montesano, R. (1982): Removal of O⁶-methylguanine from DNA by human liver fractions. *Proc. Natl. Acad. Sci. USA*, 79:5162–5165.
93. Radany, E. H., and Friedberg, E. C. (1980): A pyrimidine dimer-DNA glycosylase activity associated with the υ gene product of bacteriophage T4. *Nature*, 286:182–184.
94. Radman, M. (1976): An endonuclease from *Escherichia coli* that introduces single polynucleotide chain scissions in ultraviolet-irradiated DNA. *J. Biol. Chem.*, 251:1438–1445.
95. Rajalakshmi, S., Rao, P. M., and Sarma, D. S. R. (1982): Chemical carcinogenesis: interactions of carcinogens with nucleic acids. In: *Cancer—A Comprehensive Treatise, Vol. 1, Etiology—Chemical and Physical Carcinogenesis*, edited by Becker, F. F., pp. 335–386. Plenum Press, New York.
96. Riazuddin, S., and Lindahl, T. (1978): Properties of 3-methyladenine-DNA glycosylase from *Escherichia coli. Biochemistry*, 17:2110–2118.
97. Rogers, S. G., and Weiss, B. (1980): Exonuclease III of *Escherichia coli* K-12, an AP endonuclease. *Methods Enzymol.*, 65:201–211.
98. Samson, L., and Cairns, J. (1977): A new pathway for DNA repair in *Escherichia coli. Nature*, 267:281–283.
99. Sancar, A., and Rupert, C. S. (1978): Correction of the map location for the *phr* gene in *Escherichia coli* K-12. *Mutat. Res.*, 51:139–143.
100. Sancar, A., Clarke, N. D., Griswold, J., Kennedy, W. J., and Rupp, W. D. (1981): Identification of the *uvrB* gene product. *J. Mol. Biol.*, 148:63–76.
101. Sedgwick, B., and Lindahl, T. (1982): A common mechanism for repair of O⁶-methylguanine and O⁶-ethylguanine in DNA. *J. Mol. Biol.*, 154:169–175.
102. Seeberg, E. (1978): Reconstitution of an *Escherichia coli* repair endonuclease activity from the separated *urvA*⁺ and *urvB*⁺/*uvrC*⁺ gene products. *Proc. Natl. Acad. Sci. USA*, 75:2569–2573.
103. Seeberg, E. (1981): Multiprotein interactions in strand cleavage of DNA damaged by UV and chemicals. *Prog. Nucleic Acid Res. Mol. Biol.*, 26:217–226.

104. Setlow, R. B., and Carrier, W. L. (1964): The disappearance of thymine dimers from DNA: an error-correcting mechanism. *Proc. Natl. Acad. Sci. USA*, 51:226–231.
105. Shackelton, J., Warren, W., and Roberts, J. J. (1979): The excision of *N*-methyl-*N*-nitrosourea-induced lesions from the DNA of chinese hamster cells as measured by the loss of sites sensitive to an enzyme extract that excises 3-methylpurines but not O⁶-methylguanine. *Eur. J. Biochem.*, 97:425–433.
106. Singer, B., and Brent, T. P. (1981): Human lymphoblasts contain DNA glycosylase activity excising N-3 and N-7 methyl and ethyl purines but not O⁶-alkylguanines or 1-alkyladenines. *Proc. Natl. Acad. Sci. USA*, 78:856–860.
107. Sklar, R., and Strauss, B. (1981): Removal of O⁶-methylguanine from DNA of normal and xeroderma pigmentosum derived lymphoblastoid lines. *Nature*, 289:417–419.
108. Söderhäll, S., and Lindahl, T. (1976): DNA ligases of eukaryotes. *FEBS Letters*, 67:1–8.
109. Sutherland, B. M., Runge, P., and Sutherland, J. C. (1974): DNA photoreactivating enzyme from placental mammals. Origin and characteristics. *Biochemistry*, 13:4710–4715.
110. Sutherland, B. M., Harber, L. C., and Kochevar, I. E. (1980): Pyrimidine dimer formation and repair in human skin. *Cancer Res.*, 40:3181–3185.
111. Sutherland, B. M. (1981): Photoreactivation. *BioScience*, 31:439–444.
112. Swenberg, J. A., Bedell, M. A., Billings, K. C., Umbenhauer, D. R., and Pegg, A. E. (1982): Cell-specific differences in O⁶-alkylaguanine DNA repair activity during continuous exposure to carcinogen. *Proc. Natl. Acad. Sci. USA*, 79:5499–5502.
113. Teraoka, H., and Tsukada, K. (1982): Eukaryotic DNA ligase. *J. Biol. Chem.*, 257:4758–4763.
114. Thielmann, H. W. (1976): Carcinogen-induced DNA repair in nucleotide-permeable *Escherichia coli* cells. *Eur. J. Biochem.*, 61:501–513.
115. Thielmann, H. W., and Gersbach, H. (1978): Carcinogen-induced DNA repair in nucleotide-permeable Escherichia coli cells. *Z. Krebsforsch.*, 92:157–172.
116. Thielmann, H. W., and Hess, U. (1981): Apurinic endonuclease from *Saccharomyces cerevisiae*. *Biochem. J.*, 195:407–417.
117. Thielmann, H. W., Popanda, O., and Edler, L. (1982): XP patients from Germany: correlation of colony-forming ability, unscheduled DNA synthesis and single-strand breaks after UV damage in xeroderma pigmentosum fibroblasts. *J. Cancer Res. Clin. Oncol.*, 104:263–286.
118. Thomas, L., Yang, C.-H., and Goldthwait, D. A. (1982): Two DNA glycosylases in *Escherichia coli* which release primarily 3-methyladenine. *Biochemistry*, 21:1162–1169.
119. Tomilin, N. V., Aprelikova, O. N., and Barenfeld, L. S. (1978): Enzymes from *Micrococcus luteus* involved in the initial steps of excision repair of spontaneous DNA lesions: uracil-DNA glycosidase and apurinic endonuclease. *Nucl. Acid. Res.*, 5:1413–1428.
120. Venitt, S., and Tarmy, E. M. (1972): The selective excision of arylalkylated products from the DNA of *Escherichia coli* treated with the carcinogen 7-bromomethylbenz(a)anthracene. *Biochim. Biophys. Acta*, 287:38–51.
121. Verly, W. G., and Rassart, E. (1975): Purification of *Escherichia coli* endonuclease specific for apurinic sites in DNA. *J. Biol. Chem.*, 250:8214–8219.
122. Wacker, A., Dellweg, H., and Jacherts, D. (1962): Thymin-Dimerisierung und Überlebensrate bei Bakterien. *J. Mol. Biol.*, 4:410–412.
123. Waldstein, E. A., Peller, S., and Setlow, R. B. (1979): UV-endonuclease from calf thymus with specificity toward pyrimidine dimers in DNA. *Proc. Natl. Acad. Sci. USA*, 76:3746–3750.
124. Waldstein, E. A., Cao, E.-H., and Setlow, R. B. (1982): Adaptive resynthesis of O⁶-methylguanine-accepting protein can explain the differences between mammalian cells proficient and deficient in methyl excision repair. *Proc. Natl. Acad. Sci. USA*, 79:5117–5121.
125. Wang, T. S.-F., Sedwick, W. D., and Korn, D. (1975): Nuclear deoxyribonucleic acid polymerase. *J. Biol. Chem.*, 250:7040–7044.
126. Warner, H. R., Demple, B. F., Deutsch, W. A., Kane, C. M., and Linn, S. (1980): Apurinic/apyrimidinic endonucleases in repair of pyrimidine dimers and other lesions in DNA. *Proc. Natl. Acad. Sci. USA*, 77:4602–4606.
127. Weissbach, A., Schlabach, A., Fridlender, B., and Bolden, A. (1971): DNA polymerases from human cells. *Nature*, 231:167–170.
128. Weissbach, A. (1977): Eukaryotic DNA polymerases. *Ann. Rev. Biochem.*, 46:25–47.
129. Witkin, E. M. (1976): Ultraviolet mutagenesis and inducible DNA repair in *Escherichia coli*. *Bacteriol. Rev.*, 40:869–907.
130. Wulff, D. L., and Rupert, C. S. (1962): Disappearance of thymine photodimer in ultraviolet

irradiated DNA upon treatment with a photoreactivating enzyme from baker's yeast. *Biochem. Biophys. Res. Comm.*, 7:237–240.

131. Yoakum, G. H., and Grossman, L. (1981): Identification of *E. coli uvrC* protein. *Nature*, 292:171–173.

132. Yoshida, S., Kondo, T., and Ando, T. (1974): Multiple molecular species of cytoplasmic DNA polymerase from calf thymus. *Biochim. Biophys. Acta*, 353:463–474.

Biochemical Basis of Chemical Carcinogenesis,
edited by H. Greim, R. Jung, M. Kramer,
H. Marquardt, and F. Oesch.
Raven Press, New York © 1984.

Formation and Removal of Pyrimidine Photodimers in Human Skin Fibroblasts Irradiated with Near-Ultraviolet Light

Hugo J. Niggli and Peter A. Cerutti

*Department of Carcinogenesis, Swiss Institute for Experimental Cancer Research,
CH-1066 Epalinges s/Lausanne, Switzerland*

Near-ultraviolet light in the 290-320 nm (UV-B) region is mostly responsible for the induction of skin cancer in the human (4,35). For technical reasons a majority of studies on the formation and removal of cyclobutane-type pyrimidine dimers were carried out in the far-ultraviolet at 254 nm, however. In the present paper we review our recent comparative studies on the formation and repair of cis-syn cyclobutane-type dimers of thymine-thymine (TT) and thymine-cytosine (and cytosine-thymine) (CT) in monolayer cultures of human skin fibroblasts upon exposure to light at 254 and 313 nm. New technologies were developed for the determination of dimers in the physiologic dose range. The major improvements relative to earlier methods are the application of a more efficient procedure for the isolation of DNA (19) and the modification of the dimers by $NaBH_4$ reduction before separation by high pressure liquid chromatography (HPLC). We found that the relative amounts of specific dimers and their distribution in chromatin was wavelength dependent. These findings demonstrate that photochemical and photobiological data obtained in the far-UV cannot be simply extrapolated to the near-UV. Furthermore, we observed that the efficiency of dimerization varied with the irradiation temperature (0°C and 37°C) probably due to differences in the conformation of chromatin and DNA. Our excision repair studies at 313 nm showed that CT was removed more rapidly than TT from the DNA of confluent monolayers of human skin fibroblasts. This result is intriguing in view of the role which CT may play in UV-mutagenesis.

EFFICIENCY OF FORMATION OF THYMINE-THYMINE AND CYTOSINE-THYMINE CYCLOBUTANE-TYPE PHOTODIMERS WITH NEAR-ULTRAVIOLET LIGHT

To determine dose response curves, monolayer cultures of skin fibroblasts from a patient with Xeroderma pigmentosum of complementation group A (strain XP12BE) were labeled in their DNA with ^{3}H thymidine and irradiated with monochromatic

257

light (10 nm half-bandwidth, Kodacel filter) at 313 nm at 37°C. XPA cells are deficient in the removal of cyclobutane-type dimers, and dose-response curves which are unperturbed by excision repair were therefore obtained. TT were formed with a rate of 0.0036% and CT of 0.0044% per KJm^{-2}, respectively (Niggli and Cerutti, unpublished). Our finding that CT-dimerization was somewhat more efficient than TT-dimerization in the physiologic dose range at 313 nm is in agreement with results of Ellison & Childs (11) obtained at much higher doses with free DNA. Qualitatively similar results were also obtained by Suzuki et al. (34) with monolayers of rodent fibroblasts irradiated with a filtered sun-lamp.

In studies of the excision of UV-lesions irradiation is often carried out at 0°C in order to inhibit repair processes during irradiation on the assumption that the dimer yields are independent of the temperature. However, since intracellular DNA- and chromatin-conformation may change with temperature and since conformation may affect dimerization, we compared the efficiency of formation to TT and CT at 0°C and 37°C. Figure 1A contains the dose response curves for TT. From the slopes of the curves a rate of formation of 0.0026% per KJm^{-2} at 0°C is determined relative to 0.0036% per KJm^{-2} at 37°C, i.e., the rate at 0°C is almost ⅓ lower than at 37°C. As shown in Fig. 1B this temperature dependence on the rate of formation was even more pronounced for CT dimers, the rate at 0°C being 0.0024% per KJm^{-2} and at 37°C 0.0044% per KJm^{-2}, i.e., a difference of nearly a factor 2. It follows that overall pyrimidine dimerization at 313 nm is considerably more efficient at 37°C than at 0°C. (22). Similar results were obtained for thymine dimerization in the normal repair proficient human skin fibroblast strain 1221 (data not shown).

The notion that the observed temperature effect is due to changes in DNA- and chromatin-conformation is supported by observations reported in the literature. A similar temperature effect on TT formation in *E. coli* upon irradiation with 254 nm light has been reported (31). The comparison was between frozen cells at −79°C and unfrozen cells at 21°C with far UV-light treatment. Hosszu and Rahn (14) showed that the rate of TT formation over the range from 25 to 100°C in the native DNA was essentially temperature independent up to the melting temperature where it underwent a sharp decrease. At temperatures below 0°C the yield of TT decreased depending on the solvent used (26). Changes in DNA secondary structure have been noted as a function of temperature in the premelting zone of chromatin by circular dichroism (12,2,3). Similar results have been obtained with Raman- and absorption-spectroscopy (28). Proton nuclear magnetic resonance studies of a double helical oligonucleotide showed a sequential broadening of the resonances upon raising the temperature from 3°C to 25°C which was explained by fraying of the helix ends at premelting temperature (25). These observations indicate that DNA local structure depends on temperature (24). Temperature may also affect the conformation of histone and nonhistone proteins containing aromatic aminoacids which are known to photosensitize pyrimidine dimerization and therefore affect TPy (thymine-pyrimidine dimers) yields (15,33).

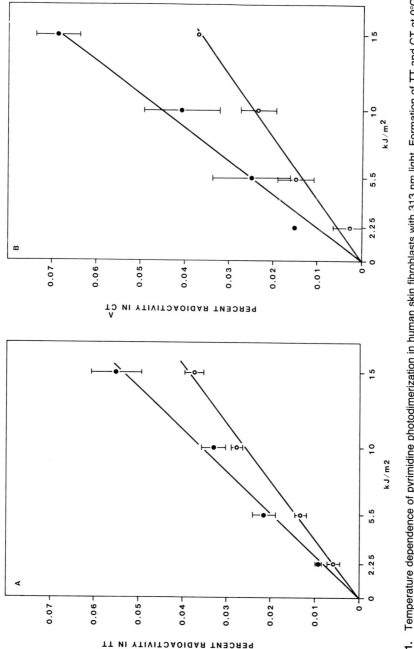

FIG. 1. Temperature dependence of pyrimidine photodimerization in human skin fibroblasts with 313 nm light. Formation of TT and CT at 0°C and 37°C in xeroderma pigmentosum fibroblasts of complementation group A (XP12BE). **A,** formation of TT at 0°C (correlation coefficient by linear regression of mean values is 0.997); *solid circle,* TT at 37°C (correlation coefficient 0.998). **B,** formation of CT at 0°C (correlation coefficient 0.995); *solid circle,* CT at 37°C (correlation coefficient 0.993). (Data from ref. 22.)

NUCLEOSOMAL DISTRIBUTION OF PYRIMIDINE PHOTODIMERS FOLLOWING FAR- AND NEAR-ULTRAVIOLET IRRADIATION

The role of the nucleosomal structure of chromatin in the formation and repair of carcinogen-induced DNA has been studied intensively over the last years. In general it has been found that bulky adducts, e.g., adducts formed by *N*-acetoxy-2-acetylaminofluorene (16,21), benzo(*a*)pyrene-diol-epoxide I (17), aflatoxin B_1 (8), and trimethylpsoralen plus light (6,37) are introduced preferentially into nucleosomal linker DNA. Where this was studied bulky adducts were also excised more efficiently from linker- than core-DNA (16,17). For ultraviolet-induced photodimers the reports in the literature did not allow it to construct a clear picture. Williams and Friedberg (38) reported random distribution of TPy between micrococcal nuclease (MN)-sensitive and -resistant DNA following irradiation of monolayer cultures of human skin fibroblasts with moderate doses of 254 nm light. In contrast, Snapka and Linn (32) observed more efficient formation of TPy in SV40 chromatin relative to free SV40 DNA by 254 nm light *in vitro*. They estimated that the rate of photodimerization was approximately 1.8 times higher in nucleosomal cores than in linker DNA. Lippke et al. (20) reported that the overall rate of pyrimidine photodimerization was about half for DNA *in situ* in human cells than for free DNA irradiated *in vitro* with 254 nm light. The lack of clear knowledge of the distribution of TPy in chromatin has hampered the interpretation of repair experiments such as studies of the distribution of MN-sensitive and -resistant repair replicated DNA patches (38,30,9,5).

In order to clarify this question we have determined the nucleosomal distribution of TT in normal human skin fibroblasts following exposure to light at 254 and 313 nm at 0°C using our new methodology. The concentration of TT was determined in total nuclear DNA and DNA extracted from purified mononucleosomes. The mononucleosomes were obtained from micrococcal nuclease treated nuclei by sucrose gradient centrifugation and contained core-DNA of 145 base pairs (b.p.) to approximately 70% and chromatosomal DNA of 165 b.p. to 30%. The TT concentration in nucleosomal linker DNA was calculated from these data (16,17). The TT contents of the acid hydrolysates of these DNA preparations were determined by HPLC as described above. Figure 2A contains dose response curves at 254 nm for TT formation. From the linear curves it is calculated that TT is formed with an efficiency of 0.0024% per Jm^{-2} both in total and mononucleosomal DNA.

Since no significant difference is observed for the TT concentrations in total- and mononucleosomal DNA it is concluded that TT distribution is random between nucleosomal core/chromatosomal-DNA and linker-DNA. Our results support those of Williams and Friedberg (38) but disagree with those of Snapka and Linn (32) who reported somewhat higher TPy concentrations in SV40 minichromosomes than in free SV40 DNA irradiated *in vitro*. However, their *in vitro* system may not be directly comparable to intracellular chromatin. While SV40 minichromosomes contain a full complement of nucleosomal cores (29) they may differ substantially from that of intracellular chromatin. The uniform nucleosomal distribution of TT in

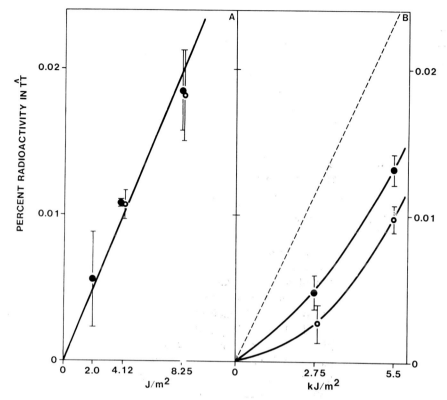

FIG. 2. Nucleosomal distribution of thymine photodimers in human skin fibroblasts following irradiation with 254 nm and 313 nm light. **A,** irradiation with 254 nm (at 0°C). *Solid circle,* total cellular DNA; *empty circle,* mononucleosomal DNA (70% 145 base pair core-DNA and 30% 165 base pair chromatosomal DNA). **B,** irradiation with 313 nm (at 0°C). *Solid circle,* total cellular DNA; *empty circle,* mononucleosomal DNA (70% 145 base pair core-DNA and 30% 165 base pair chromatosomal DNA). The dashed curve gives the concentration of TT in 47 base pair linker DNA and is calculated from the data for total- and mononucleosomal DNA. (Data from ref. 23.)

intracellular chromatin following 254 nm irradiation contrasts with the preference of a variety of bulky carcinogens to bind to linker DNA mentioned above.

Figure 2B contains the dose response curves for the induction of TT at 313 nm. In contrast to 254 nm, TT is introduced with significantly higher efficiency into total- than mononucleosomal-DNA. Since human fibroblasts possess a nucleosomal repeat of 192 b.p. (16,17) the linker DNA which connects the 145 b.p. cores is 47 b.p. in length. The ratio of the TT concentration in 47 b.p. linker- and 145 b.p. core-DNA was calculated to 4.2 at a dose of 2.75 KJm^{-2} and 2.4 at 5.5 KJm^{-2}. Since TT formation was random at 254 nm it is unlikely that differences in the conformational states of linker- and core-DNA *per se* are responsible for our results. Differences in the rates of the deactivation of the excited states responsible for dimerization or photosensitization reactions may influence the efficiency of TT formation. In particular, aromatic amino acids contained in the histones and the nonhistone proteins may photosensitize dimerization or monomerization of TT in a nonrandom fashion (15,33). The presence of increased concentrations of lesions other than TPy after 313 nm irradiation, such as single strand breaks and lesions of the 5,6-dihydroxy-dihydrothymine type (13,7,36), may affect TT yields and their distribution. It is again evident that photochemical and photobiological data obtained in the far-UV cannot be directly extrapolated to the near-UV (23).

EXCISION OF THYMINE-THYMINE AND CYTOSINE-THYMINE CYCLOBUTANE-TYPE PHOTODIMERS

The removal of TT and CT from the DNA of confluent monolayers of human skin fibroblasts was followed after they had received a dose of 10 KJm^{-2} of 313 nm light at 37°C. Within the first 8 hrs 62% CT but only 30% TT were removed from high molecular weight DNA. Excision of both types of dimers continued at a much lower rate. TT and CT were refractory to excision in a strain of Xeroderma pigmentosum fibroblasts of complementation group A (strain XP12BE) (39).

Our kinetics of dimer removal at 313 nm agree best with those of Konze-Thomas et al. (18) at 254 nm who found 70% excision in 6 hrs. Faster removal has been reported by Amacher et al. (1) while Regan et al. (27) and Ehman et al. (10) did not observe any excision. In our experience the kinetics are dose dependent even at doses which are usually not believed to lead to saturation of the repair system. No significant difference in kinetics was found at the same initial dimer concentrations regardless of whether they were induced with 254 nm or 313 nm light (equidimer doses were 8.25 Jm^{-2} of 254 nm light and 5.5 KJm^{-2} 313 nm light of 10 nm half bandwidth). Other lesions such as single-strand breaks and products of the 5,6-dihydroxy-dihydrothymine type which are induced with much higher relative efficiency at 313 nm (7) apparently have no major effect on dimer excision, therefore. It is interesting that CT were removed more rapidly than TT since they are both cis-syn cyclobutane type dimers which are expected to have similar effects on local DNA- and chromatin-conformation. It is conceivable that their removal from DNA occurs by different enzymes or that their distribution in chromatin is not the same. The latter question could not be investigated in the low dose range even with our improved methodology.

ACKNOWLEDGMENT

This work has been supported by Grant No. 3'627.80 of the Swiss National Science Foundation.

REFERENCES

1. Amacher, D. E., Elliot, J. A., and Lieberman, M. W. (1977): Differences in removal of acetyl-aminofluorene and pyrimidine dimers from the DNA of cultured mammalian cells. *Proc. Natl. Acad. Sci. USA*, 74:1553–1557.

2. Baase, W. A., and Johnson, W. C. (1979): Circular dichroism and DNA secondary structure. *Nucl. Acid. Res.*, 6:797–814.

3. Beaudette, N. V., Okabayashi, H., and Fasman, G. D. (1982): Conformational effects of organic solvents on histone complexes. *Biochem.*, 21:1765–1772.

4. Blum, H. F. (1959): *Carcinogenesis by Ultraviolet Light*. Princeton University Press, Princeton, N.J.

5. Bodell, W. J., and Cleaver, J. E. (1981): Transient conformation changes in chromatin during excision repair of ultraviolet damage to DNA. *Nucl. Acid Res.*, 9:203–212.

6. Cech, T., and Pardue, M. L. (1977): Cross-linking of DNA with trimethylpsoralen is a probe for chromatin structure. *Cell*, 11:631–640.

7. Cerutti, P. A., and Netrawali, M. S. (1979): Formation and repair of DNA damage induced by indirect action of ultraviolet light in normal and xeroderma pigmentosum skin fibroblasts. In: *Proceedings of VIth Int. Congr. of Radiat. Res., Tokyo*, pp. 423–432. Toppan Printing Co., Ltd., Tokyo.

8. Cerutti, P. A. (1982): DNA lesions: nature and genesis. In: *Chemical Carcinogenesis*, edited by Claudio Nicolini, pp. 75–92. Plenum Publishing Corp., New York.

9. Cleaver, J. E. (1977): Nucleosome structure control rates of excision repair in DNA of human cells. *Nature*, 270:451–453.

10. Ehman, U. K., Cook, K. H., and Friedberg, E. C. (1978): The kinetics of thymine dimer excision in UV-irradiated human cells. *Biophys. J.*, 22:249–264.

11. Ellison, M. J., and Childs, J. D. (1981): Pyrimidine dimers induced in escherichia coli DNA by ultraviolet radiation present in sunlight. *Photochem. Photobiol.*, 34:465–469.

12. Gennis, R. B., and Cantor, C. R. (1972): Optical studies of a conformational change in DNA before melting. *J. Mol. Biol.*, 65:381–399.

13. Hariharan, P. V., and Cerutti, P. A. (1977): Formation of products of the 5,6-dihydroxydihydro-thymine type by ultraviolet light in HeLa cells. *Biochemistry*, 16:2791–2795.

14. Hosszu, J. L., and Rahn, R. O. (1967): Thymine dimer formation in DNA between 25°C and 100°C. *Biochem. Biophys. Res. Commun.*, 29:327–330.

15. Kaneko, M., Matsuyama, A., and Nagata, C. (1979): Photosensitized formation of thymine dimers in DNA by tyramine, tyrosine and tyrosine-containing peptides. *Nucl. Acid. Res.*, 6:1177–1187.

16. Kaneko, M., and Cerutti, P. A. (1980): Excision of N-acetoxy-2-acetylaminofluorene-induced DNA adducts from chromatin fractions of human fibroblasts. *Cancer Res.*, 40:4313–4319.

17. Kaneko, M., and Cerutti, P. A. (1982): Excision of benzo(a)pyrene diol epoxide I adducts from nucleosomal DNA of confluent normal human fibroblasts. *Chem. Biol. Interactions*, 38:261–274.

18. Konze-Thomas, B., Levinson, J. W., Maher, V. M., and McCormick, J. J. (1979): Correlation among the rates of dimer excision, DNA repair replication, and recovery of human cells from potentially lethal damage induced by ultraviolet radiation. *Biophys. J.*, 28:315–326.

19. Leadon, S. A., and Cerutti, P. A. (1982): A rapid and mild procedure for the isolation of DNA from mammalian cells. *Anal. Biochem.*, 120:282–288.

20. Lippke, J. A., Gordon, L. K., Brash, D. E., and Haseltine, W. A. (1981): Distribution of UV-light induced damage in a defined sequence of human DNA: Detection of alkaline-sensitive lesions at pyrimidine nucleoside-cytidine sequences. *Proc. Natl. Acad. Sci. USA*, 78:3388–3392.

21. Metzger, G., Wilhelm, F. X., and Wilhelm, M. L. (1977): Non-random binding of a chemical carcinogen to the DNA in chromatin. *Biochem. Biophys. Res. Commun.*, 75:703–710.

22. Niggli, H. J., and Cerutti, P. A. (1983): Temperature dependence of induction of cyclobutane-type pyrimidine photodimers in human skin fibroblasts by 313 nm light. *Photochem. Photobiol.*, 37:467–469.

23. Niggli, H. J., and Cerutti, P. A. (1982): Nucleosomal distribution of thymine photodimers following far- and near-ultraviolet irradiation. *Biochem. Biophys. Res. Commun.*, 105:1215–1223.

24. Palaček, E. (1976): Premelting changes in DNA conformation. In: *Progress in Nucleic Acid Research and Molecular Biology, Vol. 18*, edited by Cohn, W. E., pp. 151–213. Academic Press, New York.

25. Patel, D. J., and Tonelli, A. E. (1974): Assignment of the proton Nmr chemical shifts of the T-N_3H and G-N_1H proton resonances in isolated AT and GC Watson-Crick base pairs in double-stranded deoxy oligonucleotides in aqueous solution. *Biopolymers*, 13:1943–1964.

26. Rahn, R. O., and Hosszu, J. L. (1968): Photoproduct formation at low temperature. *Photochem. Photobiol.*, 8:53–63.

27. Regan, J. E., Carrier, W. L., Smith, D. P., Waters, R., and Lee, W. H. (1978): Pyrimidine dimer excision in human cells and skin cancer. *National Cancer Institute Monograph*, 50:141–143.
28. Rimai, J., Maher, V. M., Gill, D., Salmeen, I., and McCormick, J. J. (1974): The temperature dependence of raman intensities of DNA. Evidence for premelting changes and correlations with ultraviolet spectra. *Biochim. Biophys. Acta*, 361:155–165.
29. Shelton, E. R., Wassarman, P. M., and DePamphilis, M. L. (1980): Structure, spacing and phasing of nucleosomes on isolated forms of mature simian virus 40 chromosomes. *J. Biol. Chem.*, 255:771–782.
30. Smerdon, M. J., Tlsty, T. D., and Lieberman, M. W. (1978): Distribution of ultraviolet-induced DNA repair synthesis in nuclease sensitive and resistant regions of human chromatin. *Biochem.*, 17:2377–2386.
31. Smith, K. C., and O'Leary, M. E. (1967): Photo-induced DNA-protein cross-links and bacterial killing: a correlation at low temperatures. *Science*, 155:1024–1026.
32. Snapka, R. M., and Linn, S. (1981): Efficiency of formation of pyrimidine dimers in SV40 chromatin in vitro. *Biochem.*, 20:68–72.
33. Sutherland, J. C., and Griffin, K. P. (1980): Monomerization of pyrimidine dimers in DNA by tryptophan-containing peptides: wave-length dependence. *Rad. Res.*, 83:529–536.
34. Suzuki, F., Han, A., Lankas, G. R., Utsumi, H., and Elkind, M. M. (1981): Spectral dependences of killing, mutation, and transformation in mammalian cells and their relevance to hazards caused by solar ultraviolet radiation. *Cancer Res.*, 41:4916–4924.
35. Urbach, F. (1975): Skin cancer and UV radiation. In: *Impacts of Climatic Change on the Biosphere, Part 1*, edited by D. S. Nachtwey, Chapter 7, pp. 19–28. Dept. of Transportation, Washington, D.C.
36. Webb, R. (1977): Lethal and mutagenic effects of near-ultraviolet radiation. In: *Photochemical and Photobiological Reviews, Vol. 2*, pp. 169–261. Plenum Press, New York.
37. Wiesehahn, G. P. Hyde, J. E., and Hearst, J. E. (1977): The photoaddition of trimethylpsoralen to drosophila melanogaster nuclei: a probe for chromatin substructure. *Biochem.*, 16:925–932.
38. Williams, J. I., and Friedberg, E. C. (1979): Deoxyribonucleic acid excision repair in chromatin after ultraviolet irradiation of human fibroblasts in culture. *Biochem.*, 18:3965–3972.
39. Niggli, H. J. and Cerutti, P. A. (1983): Cyclobutane-type pyrimidine photodimer formation and excision in human skin fibroblasts after irradiation with 313nm ultraviolet light. *Biochem.*, 22:1390–1395.

Biochemical Basis of Chemical Carcinogenesis,
edited by H. Greim, R. Jung, M. Kramer,
H. Marquardt, and F. Oesch.
Raven Press, New York © 1984.

Repair of O6-Methylguanine in DNA by Mammalian Tissues

Anthony E. Pegg

*Department of Physiology and Specialized Cancer Research Center,
The Milton S. Hershey Medical Center, The Pennsylvania State University
College of Medicine, Hershey, Pennsylvania 17033*

Alkylating agents form a major class of chemical carcinogens. These may have considerable environmental significance owing to the widespread occurrence of low levels of nitrosamines and related compounds which are converted to alkylating agents within the body. Studies of their interaction with DNA have indicated that at least 12 sites of alkylation are seen under physiologic conditions (17,21,25,28,40). Probably all of these products are subject to enzymatic repair, but discrete enzymes carrying out such repair have been characterized for only 4 of these, namely 7-methylguanine, 3-methyladenine, 3-methylguanine, and O6-methylguanine (13,14,30). The first three of these products are removed from DNA by the action of glycosylases which split the purine deoxyribose bond liberating the base and generating an AP site (apurinic site). Such reactions may be of great importance in counteracting the toxicity of alkylating agents, but do not appear to play a major role in the prevention of mutagenesis or carcinogenesis (13,14,17,21,25). Instead, there is substantial evidence that O6-methylguanine may be an important lesion in these processes and that the enzyme which repairs this product provides resistance to them. This enzyme is a transmethylase rather than a glycosylase (14,34,36). The mechanism and regulation of the repair of O6-methylguanine in *E. coli* has been extensively reviewed recently (5,14,39) and the present chapter will, therefore, be devoted exclusively to studies on mammalian cells with brief mention of the similarities and differences with the bacterial system. This article will focus on *in vitro* studies on the transmethylase, but in order to place the results in context, a brief review of studies of O6-methylguanine persistence in DNA *in vivo* is included.

PERSISTENCE OF O6-METHYLGUANINE IN DNA OF MAMMALIAN TISSUES

In rodents, the removal of O6-methylguanine from DNA is tissue specific (17,25). Liver is the most active tissue in removal and brain the least. As shown in Figure 1, rat liver cells can remove small amounts of O6-methylguanine produced by dimethylnitrosamine very rapidly so that more than 90% of the lesions are removed within 3 hrs (31). The loss of O⁶-ethylguanine produced by diethylnitrosamine is also quite rapid (29) but considerably slower than the removal of the methyl adduct (Fig. 1).

There are differences in the persistence of O⁶-methylguanine between cell types even in the same organ. In the liver, this lesion is much more long-lived in the DNA of nonparenchymal cells than in the hepatocytes (15,43).

The loss of O⁶-methylguanine from DNA appears to be saturable or inhibited after exposure to higher doses of alkylating agents (21,24,25,42). The dose required to saturate this process varies with the tissue, i.e., rat kidney is saturated at a lower level than rat liver, and the species, i.e., hamster liver is saturated at a lower level than rat liver. This correlates well with the sensitivity of these tissues to carcinogenesis by large single doses of dimethylnitrosamine which produce exclusively renal tumors in rats and yield liver tumors in hamsters.

Human fibroblasts and lymphoblast cells grown in culture have greater abilities to remove O⁶-methylguanine from their DNA than corresponding rodent cell lines (1,8,11,41). Transformed human cell lines appear to fall into at least two classes. Those designated mer⁺ (or mex⁺ according to the laboratory) are competent in catalyzing removal of O⁶-methylguanine and those designated mer⁻ are not.

The ability to remove O⁶-methylguanine from DNA in rat liver is enhanced by chronic exposure to dimethylnitrosamine (21,22), other hepatocarcinogens (24), and partial hepatectomy (37). This induction is in some ways analogous to the adaptive response in *E. coli*, but as discussed below there are also striking differences between this induction and that in bacteria. In particular, the magnitude of the enhancement in rat liver is much lower.

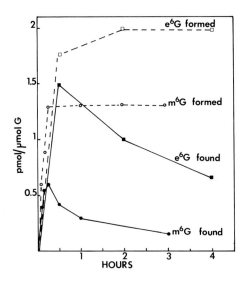

FIG. 1. Formation and loss of O⁶-methylguanine (m⁶G; circles) and O⁶-ethylguanine (e⁶G; squares) from DNA in rat liver after administration of dimethylnitrosamine (50 μg/kg) and diethylnitrosamine (500 μg/kg). Results are shown for formation *(open symbols, dotted lines)* based on the 7-alkylguanine produced and for the actual values found *(closed symbols, solid lines)*. The difference indicates the amount of O⁶-adduct removed. (Data from refs. 29 and 31.)

REMOVAL OF O⁶-METHYLGUANINE FROM DNA *IN VITRO*

Purification of Protein and Characterization of Reaction

A protein fraction carrying out the removal of O^6-methylguanine from DNA has been purified over 1000-fold from regenerating rat liver (36). This protein appears to be exactly analogous to that purified from *E. coli* in that the methyl group is transferred to a cysteine residue on the protein and that guanine is regenerated directly in the DNA (Table 1). Similar characterization of the reaction showing stoichiometry between O^6-methylguanine lost, S-methylcysteine-protein formed, and guanine produced in the DNA substrate has now been carried out not only for the rat liver and human liver proteins (34,36) as shown in Table 1, but also for the protein from other human tissues and other mammalian liver extracts (unpublished observations), and from rat kidney (35). It, therefore, appears that this mechanism is widespread. This conclusion has also been reached on the basis of stoichiometry between S-methylcysteine production and loss of O^6-methylguanine alone (4,18,44–48), but it should be noted that this is not sufficient to characterize the reaction since the guanine moiety from which the methyl group arises could also be modified in the reaction. Thus, the use of a substrate containing O^6-methyldeoxyguanosine labeled in the guanosine moiety as introduced by Mitra and colleagues (9,20) is essential for complete characterization.

The partially purified rat liver protein has been tested for substrate specificity, but only O^6-methyl- and O^6-ethyldeoxyguanosine residues in DNA were found to be substrates (36). The protein did not remove methyl groups from RNA, from O^6-methyldeoxyguanosine or O^6-methylguanosine nor did it remove methyl groups from other methylated purines in DNA. Single-stranded DNA and poly(dG.dC.m⁶dG) were substrates for the protein, but the rate of removal was slower than with double-stranded DNA. Similarly, de-ethylation of O^6-ethylguanine in DNA was considerably slower than de-methylation (36) which is in good agreement with the *in vivo* results of Fig. 1. Finally, the rate of demethylation was progressively reduced when DNA substrates with progressively lower degrees of methylation (but the same total amount of O^6-methylguanine) were used as substrates. This is probably due to the high affinity of the protein for double-stranded DNA. When a substrate containing

TABLE 1. *Characterization of reaction catalyzed by human and rat liver protein removing O⁶-methylguanine from DNA*

Source of protein	O⁶-Methylguanine lost from DNA (pmoles/mg protein)	S-methylcysteine formed in protein (pmoles/mg protein)	Guanine formed in DNA (pmoles/mg protein)
Purified rat liver	28	26	24
Crude human liver	0.70	0.61	0.59

(Data from refs. 34 and 36.)

only a few O^6-methylguanine lesions in a large amount of DNA is used, this affinity may retard the reaction by increasing the time for recognition of the substrate. The effect of DNA concentration on the rate of reaction may account for the substantial variation from one laboratory to another in the time courses reported for the action of this protein.

Saturation of Reaction

The removal of O^6-methylguanine from methylated calf thymus DNA by the rat liver protein is shown in Fig. 2. The reaction is complete within 30 minutes even though additional O^6-methylguaninae remains in the substrate and can be removed if additional protein is added. The protein itself is not unstable when incubated for 30 minutes alone without the methylated DNA substrate. These results indicate that some component of the system is used up and this appears to be the cysteine acceptor site. There is unequivocal evidence with the bacterial transmethylase that the same protein which catalyzes the transfer of the methyl group is the acceptor protein (14). This is not so firmly established with the mammalian protein which has not been purified to homogeneity, but the acceptor and transferase activity copurify over at least a 6000 fold range of purification and have a similar molecular weight of about 20,000 as judged by gel filtration (36). Irrespective of this, the stoichiometry between S-methylcysteine-protein formed and O^6-methylguanine removed (Table 1 and Fig. 2) indicates that there is little, if any, regeneration of the acceptor site *in vitro*. If this is also the case *in vivo*, it provides a clear explanation for the saturation of O^6-methylguanine repair. Such saturation would occur when the acceptor protein has been used up, and the removal rate would then reflect the synthesis or slow regeneration of this protein.

This mechanism is consistent with most of the experimental evidence including the inability to isolate transmethylase activity from rat tissues after high doses of dimethylnitrosamine (27). However, there is another factor which may also contribute to the loss of activity. As indicated in Table 2, the rat liver transmethylase protein is directly inactivated by exposure to the methylating agent, *N*-methyl-*N*-nitrosourea *in vitro*. This sensitivity to inactivation could be due to the facile reaction between the cysteine-acceptor site and the methylating agent because of the structure of the protein. It remains to be determined to what extent the inactivation of the

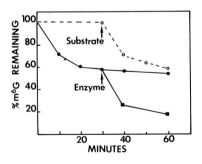

FIG. 2. Saturation of removal of O^6-methylguanine from DNA by liver protein. The enzyme protein was incubated with substrate for the times shown (●——●). At 30 min a second aliquot of protein was added to some tubes (■——■). In other tubes the enzyme was incubated without substrate for 30 min and then the DNA substrate was added (○-----○). (Data from ref. 36.)

TABLE 2. *Inactivation of rat liver O^6-methylguanine-DNA reaction with N-methyl-N-nitrosoure.*

Treatment	Transmethylase activity (pmoles removed from DNA)
None	1.18
Preincubated 30 min	1.12
Preincubated 30 min + 5 mM N-methyl-N-nitrosourea	0.13

(Data from ref. 36.)

TABLE 3. *Induction of rat liver O^6-methylguanine-DNA transmethylase*

Treatment	Number of molecules of transmethylase per cell
Control	60,000
Dimethylnitrosamine (2 mg/kg/day for 21 days)	177,000
Diethylnitrosamine (10 mg/kg/day for 7 days)	149,000
1,2-Dimethylhydrazine (3 mg/kg/day for 7 days)	176,000
N-Methyl-N-nitrosourea (10 mg/kg/day for 21 days)	57,000
Streptozotocin (30 mg/kg/day for 21 days)	53,000
Carbon tetrachloride (40 h after 1.5 ml/kg)	158,000
Thioacetamide (48 hrs after 150 mg/kg)	150,000
Partial hepatectomy (60 hrs after operation)	390,000

(Data from refs. 32 and 33 and expressed per cell using values for the number of hepatocytes per cell in ref. 10.)

protein by direct methylation could occur under physiologic conditions where there is a higher concentration of competing nucleophiles.

Induction of Activity

Many substances have now been shown to increase the content of the transmethylase in rat liver. As shown in Table 3, these include treatments with alkylating agents such as dimethylnitrosamine, diethylnitrosamine and 1,2-dimethylhydrazine (22,32,33). This induction which occurs only in the hepatocytes and not in the nonparenchymal cells (43) is in some ways comparable to the adaptive response in *E. coli* (5,39), but the magnitude is at most 3-fold whereas the bacterial transmethylase is induced by 1000-fold (14). There are other striking differences. The rat liver transmethylase is not induced by the direct acting alkylating agents, streptozotocin and N-methyl-N-nitrosourea (Table 3) which induce well in bacteria. The rat liver transmethylase is also induced by a variety of other hepatotoxins which are not methylating agents including thioacetamide and carbon tetrachloride (Table 3), aflatoxin and acetylaminofluorene (6,7). Furthermore, an even greater induction of 6 to 7 fold is produced by partial hepatectomy (Table 3).

These results raise the possibility that the apparent induction of O^6-methylguanine-DNA transmethylase in rat liver by carcinogens may be a secondary response to the tissue damage and regenerative growth. A similar induction can be demonstrated in the rat kidney in response to unilateral nephrectomy or injury with folic acid (35). The transmethylase in rat liver is also under the control of hormones; decreasing in activity in response to hypophysectomy or thyroidectomy and increasing in response to growth hormone or thyroxin. However, there is no obligatory linkage between the transmethylase activity and cell growth as the activity is below adult levels in neonatal rats and reaches adult values only by 14 days of age (35).

At present, induction of O^6-methylguanine-DNA transmethylase in mammalian cells has only been unequivocally demonstrated in the rat liver and kidney. Attempts to induce in livers of other rodents were unsuccessful (23) and although there is one report of induction by exposure to N-methyl-N'-nitro-N-nitrosoguanidine in HeLa cells (46), this experiment was carried out using a dubious assay technique which gives controversial results with other cell lines (see below). Therefore, although induction of the transmethylase clearly plays a role in limiting the build-up of O^6-methylguanine in the DNA of hepatocytes of rats treated chronically with dimethylnitrosamine or 1,2-dimethylhydrazine the generality of this phenomenon and its parallel to the adaptive response remain to be determined.

O⁶-Methylguanine-DNA Transmethylase Levels in Different Tissues and Species

As shown in Table 4, the *E. coli* transmethylase protein is present in unadapted cells at only a few copies (about 30) per cell. This number is increased to 3,000 in adapted cells and to 6,700 in a constitutive mutant (20). Rat hepatocytes contain about 60,000 molecules per cell which can be increased to about 400,000 by induction (32,33,43), but since the genome is about a thousand times greater in these cells, the total capacity to repair this lesion is considerably greater in the adapted bacteria.

Other rat cells contain considerably less of the transmethylase. Nonparenchymal cells isolated by elutriation from dispersed rat liver preparations had 12,000 molecules per cell, and this value did not increase with chronic carcinogen treatment (43). The rat kidney contained 12,000 molecules per cell and brain less than 1,500 (Table 4). [These values were obtained from estimates on total activity extracted from the tissue (27,35) and total DNA present to provide an estimate of the cell number and could mask large differences between individual cell types.]

Hamster, mouse, and guinea pig liver contained lower amounts of the transmethylase than the rat (36,42), but the human liver was substantially more active (34) and if it is assumed that this activity is limited to hepatocytes contains about 750,000 molecules per cell (Table 4). Other human cells are also more active than rodent equivalents in experiments carried out in our laboratory and elsewhere (Table 4). Waldstein et al. (44) have estimated that human lymphocytes contain 14,000 to 110,000 molecules of the protein in the unstimulated state and that this level

TABLE 4. *Estimates of the number of molecules of O^6-methyguanine-DNA transmethylase protein per cell*

Source	Number of molecules per cell	Reference no.
E. coli B/r and adaption-deficient strains	13–60	20
E. coli B/r (adapted)	3,000	9,14,20
E. coli BS21 (adaption-constitutive)	6,700	20
Rat hepatocytes (uninduced)	60,000	32,43
Rat hepatocytes (induced)	400,000	32,33
Rat liver non-parenchymal cells	5,000-12,000	43
Rat kidney	12,000	27,35
Rat kidney (induced)	31,000	35
Rat brain	<1,500	27
Hamster liver	28,000	36
Human liver	600,000-900,000	34
Human lymphocytic leukocytes	91,000-220,000	45
Human lymphocytes	14,000-140,000	44
Human fibroblasts	110,000-130,000	47
HeLa CLL2	95,000-119,000	46,47
	c100,000	19
HeLa CLL2 (induced)	320,000	46
HeLa 53	114,000	47
	<100	19
V79 hamster fibroblasts	94,000	47
	<3,000	unpublished observations, A. E. Pegg

increases to 40,000 to 140,000 after stimulation with phytohemagglutinin. In other experiments they found that human lymphocytic leukocytes (45), HeLa cells (46), and a variety of other malignant human cells and normal fibroblasts contain about 100,000 molecules of this protein (46,47). On exposure to N-methyl-N'-nitro-N-nitrosoguanine this value increased in mer$^+$ lines up to 3-fold (46,47). If this is correct, the capacity of these cells to remove O^6-methylguanine from DNA would be comparable to that of rat liver. However, there is some doubt that the assay method used by this group is satisfactory since they find no difference in the number of molecules in the mer$^+$ and mer$^-$ strains of HeLa and other cells (47) whereas other groups (19) have been unable to detect the protein in the mer$^-$ strains. Similarly, Waldstein et al. (47) report that V79 hamster fibroblasts contain 94,000 molecules of the protein per cell, but we were unable to find any activity in these cells (Table 4). Therefore, results obtained by this group require independent confirmation by other techniques and at present this is available only for the HeLa CLL2 line and the lymphocytic leukocytes which were also assayed by other methods (19,45,47).

CONCLUSIONS

At present, there is a good correlation (except for the estimates in mer$^+$ and mer$^-$ cells discussed above) between the level of the transmethylase protein detected in *in vitro* assays and in the ability of the cell to remove O^6-methylguanine from its DNA *in vivo*. In this respect, the high level of activity found in human liver is of particular interest since this organ is likely to metabolize the great majority of ingested dimethylnitrosamine and to receive most of the alkylation damage. The efficient repair of such damage could minimize the carcinogenic insult provided by low levels of exposure to this carcinogen.

The physiologic significance of the changes in the level of the rat liver transmethylase protein is at present unclear. It should be noted, however, that the assays measure only the amount of active protein. Changes in this value could be brought about by alterations in endogenous methylation of DNA which would then convert more of the protein to the methylated, inactive form. There is, at present, much interest in methylation of DNA as a means of regulating gene expression (12,38), and it has been reported that a number of hepatotoxins which are not themselves methylating agents derange cellular metabolism in such a way as to cause an appearance of O⁶-methylguanine in DNA (2,3). It is possible that the transmethylase protein plays a role in normal cellular metabolism, and further studies of the amount of this protein and the degree to which it is present in the S-methylcysteine form would be of interest. Such studies could be carried out with the aid of specific antibodies to the protein and the production of such antibodies is currently in progress.

ACKNOWLEDGMENTS

This research was supported in part by grants CA-18137 and 1P30 CA-18450 from the National Cancer Institute, DHEW.

REFERENCES

1. Ayres, K., Sklar, R., Larson, K., Lindgren, V., and Strauss, B. (1982): Regulation of the capacity for O⁶-methylguanine removal from DNA in human lymphoblastoid cells studied by cell hybridization. *Mol. Cell. Biol.*, 2:904–913.
2. Barrows, L. R., and Shank, R. C. (1981): Aberrant methylation of liver DNA in rats during hepatotoxicity. *Toxicol. Appl. Pharmacol.*, 60:334–345.
3. Becker, R. A., Barrows, L. R., and Shank, R. C. (1981): Methylation of liver DNA guanine in hydrazine hepatotoxicity: dose response and kinetic characteristics of 7-methylguanine and O⁶-methylguanine formation and persistence in rats. *Carcinogenesis*, 2:1181–1188.
4. Bogden, J. A., Eastman, A., and Bresnick, E. (1981): A system in mouse liver for the repair of O⁶-methylguanine lesions in methylated DNA. *Nucl. Acid Res.*, 9:3089–3103.
5. Cairns, J., Robins, P., Sedgwick, B., and Talmud, P. (1981): The inducible repair of alkylated DNA. *Prog. Nucleic Acid Res. Mol. Biol.*, 26:237–245.
6. Chu, Y. H., Craig, A. W., and O'Connor, P. J. (1981): Repair of O⁶-methylguanine in rat liver DNA is enhanced by pretreatment with single or multiple doses of aflatoxin B₁. *Br. J. Cancer*, 43:850–855.
7. Cooper, D. P., O'Connor, P. J., and Margison, G. P. (1982): Effect of acute doses of 2-acetylaminofluorene on the capacity of rat liver to repair methylated purines in DNA *in vivo* and *in vitro*. *Cancer Res. (in press)*.
8. Day, R. S., Ziolkowski, C. H. J., Scudiero, D. A., Meyer, S. A., Lubiniecki, A. S., Girardi, A. J., Galloway, S. M., and Bynum, G. D. (1980): Defective repair of alkylated DNA by human tumour and SV40-transformed human cell strains. *Nature*, 288:724–727.
9. Foote, R. S., Mitra, S., and Pal, B. C. (1980): Demethylation of O⁶-methylguanine in a synthetic DNA polymer by an inducible activity in *Escherichia coli*. *Biochem. Biophys. Res. Commun.*, 97:654–659.

10. Greengard, O., Federman, M., and Knox, W. E. (1972): Cytomorphometry of developing rat liver and its application to enzymatic differentiation. *J. Cell Biol.*, 52:261–272.

11. Harris, G., Lawley, P. D., and Olsen, I. (1981): Mode of action of methylating carcinogens: comparative studies of murine and human cells. *Carcinogenesis*, 2:403–411.

12. Jones, P. A., and Taylor, S. M. (1980): Cellular differentiation, cytidine analogs and DNA methylation. *Cell*, 20:85–93.

13. Karran, P., Hjelmgren, T., and Lindahl, T. (1982): Induction of a DNA glycosylase for N-methylated purines is part of the adaptive response to alkylating agents. *Nature*, 296:770–773.

14. Lindahl, T. (1982): DNA repair enzymes. *Annu. Rev. Biochem.*, 51:61–87.

15. Lindamood, III, C., Bedell, M. A., Billings, K. C., and Swenberg, J. A. (1982): Alkylation and *de novo* synthesis of liver cell DNA from C3H mice during continuous dimethylnitrosamine exposure. *Cancer Res.*, 42:4153–4157.

16. Margison, G. P. (1982): Chronic or acute administration of various dialkylnitrosamines enhances the removal of O⁶-methylguanine from rat liver DNA *in vivo*. *Chem.-Biol. Interactions*, 38:189–201.

17. Margison, G. P., and O'Connor, P. J. (1979): Nucleic acid modification by N-nitroso compounds. In: *Chemical Carcinogens and DNA*, edited by P. L. Grover, pp. 111–159. C.R.C. Press, Florida.

18. Mehta, J. R., Ludlum, D. B., Renard, A., and Verly, W. G. (1981): Repair of O⁶-ethylguanine in DNA by a chromatin fraction from rat liver: transfer of the ethyl group to an acceptor protein. *Proc. Natl. Acad. Sci.*, 78:6766–6770.

19. Mitra, S., Day, R. S., and Foote, R. S. (personal communication).

20. Mitra, S., Pal, B. C., and Foote, R. S. (1982): O⁶-Methylguanine-DNA methyltransferase in wild-type and *Ada* mutants of *E. coli*. *J. Bacteriology*, 152:534–537.

21. Montesano, R. (1981): Alkylation of DNA and tissue specificity in nitrosamine carcinogenesis. *J. Supramolec. Struc. Cell. Biochem.*, 17:259–273.

22. Montesano, R., Bresil, H., Planche-Martel, G., Margison, G. P., and Pegg, A. E. (1980): Effect of chronic treatment of rats with dimethylnitrosamine on the removal of O⁶-methylguanine from DNA. *Cancer Res.*, 40:452–458.

23. O'Connor, P. J., Chu, Y.-H., Cooper, D. P., Maru, G. B., Smith, R. A., and Margison, G. P. (1982): Species differences in the inducibility of hepatic O⁶-alkylguanine repair in rodents. *Biochimie*, 64:769–774.

24. O'Connor, P. J., and Margison, G. P. (1981): The enhanced repair of O⁶-alkylguanine in mammalian systems. In: *Chromosome Damage and Repair*, edited by E. Seeberg, and K. Kleppe, pp. 233–245. Plenum Publishing Corporation, New York.

25. Pegg, A. E. (1977): Formation and metabolism of alkylated nucleosides: possible role in carcinogenesis by nitroso compounds and alkylating agents. *Adv. Cancer Res.*, 25:195–267.

26. Pegg, A. E. (1978): Dimethylnitrosamine inhibits enzymatic removal of O⁶-methylguanine from DNA. *Nature*, 274:182–184.

27. Pegg, A. E. (1978): Enzymatic removal of O⁶-methylguanine from DNA by mammalian cell extracts. *Biochem. Biophys. Res. Commun.*, 84:166–173.

28. Pegg, A. E. (1982): Formation and removal of methylated nucleosides in nucleic acids of mammalian cells. In: *Recent Results in Cancer Research*, edited by G. Nass, vol. 84, pp. 49–62. Springer-Verlag, Berlin.

29. Pegg, A. E., and Balog, B. (1979): Formation and subsequent excision of O⁶-ethylguanine from DNA of rat liver following administration of diethylnitrosamine. *Cancer Res.*, 39:5003–5009.

30. Pegg, A. E., and Bennett, R. A. (1982): Mammalian DNA repair enzymes. In: *Enzymes of Nucleic Acid Synthesis and Processing: CRC Series on Biochemistry and Molecular Biology of the Cell Nucleus*, edited by S. T. Jacob, CRC Press, Inc., Boca Raton, Florida, pp. 179–206.

31. Pegg, A. E., and Perry, W. (1981): Alkylation of nucleic acids and metabolism of small doses of dimethylnitrosamine in the rat. *Cancer Res.*, 41:3128–3132.

32. Pegg, A. E., and Peggy, W. (1981): Stimulation of transfer of methyl groups from O⁶-methylguanine in DNA to protein in rat liver extracts in response to hepatotoxins. *Carcinogenesis*, 2:1195–1200.

33. Pegg, A. E., Perry, W., and Bennett, R. A. (1981): Partial hepatectomy increases the ability of rat liver extracts to catalyze removal of O⁶-methylguanine from alkylated DNA. *Biochem. J.*, 197:195–201.

34. Pegg, A. E., Roberfroid, M., von Bahr, C., Mitra, S., Foote, R. S., Bresil, H., Likhachev, A.,

and Montesano, R. (1982): Removal of O⁶-methylguanine from DNA by human liver fractions. *Proc. Natl. Acad. Sci.*, 74:5162–5166.

35. Pegg, A. E., and Wiest, L. (1983): Regulation of O⁶-methylguanine-DNA transmethylase activity in rat liver and kidney. *Cancer Res.*, 43:972–975.

36. Pegg, A. E., Wiest, L., Foote, R. S., Mitra, S., and Perry, W. (1983): Purification and properties of O⁶-methylguanine-DNA transmethylase from rat liver. *J. Biol. Chem.*, 258:2327–2333.

37. Rabes, H. M., Wilhelm, R., Kerler, R., and Rode, G. (1982): Dose- and cell cycle-dependent O⁶-methylguanine elimination from DNA in regenerating rat liver after [¹⁴C]dimethylnitrosamine injection. *Cancer Res.*, 42:3814–3821.

38. Razin, A., and Friedman, J. (1981): DNA methylation and its possible biological roles. *Progr. Nucleic Acid Res. Molec. Biol.*, 25:33–52.

39. Schendel, P. F. (1981): Inducible repair systems and their implications for toxicology. *CRC Crit. Rev. Toxicol.*, 8:311–362.

40. Singer, B., and Kusmierek, J. T. (1982): Chemcial mutagenesis. *Ann. Rev. Biochem.*, 52:655–693.

41. Sklar, R., Brady, K., and Strauss, B. (1981): Limited capacity for the removal of O⁶-methylguanine and its regeneration in a human lymphoma line. *Carcinogenesis*, 2:1293–1298.

42. Stumpf, R., Margison, G. P., Montesano, R., and Pegg, A. E. (1979): Formation and loss of alkylated purines from DNA of hamster tissues after administration of dimethylnitrosamine. *Cancer Res.*, 39:1041–1045.

43. Swenberg, J. A., Bedell, M. A., Billings, K. C., Umbenhauer, D. R., and Pegg, A. E. (1982): Cell specific differences in O⁶-alkylguanine DNA repair activity during continuous carcinogen exposure. *Proc. Natl. Acad. Sci.*, 79:5499–5502.

44. Waldstein, E. A., Cao, E.-H., Bender, M. A., and Setlow, R. B. (1982): Abilities of extracts of human lymphocytes to remove O⁶-methylguanine from DNA. *Mutation Res.*, 95:405–416.

45. Waldstein, E. A., Cao, E.-H., Miller, M. E., Cronkite, E. P., and Setlow, R. B. (1982): Extracts of chronic lymphocytic leukemic lymphocytes have a high level of DNA repair. *Proc. Natl. Acad. Sci.*, 79:4786–4790.

46. Waldstein, E. A., Cao, E.-H., and Setlow, R. B. (1982): Adaptive increase in O⁶-methylguanine-acceptor protein in HeLa cells following N-methyl-N'-nitro-N-nitrosoguanidine treatment. *Nucleic Acid Res.*, 10:4595–4604.

47. Waldstein, E. A., Cao, E.-H., and Setlow, R. B. (1982): Adaptive resynthesis of O⁶-methyl-guanine-accepting protein can explain the differences between mammalian cells proficient and deficient in methyl excision repair. *Proc. Natl. Acad. Sci. USA*, 79:5117–5121.

Biochemical Basis of Chemical Carcinogenesis,
edited by H. Greim, R. Jung, M. Kramer,
H. Marquardt, and F. Oesch.
Raven Press, New York © 1984.

Mechanisms of Organ-Specific Tumor Induction in the Upper Gastro-Intestinal Tract

P. Kleihues, O. Wiestler, E. Herchenhan, A. Uozumi and C. Veit

*Abteilung Neuropathologie, Pathologisches Institut,
Universität Freiburg, Federal Republic of Germany*

There is an increasing number of chemicals and industrial processes which have been positively identified as causative factors in the etiology of human cancer (9). For most of these agents their link to human disease has been established by clinical observations and epidemiologic studies. Although the usefulness of experimental carcinogenicity studies in the evaluation of potential risks to humans has often been questioned, it is noteworthy that so far all agents known to be carcinogenic in man have also been proven to induce tumors in at least one nonhuman species. One should, therefore, expect that animal experiments could guide epidemiologic research. Unfortunately, this has rarely been the case, one reason being that for many carcinogens the principal site of tumor induction varies with species, dose, route of application, and age or developmental stage. Some species also exhibit marked differences in their overall susceptibility to certain classes of chemical carcinogens. A typical example is diethylstilboestrol (DES) which before its widespread clinical use was shown to induce a high incidence of kidney tumors in hamsters. In rats, mice, and other laboratory rodents DES was not carcinogenic, but in humans, prenatal exposure was found to cause the development of clear-cell adenocarcinomas of vagina and cervix (3,11). In order to accurately predict the adverse effects of genotoxic agents in humans, the basic mechanisms underlying organ and species specificity must first be understood.

This contribution summarizes experimental data on the metabolism and reaction with cellular DNA of two carcinogenic nitroso compounds, N-nitrosomethylbenzylamine (MBN) and N-methyl-N'-nitro-N-nitrosoguanidine (MNNG). Both agents share a common ultimate carcinogen, methyl diazoniumhydroxide but differ greatly in their target organ specificity.

CARCINOMAS OF ESOPHAGUS AND FORESTOMACH INDUCED BY N-NITROSOMETHYLBENZYLAMINE

Following the pioneering work of H. Druckrey et al. (4) more than 30 nitrosamines have become known to induce a high incidence of esophageal tumors in rats.

Structure-activity studies have shown that nonsymmetrical aliphatic nitrosamines, particularly those with one methyl group are most effective. In recent years, intensive studies have been carried out to detect possible links between human esophageal cancer and nutritional exposure to MBN and related nitrosamines. Most investigations have concentrated on high risk areas in Northern China (14,16,27). MBN and a hitherto unknown *N*-nitrosation product, *N*-3-methylbutyl-*N*-1-methyl-acetonylnitrosamine, have been isolated from corn-bread contaminated with moulds commonly occurring in Linshien county, but a causal relationship with the human disease has yet to be proven (15). Fungi of the *Candida* type are frequent invaders of the esophageal epithelium of patients with early esophageal carcinoma. *Candida albicans* was found to augment the nitrosative formation of MBN when incubated with its chemical precursors, methylbenzylamine and sodium nitrite (8). In high-risk areas of Northern China domestic fowls also exhibit a high incidence of pharyngeal/esophageal cancer but several attempts to induce tumors in chickens by chronic oral administration of MBN were unsuccessful (S. H. Lu, *personal communication*).

Metabolism of MBN

The carcinogenicity of nitrosamines is based on their conversion to alkylating metabolites. Ultimate carcinogen is an alkyldiazonium hydroxide generated after enzymic hydroxylation preferentially at one of the α-carbon atoms, which acts as alkylating agent with the release of nitrogen.

To produce a methylating intermediate, hydroxylation of MBN must occur at the methylene bridge, leading to the release of benzaldehyde (Fig. 1). Alternatively, hydroxylation at the methyl group would yield a benzylating intermediate (benzyldiazonium hydroxide) and formaldehyde. *In vitro* studies with isolated microsomes have shown that both rat esophageal mucosa and rat liver are able to metabolise MBN. Hepatic microsomes oxidized MBN at the methylene bridge at a rate approximately 10-fold higher than at the methyl carbon, whereas this difference was 100-fold with microsomes isolated from esophageal mucosa (13). Accordingly, *in vivo* studies using MBN labeled with ^{14}C in either position only showed methylation of DNA purines. No benzylated bases were detectable in rat tissues (7). Autrup and Stoner (2) reported that in cultured rat esophagus the level of DNA methylation is about 100-fold higher than in human esophagus. In contrast to *in vivo* studies, these authors also noted DNA benzylation by MBN in cultured rat esophagus (at one-tenth the level of methylation), but benzylated purines were not identified. In conclusion, these studies indicate that MBN exerts its adverse biological effects *via* methylation rather than benzylation of cellular macromolecules.

Preferential Methylation of Esophageal DNA in Rats

The organ-specific carcinogenicity of MBN in rats is largely independent of the route of application. After both oral and subcutaneous administration tumors are selectively located in pharynx and esophagus (Table 1). Within 10 minutes after a

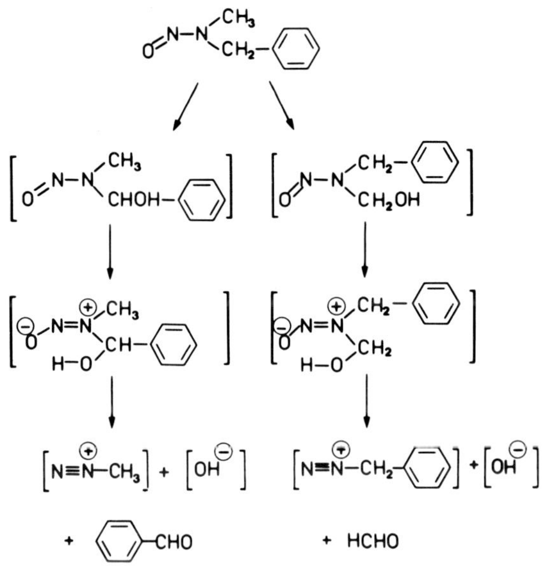

FIG. 1. Routes of metabolism involved in the bioactivation of MBN. α-C-Hydroxylation at the methylene bridge *(left)* produces methyldiazonium hydroxide and benzaldehyde whereas hydroxylation at the methyl group *(right)* would yield benzyldiazonium hydroxide and formaldehyde.

TABLE 1. *Carcinogenicity of MBN and MNNG in laboratory rodents*

Carcinogen	Species	Route of administration	Principal target tissue	Reference no.
MBN	Rat	oral (drinking water)	Esophagus	21
		s.c.	Esophagus	23
MBN	Mouse	oral (drinking water)	Esophagus, forestomach	19
		i.p.	Forestomach, lung	19
MNNG	Rat	oral (drinking water)	Glandular stomach, duodenum	24
		intragastric	Forestomach, glandular stomach	20

MBN, *N*-Nitrosomethylbenzylamine; MNNG, *N*-methyl-*N'*-nitro-*N*-nitrosoguanidine.

single i.v. dose of (^{14}C-*methyl*)MBN (2.5 mg/kg), ^{14}C-labelled metabolites (methanol, formic acid) accounted for 50% of the total radioactivity present in the esophagus, for approximately 25% in liver and forestomach, and for less than 20% in all other organs investigated (6). Four hr after the injection, methylation of purine bases in DNA was most extensive in the esophagus, followed by liver, lung and forestomach DNA (Table 2). In the remaining tissues, DNA methylation was either considerably less (kidney, glandular stomach, spleen) or not at all detectable (ileum, colon, brain). At this time, the concentration of the promutagenic base O^6-meth-

TABLE 2. *DNA methylation by N-nitrosomethylbenzylamine (MBN)*

| | Rat | | | | Mouse | | | |
| | i.v.[a] | | oral | | i.p.[b] | | oral | |
Organ	7-meG	O^6-meG	7-meG	O^6-meG	7-meG	O^6-meG	7-meG	O^6-meG
Liver	120.2	4.9	190.0	6.7	162.9	11.8	171.7	13.5
Lung	64.9	7.7	23.6	2.7	*46.1*	*4.8*	6.0	0.7
Esophagus	*344.5*	*46.1*	*404.2*	*14.6*	18.3	1.5	*289.1*	*39.1*
Forestomach	10.3	n.d.	41.5	1.8	*23.3*	*1.7*	*291.1*	*29.2*
Stomach	2.3	n.d.	5.2	0.3	2.5	n.d.	14.2	1.5
Small intestine	n.d.	n.d.	1.3	n.d.	n.d.	n.d.	3.4	n.d.
Colon	n.d.	n.d.	0.4	n.d.	4.3	n.d.	1.1	n.d.

Male Wistar rats (120–150 g) or female NMRI mice (25 g) received a single i.v., i.p. or oral (60 ppm in the drinking water) dose of (^{14}C-*methyl*) MBN (2.5 mg/kg) and were killed 4 hr later. Concentrations of methylated DNA purines are expressed as μmoles/mole guanine. For each species and mode of administration values of the respective target organ are italicized.

n.d., not detectable.

[a]Data from Hodgson et al. (6).
[b]Data from Kleihues et al. (10).

ylguanine in esophageal DNA was six times higher than in lung and nine times higher than in hepatic DNA. These data suggest that in rats the selective induction of esophageal tumors by *N*-nitrosomethylbenzylamine and related asymmetrical nitrosamines is mediated by a preferential bioactivation of the carcinogen in the target organ. Of particular interest is the observation that the extent of DNA alkylation in the esophagus is approximately 30-fold higher than in forestomach, although both tissues share an anatomically similar type of squamous epithelium.

These data suggest that of the microsomal P-450 system responsible for α-C hydroxylation subclasses may exist with a higher level in extrahepatic tissues. This view is supported by the observation of a differential sensitivity of MBN metabolism in liver and esophagus toward inhibition by disulfiram (22), and induction by phenobarbitone (13).

Following a single *oral* exposure to MBN, DNA methylation was again highest in esophagus, followed by liver, forestomach, and lung (Table 2). For obvious pharmacokinetic reasons, the concentrations of methylpurines in forestomach and liver were higher, and in lung DNA lower than after i.v. injection of a similar dose of (^{14}C-*methyl*)MBN. After oral administration, the O^6-/7-methylguanine ratio in esophageal DNA (Fig. 2) was much lower (0.036) than after i.v. injection (0.13). This difference is difficult to explain in view of the very low capacity of the esophageal mucosa for enzymatic removal of O^6-methylguanine (Table 4). From the data in Table 1 it is obvious that the route of administration has little effect on the extent of DNA methylation in the principal target organ. This is, however, different for the ring-methylated analog of MBN, *N*-nitrosomethyl(4 methyl-benzyl)amine (4-MeMBN) which is not carcinogenic after systemic administration of equimolar doses, due to the rapid formation (mainly in the liver) and excretion *via* the urine of its benzoic acid derivative.

The strong carcinogenic effect of orally administered 4-MeMBN results from direct uptake from the drinking water into the esophageal mucosa (7).

DNA Methylation by MBN in Target and Nontarget Tissues of Mice

In mice, chronic administration of MBN in the drinking water (20 ppm) causes the development of carcinomas of the esophagus and forestomach in up to 100% of experimental animals. In contrast, weekly i.p. injections (2.5 mg/kg) were found to selectively induce forestomach carcinomas and lung adenomas but no esophageal neoplasms (Table 1). We have, therefore, determined the initial extent of DNA methylation in various mouse tissues following a single i.p. injection of (^{14}C-*methyl*)MBN (10). After a survival time of 6 hr, highest concentrations of 7-methylguanine and O^6-methylguanine were present in hepatic DNA, followed by lung and forestomach, the principal target tissues for this route of administration. Lung tumors have been induced in mice by a great variety of chemical carcinogens. As with MBN such tumors are usually multiple adenomas. The present study indicates that MBN is metabolised to a significant extent in mouse lung but the level of alkylation is still 30% lower than in rats following a similar dose of MBN (Table 2). This indicates that the basic susceptibility for malignant transformation in the lung is considerably higher in mice than in rats.

DNA methylation in the esophagus was only 21% less than in forestomach. Since both tissues develop a high tumor incidence after oral administration of MBN, this observation suggests that despite their anatomic similarities the level of DNA modification required for malignant transformation differs considerably in these tissues. In the remaining organs, DNA alkylation was either considerably less (colon, glandular stomach, kidney) or not detectable (small intestine, spleen).

Administration of (^{14}C-*methyl*)MBN to mice in the drinking water led to a very high level of DNA methylation in both esophagus and forestomach (Table 2). This corresponds well with carcinogenicity studies which revealed a 100% incidence of carcinomas at these sites. On the other hand oral administration greatly reduced the extent of DNA methylation in the lung which is not a target organ for this route of application.

INDUCTION OF GASTRIC CANCER BY
N-METHYL-*N'*-NITRO-*N*-NITROSOGUANIDINE

Adjusted mortality rates of 52 countries for the year 1973 show that the incidence of gastric cancer was highest in Japan (59.6 males per 100,000) and lowest in Thailand (2.2). Since Japanese immigrants to North America rapidly acquire the low U.S. incidence (7.5), a strong environmental influence is likely to be involved. High risk factors are the custom of eating starchy foods in large amounts as a staple food, and the consumption of highly salted foods and Japanese pickles, and little animal protein and dairy products, but no chemical carcinogen has been positively

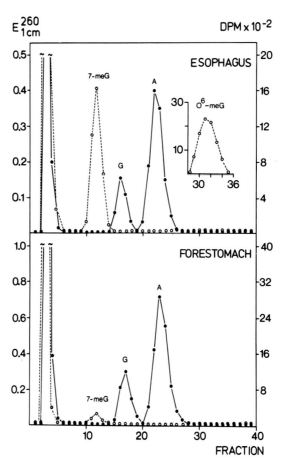

FIG. 2. Chromatographs of acid DNA hydrolysates from esophagus and forestomach of rats which after 20 hr of water withdrawal were allowed to drink approximately 5 ml of an aqueous solution containing 60 ppm (^{14}C-*methyl*)MBN (2.5 mg/kg; 17.9 mCi/mmole; survival time 4 hr). DNA was isolated from the pooled organs of 8 adult male Wistar rats and hydrolysed in 0.1 HCl (37°C; 20 hr). Neutralized hydrolysates were chromatographed on Sephasorb columns as described by Hodgson et al. (6). E^{1cm}_{260}, O---O; d.p.m., ●—●.

identified as causative agent (1). In rats, chronic administration of MNNG in the drinking water (80 ppm) causes a high incidence of carcinomas of the glandular stomach and, less frequently, of the duodenum (24,25).

Although extensive studies have been carried out on the sequential development of MNNG-induced gastric carcinomas and a variety of modulating factors (including preexisting ulcers, strain differences, partial gastrectomy and diets), little is known about the biochemical basis for preferential tumor induction in the glandular stomach. We found that after a single oral dose of (^{14}C-methyl)MNNG in the drinking water (2.5 mg/kg; 80 mg/l) the extent of DNA methylation in the target tissue exceeded that of any other segment of the gastrointestinal tract (Table 3). In glan-

TABLE 3. *DNA alkylation by MNNG and thiol concentrations in various tissues*

Organ	Methylated DNA purines		Thiol concentration (μmoles/g wt. tissue)
	7-methylguanine	O⁶-methylguanine	
Esophagus	9.9	n.d.	0.279
Forestomach	22.2	n.d.	0.119
Stomach	204.7	9.0	1.249
Duodenum	169.8	6.7	2.149
Liver	5.7	n.d.	5.003

(Data from ref. 26., with permission.)
Female Wistar rats (WIS/HAN) received a single oral dose of (^{14}C-*methyl*) MNNG (80 ppm, 2.5 mg/kg; 5 mCi/mmole) in the drinking water. After a survival time of 5 hr, DNA was isolated from the pooled organs of 8 rats, hydrolyzed and analyzed on Sephasorb HP columns. Values for methylated DNA purines are expressed as μmoles/ mole guanine. n.d., not detectable. Free thiol concentrations were determined in acid-soluble supernatants prepared from different rat organs using the Ellman procedure (5). The values shown are the mean of 5–7 rats.

TABLE 4. *Capacity of cell-free extracts for removal of O⁶-methylguanine from DNA in vitro[a]*

Organ	Pretreatment	f.moles removed/mg/30 min
Liver	—	102
	MBN[b]	216
	MNNG[c]	126
Esophagus	—	n.c.
	MBN[b]	n.c.
Gland.stomach	—	n.c.
	MNNG[c]	n.c.

n.c., not calculable
[a]Extracts from adult male Wistar rats were prepared and assayed as described by Pegg et al. (18).
[b]20 ppm in the drinking water over a period of 3 weeks.
[c]80 ppm in the drinking water over a period of 3 weeks.

dular stomach, concentrations of 7-methylguanine were 9 and 21 times higher than in DNA of forestomach and esophagus respectively. In duodenal DNA, 7-methylguanine values were only 17% lower than in the glandular stomach and this correlates with the observation that second to the glandular stomach, duodenum is a preferred site of tumor induction by MNNG in the rat. Since the bioactivation of MNNG does not require microsomal enzymes we assumed that the uptake by and the rate of decomposition in the gastric mucosa may differ from other segments of the gastrointestinal tract. Since SH-compounds, e.g., cysteine, greatly accelerate the decomposition of MNNG and the formation of its ultimate reactant, methyl-diazonium hydroxide, we determined the concentrations of thiols in target and nontarget tissues. The results shown in Table 1 reveal rather low values in esophagus and forestomach and 5- to 20-fold higher concentrations in glandular stomach and intestines. This indicates that the lack of susceptibility of esophagus and forestomach is due to their low thiol content and that after oral administration, MNNG is only bioactivated to a significant extent upon reaching the glandular stomach. A significant fraction of the carcinogen passes the stomach but decomposes in the duodenum, leaving the lower intestinal segments (jejunum, ileum, colon) largely unexposed to the parent carcinogen.

To exclude a coincidental correlation between high thiol concentrations and extensive DNA alkylation by MNNG in glandular stomach, we carried out additional experiments using a thiol blocking agent, *N*-ethylmaleimide (NEM). This compound was found to inhibit completely the thiol-mediated decomposition of MNNG *in vitro* and greatly reduce thiol concentrations *in vivo*. When MNNG was given intragastrically together with NEM (50 mg/kg), covalent binding to forestomach, glandular stomach, and upper duodenum was almost completely abolished.

Autoradiographs of the upper gastrointestinal tract (Fig. 3) showed that the distribution of (^{14}C-*methyl*)MNNG-derived radioactivity depends on the mode of ap-

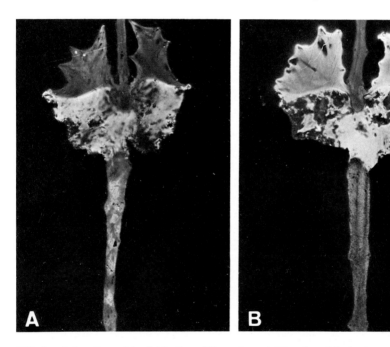

FIG. 3. Autoradiographic distribution of tissue-bound ^{14}C-radioactivity in the upper gastrointestinal tract following a single exposure to (^{14}C-*methyl*)MNNG. **A,** Following a 20 hr period of water deprivation, female Wistar rats were allowed to drink 5 ml of an aqueous solution containing ^{14}C-MNNG (80 ppm; 2.5 mg/kg; 10 mCi/mmole) and were killed 5 hr later. Alkylation *(light areas)* occurs preferentially in the glandular stomach and, to a lesser extent, in the duodenum. **B,** ^{14}C-MNNG was given as a single intragastric dose (50 μCi in 0.6 ml; 15 mCi/mmole). Labeling occurs in both forestomach and glandular stomach. (Data from ref. 26, with permission.)

plication. Following a single exposure to MNNG in the drinking water, alkylation occurred mainly in the glandular stomach and duodenum, the preferred sites of tumor induction for this route of application. When ^{14}C-MNNG was given intragastrically (by gavage), alkylation occurred in both glandular stomach and forestomach (Fig. 3), probably due to an extended period of exposure. This mode of application is indeed known to cause the induction of tumors in both glandular stomach and forestomach (20).

CONCLUSIONS

Several factors contributing to the organ-specific effects of chemical carcinogens have been identified, including tissue distribution of the parent carcinogen, bioactivation, DNA modification, DNA repair and cell turnover. Our present knowledge is insufficient to compose a unifying theory that would enable us to predict the principal target tissue and species susceptibility for methylating carcinogens but from the present and previous studies (12,17) some general conclusions can be drawn:

1. In the gastrointestinal tract of laboratory rodents, incidence and location of tumors closely correlate with the initial extent of DNA methylation. This is particularly true for the promutagenic base O^6-methylguanine. However, the extent of DNA modification required to produce a certain tumor incidence is not identical in each tissue and species.

2. High levels of DNA alkylation in specific sites can result from a variety of factors, including preferential bioactivation in the target tissue (MBN), accelerated decomposition mediated by cellular thiols (MNNG) and insufficient systemic distribution (first-pass-effect) of the parent carcinogen.

3. O^6-Methylguanine can be enzymically removed from DNA and in several rat tissues tumor induction has been shown to correlate with a repair deficiency in the target organ (17). However, species and strain differences in the response to methylating carcinogens are not paralleled by differences in the repair capacity for O^6-methylguanine. In the gastrointestinal tract of rats the capacity for enzymic removal of O^6-methylguanine is very low (when measured *in vitro*, Table 4) and apparently noninducible.

ACKNOWLEDGMENT

This work was supported by grants from the Deutsche Forschungsgemeinschaft (SFB 31) and Bundesministerium Forschung und Technologie (CMT 15).

REFERENCES

1. Aoki, K. (1980): Epidemiology of Gastric Cancer, with Reference to Etiology. *Igan to Shidan Kenshin*, 48:44–54.
2. Autrup, H., and Stoner, G. D. (1982): Metabolism of N-Nitrosamines by Cultured Human and Rat Esophagus. *Cancer Res.*, 42:1307–1311.

3. Bibbo, M. (1979): Transplacental Effects of Diethylstilbestrol. In: *Current Topics in Pathology, Vol. 66 (Perinatal Pathology)*, edited by E. Grundmann, pp. 191–212. Springer Verlag, Berlin-Heidelberg-New York.

4. Druckrey, H., Preussmann, R., Ivanković, S., and Schmähl, D. (1967): Organotrope carcinogene Wirkungen bei 65 verschiedenen N-Nitroso-Verbindungen an BD-Ratten. *Z. Krebsforsch.*, 69:103–201.

5. Ellman, G. L. (1959): Tissue Sulfhydryl Groups. *Arch. Biochem. Biophys.*, 82:70–77.

6. Hodgson, R. M., Wiessler, M., and Kleihues, P. (1980): Preferential methylation of target organ DNA by the oesophageal carcinogen N-Nitrosomethylbenzylamine. *Carcinogenesis*, 1:861–866.

7. Hodgson, R. M., Schweinsberg, F., Wiessler, M., and Kleihues, P. (1982): Mechanism of Esophageal Tumor Induction in Rats by N-Nitrosomethylbenzylamine and Its Ring-methylated Analog N-Nitrosomethyl(4-methyl-benzyl)amine. *Cancer Res.*, 42:2836–2840.

8. Hsia, C.-C., Sun, T.-T., Wang, U.-U., Anderson, L. M., Armstrong, D., and Good, R. A. (1981): Enhancement of formation of the esophageal carcinogen benzylmethylnitrosamine from its precursors by Candida albicans. *Proc. Natl. Acad. Sci. USA*, 78:1878–1881.

9. IARC Working Group (1980): An Evaluation of Chemicals and Industrial Processes Associated with Cancer in Humans Based on Human and Animal Data: IARC Monographs Volumes 1 to 20. *Cancer Res.*, 40:1–12.

10. Kleihues, P., Veit, C., Wiessler, M., and Hodgson, R. M. (1981): DNA methylation by N-nitrosomethylbenzylamine in target and non-target tissues of NMRI mice. *Carcinogenesis*, 2:897–899.

11. Kleihues, P. (1982): Developmental Carcinogenicity. In: *Developmental Toxicology*, edited by K. Snell, pp. 211–246. Croom Helm, London.

12. Kleihues, P., Hodgson, R. M., Veit, C., Schweinsberg, F., and Wiessler, M. (1983): DNA modification and repair in vivo: Towards a biochemical basis of organ-specific carcinogenesis by methylating agents. In: *Organ and Species Specificity in Chemical Carcinogenesis*, edited by R. Langenbach, S. Nesnow and J. M. Rice, pp. 509–528. New York: Plenum Publishing Corp. *(in press)*.

13. Labuc, G. E., and Archer, M. C. (1982): Esophageal and Hepatic Microsomal Metabolism of N-Nitrosomethylbenzylamine and N-Nitrosodimethylamine in the Rat. *Cancer Res.*, 42:3181–3186.

14. Li, M., Li, P., and Li, B. (1980): Recent Progress in Research on Esophageal Cancer in China. *Adv. Cancer Res.*, 33:173–249.

15. Lu, S. H., Camus, A.-M., Ji, C., Wang, Y. L., Wang, M. Y., and Bartsch, H. (1980): Mutagenicity in Salmonella typhimurium of N-3-methylbutyl-N-1-methyl-acetonyl-nitrosamine and N-methyl-N-benzylnitrosamine, N-nitrosation products isolated from corn-bread contaminated with commonly occurring moulds in Linshien county, a high incidence area for oesophageal cancer in Northern China. *Carcinogenesis*, 1:867–870.

16. Lu, S. H., and Lin, P. (1982): Recent research on the etiology of esophageal cancer in China. *Z. Gastroenterologie*, 20:361–367.

17. O'Connor, P. J. (1981): Interaction of Chemical Carcinogens with Macromolecules. *J. Cancer Res. Clin. Oncol.*, 99:167–186.

18. Pegg, A. E., Perry, W., and Bennett, R. A. (1981): Effect of partial hepatectomy on removal of O^6-methylguanine from alkylated DNA by rat liver extracts. *Biochem. J.*, 197:195–201.

19. Sander, J., and Schweinsberg, F. (1973): Tumorinduktion bei Mäusen durch N-Methylbenzylnitrosamin in niedriger Dosierung. *Z. Krebsforsch.*, 79:157–161.

20. Schoental, R. (1966): Carcinogenic Activity of N-Methyl-N-nitroso-N'-nitroguanidine. *Nature (London)*, 209:726–727.

21. Schweinsberg, F., Schott-Kollat, P., and Bürkle, G. (1977): Veränderung der Toxizität und Carcinogenität von N-Methyl-N-nitrosobenzylamin durch Methylsubstitution am Phenylrest bei Ratten. *Z. Krebsforsch.*, 88:231–236.

22. Schweinsberg, F., and Bürkle, V. (1981): Wirkung von Disulfiram auf die Toxizität und Carcinogenität von N-Methyl-nitrosobenzylamin bei Ratten. *J. Cancer Res. Clin. Oncol.*, 102:43–47.

23. Stinson, S. F., Squire, R. A., and Sporn, M. B. (1978): Pathology of esophageal neoplasms and associated proliferative lesions induced in rats by N-methyl-N-benzylnitrosamine. *J. Natl. Cancer Inst.*, 6:1471–1475.

24. Sugimura, T., and Fujimura, S. (1967): Tumour Production in the Glandular Stomach of Rat by N-Methyl-N'-nitro-N-nitrosoguanidine. *Nature (Lond.)*, 216:943–944.
25. Sugimura, T., Fujimura, S., and Baba, T. (1970): Tumor Production in the Glandular Stomach and Alimentary Tract of the Rat by N-Methyl-N'-nitro-N-nitrosoguanidine. *Cancer Res.*, 30:455–465.
26. Wiestler, O., von Deimling, A., Kleihues, P., and Kobori, O. (1983): Location of N-methyl-N'-nitro-N-nitrosoguanidine—induced gastrointestinal tumors correlates with thiol distribution. *Carcinogenesis*, 4:879–883.
27. Yang, C. S. (1980): Research on Esophageal Cancer in China: a Review. *Cancer Res.*, 40:2633–2644.

Biochemical Basis of Chemical Carcinogenesis,
edited by H. Greim, R. Jung, M. Kramer,
H. Marquardt, and F. Oesch.
Raven Press, New York © 1984.

Differential DNA Alkylation, Repair and Replication in Hepatocarcinogenesis

J. A. Swenberg, J. G. Lewis, M. A. Bedell, K. C. Billings,
M. C. Dyroff, and C. Lindamood III

*Chemical Industry Institute of Toxicology, Department of Pathology,
Research Triangle Park, NC 27709*

Presently, the long-term animal bioassay represents one of the major tools employed in drug and chemical safety evaluation for assessing a chemical's carcinogenic potential. A recent survey of such studies conducted by the NTP/NCI bioassay program showed that rodent liver tumors were responsible for 61% of the positive studies (7). Because of this dominance, we began a series of research studies aimed at gaining a better understanding of the mechanisms involved in hepatocarcinogenesis. Previous investigations had relied primarily on biochemical or autoradiographic data obtained from whole liver. Such data is heavily biased toward effects on hepatocytes, the predominant cell type of the liver. However, hepatocarcinogenesis frequently involves other cell types such as endothelial cells, bile duct cells, and Kupffer cells. Effects of chemicals on these minority cell populations of the liver are easily masked in whole liver studies. If critical mechanisms in hepatocarcinogenesis are to be identified, it is imperative that such studies compare and contrast biochemical changes in target and nontarget cells of the target organ. Quantitative relationships that hold up within the target organ could also be contrasted with nontarget tissues. A second major objective of these investigations was to examine the effects of chronic administration of the test substance, since this is the dosing regimen usually employed in carcinogen bioassays. In order to accomplish this, several chemicals that primarily induce either hepatocellular carcinomas or angiosarcomas of rodent liver following chronic administration were selected. These included 1,2-dimethylhydrazine (SDMH), dimethylnitrosamine (DMN), diethylnitrosamine (DEN), dinitrotoluene (DNT) and 2-acetylaminofluorene (2-AAF).

MECHANISMS INVOLVED IN THE INDUCTION
OF ANGIOSARCOMAS

Chronic administration of methylating agents requiring biotransformation frequently results in the induction of angiosarcomas in rats and mice. Our initial studies utilized ^{14}C-SDMH administered by gavage at 3 mg/kg to BD-IX rats (2). Two hours after carcinogen administration the animals were anesthetized and their livers perfused with collagenase. The mixed liver cell suspension obtained was then separated into hepatocytes and nonparenchymal cells (NPC) using centrifugal elutriation. The NPC population contained endothelial cells and Kupffer cells. DNA isolated from the two cell populations had similar initial amounts of O^6-methylguanine (O^6MG) and N-7-methylguanine (7MG) with O^6/N-7 ratios of 0.08 to .09. In contrast, 24 hrs after a single administration of ^{14}C-SDMH the hepatocytes had only one-tenth the initial amount of O^6MG, whereas the NPC still had more than half of this promutagenic lesion. This cell type difference was even greater in rats given a second dose of ^{14}C-SDMH 24 hrs after the first and killed 24 hrs later (2). The O^6/N-7 ratios differed by a factor of 28, indicating selective repair of O^6MG by the hepatocytes. Furthermore, there was selective incorporation of radioactivity into the normal purine bases of NPC DNA, suggesting selective increases in cell proliferation by the target cells. Thus, the target cells for angiosarcoma induction were accumulating O^6MG and replicating, providing opportunity for mispairing resulting in GC→AT transitions, while the hepatocytes were neither accumulating O^6MG nor replicating.

Subsequent studies on SDMH utilized continuous administration of 30 ppm SDMH in the drinking water to F-344 rats. O^6MG and 7MG concentrations in DNA from the two cell populations were determined using high performance liquid chromatography and fluorescence or UV detection, respectively (1). Hepatocyte O^6MG concentrations were highest after only one day's exposure and decreased rapidly during the first 3 to 4 days to about 4 pmole/mg DNA. O^6MG assumed even lower concentrations in hepatocytes after 16 and 28 days, averaging only 1 pmole/mg DNA. The opposite trend was apparent in the NPC. O^6MG accumulated during the first 8 days of exposure, reaching nearly 60 pmole/mg DNA. This peak was followed by a decrease that plateaued between 16 and 28 days at about 15 pmole/mg DNA. Such cell specific differences were not apparent for the major alkylation product, 7MG. Concentrations of 7MG increased rapidly in hepatocytes and NPC during the first 3 to 4 days of administration, after which similar steady state levels were maintained (1). The rapid decline in hepatocyte O^6MG concentrations, even though new O^6MG was being formed each time the rat ingested SDMH, suggested enhanced repair capacity. Subsequent investigations clearly demonstrated that control hepatocytes had about 5 times more O^6-alkylguanine alkyl acceptor protein activity than did NPC and that this high level of activity was enhanced 2 to 3 fold during continuous administration of SDMH (10). In contrast, O^6-alkylguanine alkyl acceptor protein activity was decreased in NPC during the period of rapid O^6MG accumulation and then returned to control levels.

More recently, the NPC have been further separated into Kupffer and endothelial cells (4). Continuous administration of 30 ppm SDMH for up to 16 days resulted in high concentrations of 7MG in hepatocytes and Kupffer cells, but only half this amount in endothelial cells. However, exposure of rats to SDMH resulted in high concentrations of O^6MG in endothelial cells, intermediate amounts in Kupffer cells and rapid removal from hepatocytes. *In vitro* exposure to SDMH resulted in similar cytotoxicity curves for cultured hepatocytes and Kupffer cells, whereas no cytotoxicity was apparent in endothelial cells. Collectively, these data suggest that both hepatocytes and Kupffer cells can activate SDMH, while endothelial cells probably acquire an active intermediate from neighboring hepatocytes and Kupffer cells. That endothelial cells are markedly deficient in O^6MG repair is evidenced by the fact that they developed $O^6/N7$ ratios 20 times higher than hepatocytes or Kupffer cells after just 4 days exposure. Endothelial cells became more proficient at removing O^6MG during the second week of exposure, but maintained $O^6/N-7$ ratios 30 times greater than hepatocytes and 4 times greater than Kupffer cells.

Cell replication was also investigated in NPC and hepatocytes of rats exposed to 30 ppm SDMH in the drinking water for up to 28 days (3). SDMH exposure caused a marked mitogenic response in NPC between 4 and 28 days, with a 28-fold increase in *de novo* DNA synthesis compared to controls. Increases were also noted in hepatocytes; the extent, however, was much less. Similar investigations on Kupffer and endothelial cells demonstrated that both cell types had marked increases in tritiated thymidine incorporation (4).

A similar model exists in C3H mice exposed to 10 ppm DMN in the drinking water, where a high incidence of vascular tumors of the liver is induced. Under these conditions, progressive increases in O^6MG and *de novo* DNA synthesis occurred in NPC (6). 7MG concentrations were similar in NPC and hepatocytes, while hepatocyte O^6MG remained at about 4 pmole/mg DNA throughout a 32 day exposure. Hepatocytes had about a 3-fold increase in *de novo* DNA synthesis throughout the exposure period. These data indicated that the mouse hepatocyte O^6MG response to exposure was markedly different than that of the rat. Subsequent studies on the O^6-alkylguanine alkyl acceptor protein demonstrated no enhancement of activity during the 32 day exposure (5). This clearly demonstrates that neither cell proliferation nor the presence of O^6MG are adequate to induce this repair activity in mouse hepatocytes.

Thus, in both continuous exposure models of angiosarcoma, there was a much greater probability for GC→AT transitions due to O^6MG mispairing during cell replication in the target cell population, the NPC. Hepatocytes exhibited rapid repair of O^6MG and a lesser mitogenic response to exposure, providing a much smaller opportunity for mutation. It therefore appears that O^6MG represents the predominant promutagenic lesion responsible for the initiation of angiosarcomas by methylating agents. Conversely, O^6MG appears to be much less important for initiating hepatocytes, due to rapid repair and less cell replication.

MECHANISMS INVOLVED IN THE INDUCTION OF HEPATOCELLULAR CARCINOMAS

At the same time the previous studies on SDMH were being conducted, comparison investigations were run on DEN. When Fischer-344 rats are exposed to 40 ppm DEN in the drinking water, nearly 100% develop hepatocellular carcinomas (12). DNA from hepatocytes and NPC of rats exposed to DEN for up to 28 days contained minimal amounts of 7-ethylguanine (7EG) and O^6-ethylguanine (O^6EG)

with most samples being below the limits of detection (1 pmole O^6EG/injection and 10 pmole 7EG/injection). Hepatocytes and NPC exhibited a similar increase in *de novo* DNA synthesis, except that the increase in hepatocytes preceded that in NPC (3). Since this exposure protocol is extremely efficient for initiating hepatocytes, it appears likely that promutagenic lesions other than O^6EG may play major roles in hepatocyte initiation. A prominent candidate is O^4-ethylthymine, an alkylated base with a reported half-life of 19 days (8). The fluorescence HPLC analysis system utilized for O^6MG is not suitable for quantifying this adduct, so other methods such as radioimmunoassay or ^{32}P-postlabeling will have to be used.

Cell specificity in chemical carcinogenesis is not only dependent on DNA repair and replication, however, since different cell types have different capacities for metabolism. Hepatocytes can metabolize many chemicals to reactive intermediates, leading to selective exposure of hepatocyte DNA to ultimate carcinogens. Data in support of this concept for cell specificity have been obtained for 2-AAF and DNT.

We have utilized the cell separation methods referred to above to compare binding of carcinogen adducts to DNA of hepatocytes and NPC following administration of equimolar doses of AAF or N-OH-AAF (11). An assessment of the binding of [ring-^{3}H]-AAF to DNA of hepatocytes and NPC following a single i.p. injection demonstrated that hepatocytes had 2.7 times more carcinogen adducts per milligram DNA than NPC at the time of peak binding. Removal of carcinogen adducts was similar over a 72 hr time course. Analogous studies with [ring-^{3}H]-N-OH-AAF showed no significant difference in the amount of carcinogen bound or removed per milligram of hepatocyte and NPC DNA. When these data are adjusted for the amount of DNA at risk for the two cell populations, the results clearly show that the amount of carcinogen bound to the DNA of target cells, i.e., hepatocytes, is much greater. This cell specificity is greatest for the procarcinogen, AAF, suggesting that hepatocytes have greater metabolic competence for N-hydroxylating AAF. Although similar amounts of N-OH-AAF covalent binding were present per mg DNA in both cell types, the total amount bound to hepatocellular DNA versus NPC DNA was considerably greater. Thus, cell specificity in N-OH-AAF binding to DNA would still favor the induction of hepatocellular tumors.

An analogous situation exists for 2,6-DNT, a potent hepatocarcinogen in rats (11). Hepatocytes had greater covalent binding to their DNA than did NPC. Furthermore, the amount bound to hepatocyte DNA increased with repetitive dosing, whereas no accumulation occurred in NPC DNA.

CONCLUSIONS

Tissue and cell specificity in chemical carcinogenesis is dependent on a multiplicity of factors including the dose and route of exposure, absorption and distribution, the requirement for and site of biotransformation, chemical reactivity with DNA, the cellular capacity for repairing promutagenic DNA lesions, and the amount of cell replication that takes place prior to such repair. Expression of these early events in chemical carcinogenesis may be further complicated by exposure to promoting agents and toxins that selectively expand populations of initiated cells.

Cellular tropism of specific chemicals will be influenced to different degrees by these factors. For example, high doses of alkylating agents can saturate the efficient hepatocyte O^6-alkylguanine alkyl acceptor protein repair system, resulting in a greater likelihood of replication of a damaged template and resultant fixation of GC→AT transitions. Compensatory cell proliferation following selective toxicity is also dependent on dose. Both the magnitude of dose and concommitant exposure to other agents can influence the site of biotransformation. Low oral doses of DMN are exclusively metabolized in the liver, whereas higher doses are activated in the kidney. Selenium can selectively decrease SDMH metabolism in liver, resulting in increased alkylation of other tissues.

Metabolic differences between male and female rats result in greater covalent binding and subsequent tumor formation in males with AAF and DNT. The metabolic competence of different cell populations within the target organ affects the extent of DNA adduct formation as well as toxicity-induced compensatory cell proliferation. This usually results in greater adduct formation in hepatocytes, both in terms of adducts per mg DNA and adducts per total cell population. Removal of covalently bound AAF was similar in hepatocytes and NPC, whereas major differences were apparent for removal of O^6-alkylguanine. In the latter case, cell specificity is also dependent on chemical reactivity with DNA. For example, the major promutagenic lesion induced in DNA by SN_1 methylating agents is O^6MG. O^6MG will therefore represent the major lesion responsible for initiation in those cell types, such as liver NPC and neuroglial cells, that have low to moderate O^6-alkylguanine alkyl acceptor protein activity. In contrast, ethylating agents produce a greater proportion of promutagenic O-alkylated pyrimidines relative to O-alkylation of guanine. These O-alkylated pyrimidines are removed from hepatocyte DNA much more slowly (8,9), so that during chronic exposure they provide increasing numbers of templates for mutations in cells that have high O^6-alkylguanine alkyl acceptor protein activity and efficient removal of O^6-alkylguanine.

Finally, the importance of cell replication in chemical carcinogenesis must be kept in mind. Mutations in a given cell population are believed to result from miscoding of promutagenic damage in the parental strand during DNA replication. Mutations that are fixed in the daughter strand are amplified in succeeding generations through cell replication. Amplification can occur at an enhanced rate due to selective cytotoxicity or specific promotion by the carcinogen, or by exposure to other agents. Understanding a process as complex as chemical carcinogenesis will require quantification of these individual components at the cellular level.

REFERENCES

1. Bedell, M., Lewis, J. G., Billings, K. C., and Swenberg, J. A. (1982): Cellular specificity in hepatocarcinogenesis: O^6-methylguanine preferentially accumulates in target cell DNA during continuous exposure of rats to 1,2-dimethylhydrazine. *Cancer Res.*, 42:3079–3083.
2. Lewis, J. G., and Swenberg, J. A. (1980): Differential repair of O^6-methylguanine in DNA of rat hepatocytes and nonparenchymal cells. *Nature*, 288:185–187.
3. Lewis, J. G., and Swenberg, J. A. (1982): The effect of 1,2-dimethyl hydrazine and diethylnitro-

samine on cell replication and unscheduled DNA synthesis in target and nontarget cell populations in rat liver following chronic administration. *Cancer Res.*, 42:89–92.

4. Lewis, J. G., and Swenberg, J. A. (1983): The kinetics of DNA alkylation, repair and replication in hepatocytes, Kupffer cells, and sinusoidal endothelial cells in rat liver during continuous exposure to 1,2-dimethyl hydrazine. *Carcinogenesis*, 4:529–536.

5. Lindamood, C., Bedell, M. A., Billings, K. C., Dyroff, M. C., and Swenberg, J. A. (1983): O⁶-alkylguanine akyl acceptor protein activity in hepatocytes of C3H and C57BL mice during dimethylnitrosamine exposure. *Chem.-Biol. Interact.*, 45:382–386.

6. Lindamood, C., Bedell, M. A., Billings, K. C., and Swenberg, J. A. (1982): Alkylation and *de novo* DNA synthesis of liver cell DNA of C3H mice during continuous dimethylnitrosamine exposure. *Cancer Res.*, 42:4153–4157.

7. NTP/NCI Bioassay Program review. Board of Scientific Counselors meeting, March 10–12, 1982.

8. Scherer, E., Timmer, A. P., and Emmelot, P. (1980): Formation by diethylnitrosamine and persistence of O⁴-ethylthymidine in rat liver DNA. *Cancer Lett.*, 10:1–6.

9. Singer, B., Spengler, S., and Bodell, W. J. (1981): Tissue-dependent enzyme-mediated repair or removal of O-ethylpyrimidines and ethyl purines in carcinogen-treated rats. *Carcinogenesis*, 2:1069–1073.

10. Swenberg, J. A., Bedell, M. A., Billings, K. C., Umbenhauer, D. R., and Pegg, A. E. (1982): Cell-specific differences in O⁶-alkylguanine DNA repair activity during continuous carcinogen exposure. *Proc. Natl. Acad. Sci. USA*, 79:5499–5502.

11. Swenberg, J. A., Rickert, D. E., Baranyi, B. L., and Goodman, J. I. (1983): Cell specificity in DNA binding and repair of chemical carcinogens. *Environ. Health Perspectives*, 49:155–163.

12. Weisburger, J. H., Madison, R. M., Ward, J. M., Viguera, C., and Weisburger, E. K. (1975): Modification of diethylnitrosamine liver carcinogenesis with phenobarbital but not with immunosuppression. *J. Natl. Cancer Inst.*, 54:1185–1188.

Biochemical Basis of Chemical Carcinogenesis,
edited by H. Greim, R. Jung, M. Kramer,
H. Marquardt, and F. Oesch.
Raven Press, New York © 1984.

Summary and Conclusions

H. Greim

Department of Toxicology, Institute for Biochemistry and Toxicology,
Gesellschaft für Strahlen- und Umweltforschung
D-8042 Neuherberg-München, Federal Republic of Germany

Three main topics have been discussed during the past few days of our workshop:

1. The metabolic control of ultimate carcinogens with regard to activation, inactivation and sequestration;
2. The mechanisms of action of chemical carcinogenesis; and
3. Adduct formation of ultimate carcinogens with DNA and repair.

The three topics have been chosen to define the status of information on the mechanisms involved in chemical carcinogenesis. This provides information whether a direct correlation between the dose and the carcinogenic effect of a chemical is to be expected or whether certain cellular responses suggest a deviation from linearity, especially at the low-dose range. Therefore, the main aspect of this conclusion is to stress those points raised in the different contributions and discussions, which may indicate mechanisms suggesting thresholds at which the dose-effect relation deviates from linearity.

ROLE OF METABOLISM

The first session dealt with the metabolic control of the ultimate carcinogens regarding activation, inactivation and sequestration.

The major metabolic inactivation mechanisms such as GSH-conjugation by GSH-S-transferases, glucuronidation and sulfation, the epoxide hydrolase and the dihydrodiol dehydrogenase have been presented. The efficiencies of these reactions have been exemplified by the specific metabolism of aromatic amines, amides, aflatoxin, and diethylstilbestrol. Species differences in the sensitivity towards chemical carcinogens and organ-specificities became explainable by demonstrating species- and organ-specificities in Phase I or Phase II activities, including human tissues.

In context with the multistep process involved in chemical hepatocarcinogenesis, attention has been focussed on the possibility that different metabolites, generated from procarcinogens such as acetylaminofluorene, may influence different stages of carcinogenesis. The sulfate ester of the *N*-hydroxy derivative seems to be associated with hepatotoxicity and promotion, whereas deacetylation-3 mediated by an acyltransferase seems to be the prerequisite for initiation.

Studying Phase I and Phase II enzyme activities in human tissue and in outbred animals revealed large interindividual differences which are not present in inbred strains. These differences are mostly neglected in extrapolation from inbred animal experiments to the heterogenous populations of man.

Very helpful in the evaluation of mutagenicity studies on nitro compounds has been the identification of a multiplicity of bacterial nitroreductases, which are also present in mammalian cells (McCoy, chapter 8), although with differing qualitative and quantitative activities. This work will help to detect risky nitrocompounds which are present in a wide variety of complex mixtures, especially in diesel emissions.

Although presently available information on Phase I and Phase II reactions of chemical carcinogens provides excellent tools to understand the different quantitative effects in species and in the different organs, they obviously do not provide a general rational basis for a threshold effect of the ultimate carcinogens formed or left over in the presence of a potent inactivation mechanism. From enzyme kinetic considerations all these reactions are subjected to quasi first order kinetics with the consequence of a linear correlation between the metabolically inactivated product versus the unmetabolized substrate, especially in the lower dose range. Thus, in general, the extent of metabolic conversion to less active metabolites will only determine the slope of the dose:effect curve, but does not suggest deviation from linearity.

However, some data indicate that a nonlinear dose-effect correlation may exist. An example is the situation when two enzymes with different K_M values metabolize the same substrate as is the case of phenols (Bock, chapter 4). At low doses, they are preferentially inactivated by the sulfotransferases which have low K_M values. With increasing concentrations this enzyme becomes saturated and the phenols become substrates of the glucuronosyl transferases having higher K_M values. A change in the dose-effect curve is the consequence.

The second example has been given by Dr. Watanabe on the p-phenyl-phenol. Similar to paracetamol, this chemical is subjected to sulfation and glucuronidation. With increasing doses both enzymes become saturated with the result of increasing formation of the dihydroxy-compound via monooxygenase activity. At the same time, dihydroxy-sulfate esters appear in the urine which seems to correlate with a steep increase in bladder tumor rate.

Regardless of the mechanisms involved, one can fully agree that in such instances a drastic decrease in the tumor incidence at low doses is to be anticipated.

Many of the data presented in this volume have been obtained from *in vitro* experiments with mammalian cell cultures.

Although the genetic system, membranes, energy supply, and synthesis of macromolecules seem to represent the situation *in vivo*, metabolic capacity, especially the ratio between activating and inactivating metabolism, in most of these cells is altered or even absent. This should encourage further work to establish cell lines with intact metabolic capacities similar to primary cells.

FATE OF DNA ADDUCTS

The multistage process of chemical carcinogenesis is initiated by the interaction of the ultimate carcinogens with the DNA. Although increasing information on the structural characterization of the DNA lesions became available by the introduction of highly sophisticated analytical procedures, detailed analysis has only been performed with a few carcinogens. These investigations indicate that many factors such as persistence of the lesion, status of cell proliferation, and saturation of repair capacity, affect the initiation process. Many of these factors have been presented in this volume.

A major initiating effect of methylating agents is supposed to be O^6-methylation of guanine. Very interesting and important for the discussion of threshold levels is that the methyl group can be removed and the base restored to normality. Of utmost importance is that this process is dose-dependent and saturable and, consequently, more efficient at low doses than at high doses. This has been demonstrated for methyl-groups after such as dimethylnitrosamine treatment as well as for ethyl groups, which are removed at a slower rate (Pegg, Chapter 24). Saturation of this process is to be expected. Removal is faster in rat than in mouse and exceeds both in human tissues. It can be induced in animal experiments after several weeks' treatment with methylating agents.

Since the removal of the methyl group is mediated via a protein, which accepts the methyl group with its cystein acceptor from the O^6-position of the guanine, the limiting step in this reaction is the removal of the methyl group from the cystein receptor. Thus, at low doses of a methylating agent as long as this receptor is not saturated, relatively more demethylation of the DNA occurs than at high saturating doses. This again indicates a change in the slope of the dose-effect curve.

In addition to dose-dependency of the removal of methyl groups, the extent of repair is influenced by the time between damage and the onset of cell replication (Maher, Chapter 15). Cells which have been prevented from replication can tolerate higher UV-doses than replicating cells, as determined by measuring cytotoxicity, mutagenicity, and transformation. This indicates that, with sufficient time, excision repair—at least in case of UV-induced dimers—removes essentially all or most of the potentially cytotoxic and mutagenic lesions. Similar results have been obtained with chemical carcinogenesis. Again, the time required for biological recovery was closely related with the length of time needed for excision repair synthesis.

Efficient removal, however, in the metabolically active epitheloid human cells A 549 occurred only during 24 hrs after treatment. Additional removal was slow and a sizable amount remained in the DNA during further incubation. Similarly, a sizable fraction of BP-induced lesion persisted over several generations in the tumor cell line A 549 of human lung. The cells possessed only limited capacity for removal of covalent DNA benzo(*a*)pyrene adducts although excision repair capacity was not saturated. It is open whether the cells lose their capacity for removal of BP-adducts during continued posttreatment incubation or whether the adducts become part of a DNA portion which cannot be repaired, possibly because the lesions are bypassed by the DNA replication enzymes at late stages of posttreatment incubation.

However, many questions on the functions of these persistent lesions remain open; for example, do they relate to the DNA which can be isolated from tumor cell lines and which is able to transform nontumor cells? These oncogenes can act across species barriers and may also act across tissue barriers as shown in cell lines obtained from different organs. They seem to derive via somatic mutation from sequences that exist in the normal genome. The successful attempts to localize these lesions within the genes have been presented in the exciting discussion by Dr. Weinberg (Chapter 14, this volume). Although it presently remains unknown how these point mutations have been induced in the oncogene, Weinberg's work strongly indicates that qualitative rather than quantitative aspects are of significance in the initiation process.

Qualitative aspects of the initiation process have also been indicated by Neumann (Chapter 6, this volume) demonstrating that in the case of transacetaminidostilbene the nontarget tissues liver and kidney not only revealed the greatest initial DNA binding, but these tissues also accumulated these lesions to a greater extent than the DNA in the target organ, the zymbals gland.

Furthermore, this at least questions the relevance of determining the extent of DNA-binding either to determine binding indices to define the relative potency of carcinogens or to exclude genetic activity of a chemical.

ROLE AND MECHANISMS OF TUMOR PROMOTERS

Several very interesting contributions to studies on the membrane effects of tumor-promoting and -transforming agents have been made. Several chemicals such as the phorbol esters and the indole alkaloid teleocidin seem to exert their transforming effects by disturbing membrane function and structure. They share certain structural features in their hydrophobic carbonyl- and hydroxymethyl residues attached to their respective ring systems which seem to define their ability to interact with the binding of the epidermal growth factor and the specific high affinity receptors at the cell surface. At the same time many biochemical changes such as disturbance of phospholipid metabolism or mitochondrial respiration and others can be observed. In addition to similarities of the carbonylhydroxymethyl residues, model building studies also revealed certain similar conformational features of the phorbol esters and teleocidine. It is suggested that other naturally occurring or synthetic compounds have similar features and share tumor-promoting activity when they also bind to the membrane. Such chemicals may have a broad significance in tumor promotion.

Interestingly, other tumor promotors such as benzo(a)pyrene, dimethylbenzanthracene, the naphthoflavones, and 3-methylcholanthrene which, at the same time, are well-known cytochrome $P-450_1$ inducers, also inhibit binding of the epidermal growth factor. However, this inhibition which has been determined in mouse embryo fibroblasts, does not occur immediately but with a time lag of a maximum of 24 hrs. It is speculated that these inducing agents act indirectly, for example via cytoplasmic and nuclear events or by metabolites. Since TCDD and phenobarbital do not exert this effect, the relevance of the delayed disturbance of epidermal growth factor binding by cytochrome P-450-inducers remains obscure. The many factors involved in the transformation have been discussed in chapters 16–20.

Although many details have been presented there is still no generally valid concept of the membranous effects of tumor promoting agents. Furthermore, little emphasis has been laid on the dose-dependency of these effects. Thus, a no-effect level of tumor-promoting agents has to be verified.

Transforming growth factors that interact with highly specific alpha- and beta-receptors have been isolated from the supernatant fluids of tumor cells growing in cultures and from several tissues. The effectors of the alpha-receptor are proteins of a molecular weight of about 6000. Purification further revealed that they slightly differ in structure from the epidermal growth factor but that there is a considerable sequence homology of the transforming growth factors isolated from tumors of different species and from virus-transformed cells. The effectors of the beta-receptor have been isolated from different normal and neoplastic tissues. Both tumor growth factor species must occupy their specific receptors when the transforming cell gains growth independence.

Whether the retinoids inhibit tumor formation by directly interfering with the membranous transforming mechanism or via cytoplasmatic or nuclear events modifying gene expression is unclear. They inhibit chemical induced cell transformation and prevent experimental cancers in different organs such as bladder, liver, pancreas, and others. Why selenium and superoxide dismutase, which scavenge free radicals and block lipid peroxidation, inhibit transformation is presently unknown. This will become a promising field of research because reactive oxygen species which induce lipid peroxidation are constantly formed in the cell.

FINAL CONCLUSIONS

From the perspective of a toxicologist several points became apparent. It has been confirmed that there is no commonly valid approach to evaluate the risk of a chemical carcinogen. Carcinogens act through different mechanisms and induce different cellular responses, which, in a few cases, may be thresholded. Thus, to provide a sound basis for extrapolation from high to low doses, as much information as possible on each chemical is required. This includes metabolic activation and inactivation in different organs and the target organ, interference with DNA, repair, promotion, and transforming capabilities in different species and over a wide range of concentrations.

Only this will permit rational extrapolation of the high doses frequently used in animal experiments to low doses of human exposure and determine whether a linear dose-effect curve is to be anticipated or if a deviation from linearity can be suggested.

Subject Index

Subject Index

2-Acetamidofluorene (AAF)
  as carcinogen, 35–38,47–50
  cytochrome P-450 and, 47–50
  DNA damage by, 35–36,42
  hydroxylation of, 47–49
  liver tumors and, 35–36,38–39
  metabolism of, 47–50
  as mutagen, 48,51–53
2-Acetamidophenanthrene (AAP)
  DNA binding, 35–36,42
  mammary tumors and, 35–36
2-Acetylaminofluorene (2-AAF), tumor
    induction by, 287, 290–291,293
Adipocytes, differentiation of, 167–169
Aflatoxin
  GSH conjugation of, 6,10
  liver and, 10
Aflatoxin B$_1$ (AFB$_1$)
  DNA binding of, 33–35,124,126
  epoxide of, 34
  GSH-S-transferase and, 34
  liver tumors and, 33
  metabolism of, 33–35
Ah receptor
  cytochrome P-450 and, 90
  enzyme induction and, 89–90
Aldrin epoxidases, induction of, 83–84
Alkylation
  differential DNA, 287
  of DNA, 249–250
  in DNA repair, 265
  MBN and, 283
  MNNG and, 283
2-Aminofluorene
  DNA binding of, 125
  metabolism of, 62–63
Anchorage dependency
  neoplastic transformation and,
    170–171,177
  tumorigenicity and, 152,154–155
Angiosarcomas
  induction of, 287–289

SDMH and, 287–289
Aplysiatoxin
  stereochemistry of, 199–200
  as tumor promoter, 198–199
Aromatic amines, carcinogenesis and,
    35–38,42,47–57
Aryl hydrocarbon hydroxylase (AHH)
  in cells in culture, 78–79,124–125
  induction of, 78–79
  interindividual differences in, 131
  in tumor cells, 78–79
Arylhydroxlamines
  DNA adducts of, 57,60
  mutagenicity of, 62
  nitroarenes and, 57,60

Benzanthracene, enzyme induction by,
    83–85
Benzene dihydrodiol, as substrate for
    DD, 25
Benzoflavone, EH activation of,
    110–111,116,118
Benzo(a)pyrene (BP)
  cytochrome P-450 and, 15–17
  DNA binding of, 9,124–130,295
  EH and, 111,113
  epoxides of, 6–7,14,27–28
  exogenous chemical modification of,
    125,128
  glucuronidation of, 14,16–17,20
  GSH-S-transferase inactivation, 6–11
  GTS and, 14–15
  interindividual differences to,
    130–133
  metabolites of, 14–15,124–130
  mutagenicity of, 16–17,26
  oxidation of, 14,79
  protein kinases and, 201
  species differences to, 125–130
  tissue distribution of metabolites,
    128–129

299